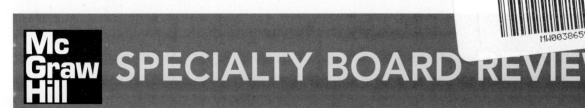

SPECIALTY BOARD REVIEW

Pain Medicine

Salahadin Abdi, MD, PhD
Professor and Chief
University of Miami Pain Center
Department of Anesthesiology, Perioperative Medicine and Pain Management
LM Miller School of Medicine
Miami, Florida

Pradeep Chopra, MD, MHCM
Assistant Professor (Clinical)
Department of Medicine, The Warren Alpert Medical School of Brown University
Providence, Rhode Island
Assistant Professor (Adj) of Anesthesiology
Boston University School of Medicine
Boston, Massachusetts

Howard Smith, MD
Associate Professor of Anesthesiology, Internal Medicine, and Physical Rehabilitation & Medicine
Academic Director of Pain Management
Albany Medical College
Department of Anesthesiology
Albany, New York

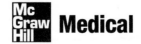 **Medical**

New York Chicago San Francisco Lisbon London Madrid Mexico City
New Delhi San Juan Seoul Singapore Sydney Toronto

McGraw-Hill Specialty Board Review:
Pain Medicine

Copyright © 2009 by The McGraw-Hill Companies, Inc. All rights reserved. Printed in the United States of America. Except as permitted under the United States Copyright Act of 1976, no part of this publication may be reproduced or distributed in any form or by any means, or stored in a data base or retrieval system, without the prior written permission of the publisher.

1 2 3 4 5 6 7 8 9 0   QPD/QPD   12 11 10 9

ISBN 978-0-07-144344-9
MHID 0-07-144344-4

Notice

Medicine is an ever-changing science. As new research and clinical experience broaden our knowledge, changes in treatment and drug therapy are required. The authors and the publisher of this work have checked with sources believed to be reliable in their efforts to provide information that is complete and generally in accord with the standards accepted at the time of publication. However, in view of the possibility of human error or changes in medical sciences, neither the authors nor the publisher nor any other party who has been involved in the preparation or publication of this work warrants that the information contained herein is in every respect accurate or complete, and they disclaim all responsibility for any errors or omissions or for the results obtained from use of the information contained in this work. Readers are encouraged to confirm the information contained herein with other sources. For example and in particular, readers are advised to check the product information sheet included in the package of each drug they plan to administer to be certain that the information contained in this work is accurate and that changes have not been made in the recommended dose or in the contraindications for administration. This recommendation is of particular importance in connection with new or infrequently used drugs.

Cover Photo: Person with back pain
Credit: © Don Carstens/Artville

This book was set in Palatino by International Typesetting and Composition.
The editors were Marsha S. Loeb and Cindy Yoo.
The production supervisor was Catherine Saggese.
Project management was provided by Somya Rustagi, International Typesetting and Composition.
The cover series designer was Aimee Davis.
Quebecor World Dubuque was printer and binder.

This book is printed on acid-free paper.

Cataloging-in-Publication Data for this book is on file with the Library of Congress.

We dedicate this book
to our patients whom we are honored to serve
and
to our families for their love and support.

Dr. Chopra also dedicates this book to Shalini and Neil Chopra.

Contents

Contributors

Salahadin Abdi, MD, PhD
Professor and Chief, Department of Anesthesia
Preoperative Medicine and Pain Management
LM Miller School of Medicine
Miami, Florida
Chapter 4, Pharmacology

Ivan Antonevich, MD
Assistant Professor
Department of Anesthesiology
Pain Medicine and Perioperative Care
University of Miami
Miller School of Medicine
Miami, Florida
Chapter 6, Types of Pain

Carlos A. Buxo, MD
Department of Anesthesiology
University of Puerto Rico, School of Medicine
Bayamon, Puerto Rico
Chapter 10, Interdisciplinary Pain Management

Lucy L. Chen, MD
Instructor
Department of Anesthesia and Critical Care
Harvard Medical School
Boston, Massachusetts
Chapter 9, Complementary and Alternative Medicine

Pradeep Chopra, MD
Assistant Professor (Clinical)
Department of Medicine
Boston University School of Medicine
The Warren Alpert Medical School
Providence, Rhode Island
Chapter 1, Anatomy

Steven P. Cohen, MD
Assistant Professor
Department of Anesthesiology
John Hopkin School of Medicine and Walter Reed
    Army Medical Center
Baltimore, Maryland
Chapter 5, Diagnosis of Pain States

Alane B. Costanzo, MD
Pain Fellow
Department of Anesthesiology and Pain Medicine
Harvard Medical School/Beth Israel Deaconess
    Medical Center
Brookline, Massachusetts
Chapter 6, Types of Pain

Ezekiel Fink, MD
Clinical Instructor
David Geffen School of Medicine at University of
    California, Los Angeles (UCLA)
Los Angeles, California
Chapter 3, Pathophysiology

Asteghik Hacobian, MD
Pain Management Specialist
Interventional Spine Medicine
Barrington, New Hampshire
Chapter 7, Pain Assessment

Robert W. Irwin, MD
Assistant Professor
Department of Rehabilitation Medicine
Miller School of Medicine
University of Miami
Miami, Florida
Chapter 15, Rehabilitation

Ronald J. Kulich, PhD
Associate Professor
Department of General Dentistry/Craniofacial Pain
  and Headache Center
Tufts University School of Dental Medicine
Boston, Massachusetts
Chapter 11, Behavioral and Psychological
  Aspects of Pain

David Lindley, DO
Assistant Professor
Department of Anesthesiology
Critical Care Medicine and Pain Management
University of Miami
Miami, Florida
Chapter 8, Pain Management Techniques

Laxmaiah Manchikanti, MD
Chief Executive Officer and Chairman of the Board,
  ASIPP and SIPMS
Medical Director, Pain Management Center of Paducah
Paducah, Kentucky
Chapter 12, Drug abuse and Addiction
Chapter 13, Cost, Ethics and Medico-legal aspects in
  Pain Medicine
Chapter 14, Compensation and Disability Assessment

Muhammad A. Munir, MD
Director
Department of Inventional Pain Management
Southwest Ohio Pain Institute
West Chester, Ohio
Chapter 5, Diagnosis of Pain States

Annu Navani, MD
Medical Director
Comprehensive Pain Management Center
San Jose, California
Adjunct Clinical Assistant Professor
Stanford University School of Medicine
Stanford, California
Chapter 5, Diagnosis of Pain States

Vikram B. Patel, MD
President and Medical Director
ACMI Pain Care
Algonquin, Illinois
Chapter 2, Physiology

Mark A. Quintero, MD
Pain Fellow
Department of Anesthesiology
Perioperative Medicine and Pain Management
University of Miami Miller School of Medicine
Miami, Florida
Chapter 6, Types of Pain
Chapter 8, Pain Management Techniques
Chapter 4, Pharmacology

Andrew L. Sherman, MD
Associate Professor of Rehabilitation Medicine
Miller School of Medicine
University of Miami
Miami, Florida
Chapter 15, Rehabilitation

Howard Smith, MD
Associate Professor
Anesthesiology, Internal Medicine, and Physical
  Rehabilitation and Medicine
Department of Anesthesiology
Albany Medical College
Albany, New York
Chapter 4, Pharmacology
Chapter 5, Diagnosis of Pain States

Milan P. Stojanovic, MD
Massachusetts General Hospital
Harvard Medical School
Boston, Massachusetts
Chapter 8, Pain Management Techniques

Ricardo Vallejo, MD, PhD, FIPP
Director of Research
Millennium Pain Center
Adjunct Professor Biology Department,
  Illinois State University
Bloomington-Normal, Illinois
Chapter 6, Types of Pain

Preface

As the number of medical organizations offering pain examinations increase, the need for well-selected collection of questions with detailed but concise explanations became apparent. Consequently, we have tried to make this book a reasonably complete source of "board-type information" and a "one-stop shop" to practice questions for all the major examinations with included answers and suggested reading so that the reader does not need to use other sources for explanation of the answers.

It is our hope that this book will serve as a source of knowledge refreshment so that readers can get a feel for which pain medicine topics they know well, and which they may need to become more familiar with. We would also like to emphasize our message what this book is about, namely, it helps our readers not only to practice answering questions in efforts to pass their Pain Medicine boards, but most importantly, to truly learn and understand the various pain topics as presented here. Medicine is an ever changing science, for the most up-to-date information readers are advised to consult current literature. Any suggestions for future editions are always welcome.

Acknowledgments

We would like to thank the publishers for their encouragement and assistance in completing this work. We would like to thank all the contributors for their hard work and willingness to contribute to this book.

CHAPTER 1

Anatomy
Questions

DIRECTIONS (Questions 1 through 45): Each of the numbered items or incomplete statements in this section is followed by answers or by completions of the statement. Select the ONE lettered answer or completion that is BEST in each case.

1. Nutrition to the lumbar intervertebral disc is from the

   (A) posterior spinal artery
   (B) internal iliac artery
   (C) lumbar artery
   (D) anterior spinal artery
   (E) abdominal aorta

2. A 65-year-old man presents with symptoms of pain in the cervical region. He also complains of radiation of his pain along the lateral part of his right forearm. He has a magnetic resonance imaging (MRI) of the cervical region with evidence of a herniated disc between the fifth and the sixth cervical vertebra. The nerve root that is most likely compressed is

   (A) fourth cervical nerve root
   (B) fifth cervical nerve root
   (C) sixth cervical nerve root
   (D) seventh cervical nerve root
   (E) first thoracic nerve root

3. The most common presenting symptom of rheumatoid arthritis is

   (A) pain in the small joints of the hand
   (B) neck pain
   (C) knee pain
   (D) low back pain
   (E) hip pain

4. The usual site of herniation of a cervical intervertebral disc is

   (A) posterior
   (B) lateral
   (C) posterolateral
   (D) anterior
   (E) anterolateral

5. The carotid tubercle (Chassaignac tubercle) is located at the

   (A) transverse process of the C6 vertebra
   (B) facet joint of the C5 and C6 vertebra
   (C) facet joint of the C6 and C7 vertebra
   (D) transverse process of the C7 vertebra
   (E) transverse process of the C5 vertebra

6. The stellate ganglion is located

   (A) anterior to the transverse process of the C6 vertebra
   (B) posterior to the subclavian artery
   (C) anterior to the transverse process of the C5 vertebra
   (D) anterior to the neck of the first rib and the transverse process of the C7 vertebra
   (E) anterior to the transverse process of the first thoracic vertbra

7. Features of Horner syndrome consist of the following, EXCEPT

   (A) ptosis
   (B) anhydrosis
   (C) miosis
   (D) enophthalmos
   (E) mydriasis

8. A 35-year-old woman with Complex Regional Pain Syndrome type I of the right upper extremity develops miosis, ptosis, and enophthalmos after undergoing a stellate ganglion block. She does not notice any significant pain relief. No significant rise in skin temperature was recorded in the right upper extremity. What is the most likely cause?

   (A) Inadequate concentration of the local anesthetic
   (B) Intravascular injection
   (C) Subarachnoid block
   (D) Anomalous Kuntz nerves
   (E) Inadvertent injection of normal saline

9. The greater occipital nerve is a branch of

   (A) posterior ramus of C2
   (B) posterior ramus of C1
   (C) anterior ramus of C1
   (D) anterior ramus of C2
   (E) trigeminal nerve

10. A 66-year-old woman presents with pain in the posterior cervical region for the last 1 year. It radiates to the right shoulder, lateral upper arm, and right index finger. She also complains in the medial part of the right scapula and anterior shoulder. On physical examination, she has numbness to the index and middle fingers of the right hand and weakness of the triceps muscle. The most likely cause of her pain is

    (A) herniated nucleus pulposus of the C5 to C6 disc causing compression of the C5 nerve root
    (B) herniated nucleus pulposus of the C5 to C6 disc causing compression of the C6 nerve root
    (C) herniated nucleus pulposus of the C6 to C7 disc causing compression of the C7 nerve root
    (D) herniated nucleus pulposus of the C6 to C7 disc causing compression of the C6 nerve root
    (E) muscle spasm

11. Blood supply to the spinal cord is by

    (A) two posterior spinal arteries and two anterior spinal arteries
    (B) two posterior spinal arteries and one anterior spinal artery
    (C) branches of the lumbar arteries
    (D) radicularis magna (artery of Adamkiewicz) and two posterior spinal arteries
    (E) internal iliac arteries

12. The most common origin of the artery of Adamkiewicz is

    (A) between T4 and T6
    (B) at T7
    (C) between T8 and L3
    (D) at L4
    (E) at L5

13. The most common location of the dorsal root ganglion is

    (A) medial to the pedicle within the lateral recess
    (B) inferolateral to the pedicle
    (C) lateral to the superior articular facet of the corresponding vertebra
    (D) directly below the pedicle
    (E) medial to the superior articular facet of the corresponding vertebra

14. Absolute central lumbar spinal stenosis is defined as

    (A) less than 8 mm diameter
    (B) less than 10 mm diameter
    (C) less than 12 mm diameter
    (D) pain at rest
    (E) pain with ambulation

15. The principal action of the quadratus lumborum muscle is

    (A) lateral flexion of the lumbar spine
    (B) axial rotation of the lumbar spine
    (C) extension of the lumbar spine

(D) fixation of the 12th rib during respiration

(E) forward flexion of the lumbar spine

16. The following structure passes under the inguinal ligament:

(A) Inferior epigastric artery
(B) Lateral femoral cutaneous nerve
(C) Obturator nerve
(D) Intra-articular nerve of the hip joint
(E) Sciatic nerve

17. The structure that passes under the flexor reticulum of the wrist is

(A) median nerve
(B) radial nerve
(C) ulnar nerve
(D) anterior interosseous nerve
(E) extensor digitorum longus

18. A boxer complains of pain in his hand after punching a bag. What is the most likely cause?

(A) Avulsed ulnar ligament
(B) Scaphoid fracture
(C) Fracture of distal radius
(D) Metacarpal fracture
(E) Dislocation of the fifth proximal interphalangeal joint

19. In the dorsal horn of the spinal cord:

(A) Cells from lamina I and II project to the hypothalamus
(B) Stimulation of lamina I and II produces pain
(C) Lamina I and II are found in the thoracic segment of the spinal cord only
(D) Discharge from lamina I and II decreases as a noxious stimulus increases
(E) Wide dynamic range (WDR) neurons are located predominantly in lamina I and II

20. In case of an injury of a peripheral nerve:

(A) Wallerian degeneration of the proximal nerve occurs
(B) The rate of regeneration is 1 mm/d

(C) Sensory nerves regenerate faster than motor nerves
(D) An inflammatory response occurs
(E) Regeneration of the nerves is faster in the central nervous system than the peripheral nervous system

21. Neuropraxia is

(A) anatomical disruption of a nerve
(B) loss of conduction of a nerve
(C) pain due to peripheral nerve injury
(D) muscle tremor
(E) increased conduction of a nerve

22. The following are true about pain, EXCEPT

(A) transmitted faster through C fibers
(B) some pain may travel through the dorsal column
(C) μ-receptors when stimulated in the brain produce analgesia
(D) intractable pain due to cancer cannot be effectively treated by hypophysectomy
(E) transmitted slower through C fibers

23. A-δ fibers:

(A) Are unmyelinated
(B) Are low-threshold mechanoreceptors
(C) Increase their firing as the intensity of the stimulus increases
(D) Do not respond to noxious stimuli
(E) Are thick nerves

24. All of the following statements are true regarding fentanyl as a good agent for transdermal use, EXCEPT

(A) low molecular weight
(B) adequate lipid solubility
(C) high analgesic potency
(D) low abuse potential
(E) high molecular weight

25. All of the following agents are α_2-agonists, EXCEPT

(A) clonidine
(B) antipamezole
(C) tizanidine
(D) dexmedetomidine
(E) baclofen

26. The antidepressant with the lowest sedation side effect is

(A) desipramine
(B) trazodone
(C) nortriptyline
(D) maprotiline
(E) amitriptyline

27. Methadone in addition to being a μ-receptor agonist has been proposed to also act as a

(A) cyclooxygenase 2 (COX-2) inhibitor
(B) sodium-channel blocker
(C) *N*-methyl-D-aspartate (NMDA) receptor antagonist
(D) δ-receptor agonist
(E) α_2-agonist

28. The beneficial effects of epidural administration of steroids have been attributed to all of the following, EXCEPT

(A) inhibit phospholipase A2
(B) improve microcirculation around the nerve root
(C) NMDA antagonist
(D) block conduction of nociceptive C nerve fibers
(E) μ-receptor agonist

29. A 22-year-old healthy woman with a history for migraine headaches develops an intense frontal headache after eating ice cream at a party. The pain is sharp and intense. What is the most likely diagnosis?

(A) Frontal sinusitis
(B) Cold stimulus headache
(C) Conversion headache

(D) Chronic paroxysmal hemicranias
(E) Aneurysm

30. An 18-year-old woman presents with frequent headaches, each lasting for several days. She has to take time off from school. She describes them as throbbing, localized to the temporal region. They are associated with nausea and vomiting, sensitivity to sound and light. A recent MRI was normal. A diagnostic lumbar puncture done was normal. The most probable cause of her headaches is

(A) migraine without aura
(B) postdural puncture headache
(C) tension-type headache
(D) temporal arteritis
(E) malingering

31. The cricoid cartilage corresponds with the following vertebra:

(A) C3
(B) C4
(C) C5
(D) C6
(E) C7

32. Rotation of the cervical spine occurs at

(A) atlantooccipital joint
(B) atlantoaxial joint
(C) atlantofacet joint
(D) cervical-facet joints at C2-C3
(E) cervical-facet joints at C3-C4

33. The nucleus pulposus in the cervical spine is absent after the age of

(A) 20 years
(B) 40 years
(C) 50 years
(D) 60 years
(E) 70 years

34. Kuntz nerves are a contribution from

    (A) the C5 sympathetic fibers to the upper extremity
    (B) the C6 sympathetic fibers to the upper extremity
    (C) the T1 sympathetic fibers to the upper extremity
    (D) the T2 sympathetic fibers to the upper extremity
    (E) the C7 sympathetic fibers to the upper extremity

35. Achilles reflex is diminished when the following nerve root is affected:

    (A) L3
    (B) L4
    (C) L5
    (D) S1
    (E) L2

36. The dermatome corresponding to the area over the medial malleolus is

    (A) L4
    (B) L5
    (C) S1
    (D) S2
    (E) L3

37. The medial branch of the dorsal rami innervates the following

    (A) multifidus muscle
    (B) subarachnoid mater
    (C) ligamentum flavum
    (D) quadratus lumborum muscle
    (E) piriformis muscle

38. The psoas major muscle is

    (A) flexor of the spine
    (B) flexor of the hip
    (C) inserts into the greater trochanter of the femur
    (D) axial rotator of the lumbar spine
    (E) extensor of the spine

39. The principal action of the piriformis muscle is

    (A) lateral flexion of the hip
    (B) external rotation of the femur
    (C) extension of the hip
    (D) internal rotation of the femur
    (E) knee flexion

40. The lumbar facet joint is innervated by

    (A) branches from the dorsal ramus at the same level and level above
    (B) branches from the dorsal ramus at the same level and level below
    (C) branches from the dorsal ramus at the same level
    (D) branches from the dorsal ramus at the level below and level above
    (E) corresponding spinal nerve root

41. The lumbar facet joints are oriented:

    (A) In coronal plane
    (B) In a sagittal plane
    (C) 45° off the saggital plane
    (D) 20° off the coronal plane
    (E) 20° off the saggital plane

42. The nerve involved in meralgia paresthetica is

    (A) lateral femoral cutaneous nerve
    (B) medial femoral cutaneous nerve
    (C) femoral nerve
    (D) obturator nerve
    (E) Inguinal nerve

43. The lumbar sympathetic chain lies

    (A) anterior to the transverse process of the lumbar vertebra
    (B) anterolateral border of the lumbar vertebral bodies
    (C) anteriorly over the lumbar vertebral bodies
    (D) posteriorly to the abdominal aorta
    (E) posteriorly to the inferior vena cava

44. A 56-year-old man presents with pain in the left flank. He gives a history of a rash for 1 week. The pain is burning in character and is sensitive to touch. He most likely has

    (A) costochondritis
    (B) herpes zoster
    (C) fractured left rib
    (D) postherpetic neuralgia
    (E) angina pectoris

45. Pain in the gluteal region produced by hip flexion, adduction, and internal rotation is caused by

    (A) sacroiliac joint
    (B) obturator muscle
    (C) hip joint
    (D) piriformis muscle
    (E) gluteus medius

Answers and Explanations

1. **(C)** The lumbar arteries supply the vertebrae at various levels. Each lumbar artery passes posteriorly around the related vertebra and supplies branches into the vertebral body. The terminal branches form a plexus of capillaries below each endplate. The disc is a relatively avascular structure. Nutrition to the disc is by diffusion from the endplate capillaries and blood vessels in the outer annulus fibrosus. Passive diffusion of fluids into the proteoglycan matrix is further enhanced by repeated compression of the disc by repeated flexion-extension of the spine associated with activities of daily living which pumps fluid in and out of the disc. The abdominal aorta does not provide any direct blood supply to the intervertebral disc.

2. **(C)** Disc herniations in the cervical region are relatively less common than the lumbar region. In the cervical region the C5, C6, and C7 intervertebral disc are most susceptible to herniation. The C6 and C7 intervertebral disc herniation is the most common cervical disc herniations. In the cervical region each spinal nerve emerges above the corresponding vertebra. An intervertebral disc protrusion between C5 and C6 will compress the sixth cervical spinal nerve. There are seven cervical vertebra and eight cervical spinal nerves. These patients characteristically present with pain in the lower part of the posterior cervical region, shoulder, and in the dermatomal distribution of the affected nerve root.

3. **(B)** Neck pain is the most common presenting symptom of rheumatoid arthritis (RA). Approximately 50% of the head's rotation is at the atlantoaxial joint, the rest is at the subaxial cervical spine. The atlantoaxial joint complex is made up of three articulations. The axis articulates with the atlas at the two facet joints laterally and another joint posterior to the odontoid process. A bursa separates the transverse band of the cruciate ligament from the dens. RA affects all three joints. The articulations formed by the uncinate processes, also known as the joint of Luschka, are not true joints and do not have synovial membrane. Hence, they are not subject to the same changes as seen in RA.

   RA is an inflammatory polyarthritis that typically affects young to middle-aged women. They present with a joint pain and stiffness in the hands. Typically the first metacarpophalangeal joint is affected whereas in osteoarthritis the carpometacarpal joint is affected. They have a history for morning stiffness. Almost 80% of these patients have a positive rheumatoid factor.

4. **(C)** The uncinate processes are bony protrusions located laterally from the C3 to C7 vertebrae. They prevent the disc from herniating laterally. The posterior longitudinal ligament is the thickest in the cervical region. It is four to five times thicker than in the thoracic or lumbar region. The nucleus pulposus in the cervical disc is present at birth but by the age of 40 years it practically disappears. The adult disc is desiccated and ligamentous. It is mainly composed of fibrocartilage and hyaline cartilage. After the age of 40 years, a herniated cervical disc is never seen because there is no nucleus pulposus. The most common cervical herniated nucleus pulposus (HNP) occurs at C6 to C7 (50%) and is followed by C5 to C6 (30%).

5. **(A)** The carotid tubercle (Chassaignac tubercle) lies 2.5 cm lateral to the cricoid cartilage. It lies over the transverse process of the C6 vertebra and can be easily palpated anteriorly. The carotid tubercle is an important landmark for stellate ganglion blocks.

6. **(D)** The stellate ganglion is the inferior cervical ganglion. The cervicothoracic ganglion is frequently formed by the fusion of the inferior cervical ganglion and the first thoracic ganglion. It is located anteriorly on the neck of the first rib and the transverse process of the C7 vertebra. It is oval in shape and 1" long by 0.5" wide. The ganglion is bound anteriorly by the subclavian artery, posteriorly by the prevertebral fascia and the transverse process, medially by the longus colli muscle, and laterally by the scalene muscle. The classical stellate ganglion block is done one level above the location of the stellate ganglion (it lies at the C7 level and the block is done at the C6 level). Typically the classical stellate ganglion block is performed with the patient supine, however, immediately after the block the patient is repositioned to a sitting position. The vertebral artery travels anteriorly over the stellate ganglion at C7 but at C6 the artery moves posteriorly. Incidence of phrenic nerve block is almost 100%.

7. **(B)** Horner syndrome consists of ptosis (drooping of the upper eyelid), miosis, (constriction of the pupil) and enophthalmos (depression of the eyeball into the orbit) only. Anhydrosis, nasal congestion, flushing of the conjunctiva and skin, and increase in temperature of the ipsilateral arm and hand are not features of Horner syndrome.

   The cervical portion of the sympathetic nervous system extends from the base of the skull to the neck of the first rib, it then continues as the thoracic part of the sympathetic chain. The cervical sympathetic system consists of the superior, middle, and inferior ganglia. In most people the inferior cervical ganglia is fused with the first thoracic ganglia to form the stellate ganglion. It lies over the neck of the first rib and the transverse process of C7, behind the vertebral artery.

8. **(D)** The sympathetic supply to the upper extremity is through the grey rami communicantes of C7, C8, and T1 with occasional contributions from C5 and C6. This innervation is through the stellate ganglion. Blocking the stellate ganglion would effectively cause a sympathetic denervation of the upper extremity.

   In some cases the upper extremity maybe supplied by the T2 and T3 grey rami communicantes. These fibers do not pass through the stellate ganglion. These are Kuntz fibers and have been implicated in inadequate relief of sympathetically maintained pain despite a good stellate ganglion block. These fibers can be blocked by a posterior approach.

   Successful block of the sympathetic fibers to the head is indicated by the appearance of Horner syndrome. Successful block of the sympathetic block of the upper extremity is indicated by a rise in skin temperature, engorgement of veins on the back of the hand, loss of skin conductance response and a negative sweat test.

   Alternatively, it is conceivable that the patient has sympathetic independent pain.

9. **(A)** The skin over the posterior part of the neck, upper back, posterior part of the scalp up to the vertex is supplied segmentally by the posterior rami of the C2 to C5. The greater occipital nerve is a branch of the posterior of ramus of C2. The lesser occipital nerve is a branch of the posterior ramus of C2 and C3. Headaches due to occipital neuralgia are characterized by either continuous pain or paroxysmal lancinating pain in the distribution of the nerve. The etiology of occipital neuralgia is compression of the C2 nerve root, migraine, or nerve entrapment. An occipital nerve block maybe performed as a diagnostic or therapeutic measure. The trigeminal nerve does not contribute to the greater occipital nerve.

10. **(C)** The pattern of pain helps identify the cervical disc causing the most problems. HNP are more common in the lumbar region. The cervical nerve roots exit above the vertebral body of the same segment. The C7 nerve root exits between the C6 to C7 vertebra.

11. **(B)** The blood supply to the spinal cord is primarily by three longitudinally running arteries—two posterior spinal arteries and one anterior spinal artery.

The anterior spinal artery supplies approximately 80% of the intrinsic spinal cord vasculature. It is formed by the union of a branch from the terminal part of each vertebral artery. It actually consists of longitudinal series of functionally individual blood vessels with wide variation in lumen size and anatomic discontinuations.

The spinal cord has three major arterial supply regions: C1 to T3 (cervicothoracic region), T3 to T8 (midthoracic region), and T8 to the conus (thoracolumbar region). There is a poor anastomosis between these three regions. As a result the blood flow at the T3 and T8 levels is tenuous. In spinal stenosis, especially in the lower cervical region, the anterior spinal artery may be compressed by a dorsal osteophyte and a HNP leading to the anterior spinal syndrome (loss of motor function).

There are two posterior spinal arteries that arise from the posterior inferior cerebellar arteries.

The three longitudinal arteries are reinforced by "feeder" arteries. They are spinal branches of the cervical, vertebral posterior intercostal, lumbar, and lateral sacral arteries. Approximately six or seven of these contribute to the anterior spinal artery and another six or seven to the posterior spinal arteries, but at different levels. The largest of these arteries is known as the radicularis magna or the artery of Adamkiewicz.

12. **(C)** The artery of Adamkiewicz originates on the left between the T8 and L3 level in most cases. This is the largest of the feeder arteries that supplies the anterior spinal artery. The artery of Adamkiewicz enters through an intervertebral foramen between T8 and L3 to supply the lumbar enlargement.

In a small percentage of cases (15%) the take off is higher at T5. In this case a slender contribution from the iliac artery enlarges to compensate for the increased blood flow to the lumbar portion of the cord and the conus.

The cervical portion up to the upper thoracic region, the anterior spinal artery receives contributions from the subclavian arteries. By the time the blood reaches the T4 segment it becomes tenuous. Although, the T4 to T9 area of

the spinal cord receives blood from the feeder vessels, it is relatively small.

13. **(D)** In approximately 90% of cases the DRG lies in the middle zone of the intervertebral foramen, directly below the pedicle. In approximately, 8% of cases it is inferolateral and in 2% of cases it is medial to the pedicle. The center of the DRG lies over the lateral portion of the intervertebral disc in some cases. Its size increases from L1 to S1 and then progressively decreases till S4. The DRG at S1 is 6 mm in width.

The DRG contains multiple sensory cell bodies. It is the site for production of neuropeptides: substance P, enkephalin, VIP (vasoactive intestinal peptides), and other neuropeptides.

The DRG is a primary source of pain when it undergoes mechanical deformity as by an osteophyte, HNP, or stenosis. It also produces pain when it undergoes an inflammatory process either by infection or chemical irritation from a herniated nucleus pulposus, release of local neuropeptides or local vascular compromise.

14. **(B)** The spinal canal is nearly round in shape; it is 12 mm or more in the anteroposterior diameter. Relative stenosis is defined as midline sagittal diameter of < 12 mm. The reserve capacity is reduced and any small disc herniation and mild degenerative changes may cause symptoms. Absolute stenosis is defined as a sagittal diameter < 10 mm.

15. **(D)** The principal action of the quadratus lumborum (QL) muscle is to fix the 12th rib during respiration. It is a weak lateral flexor of the lumbar spine. The QL is a flat rectangular muscle that arises below from the iliolumbar ligament and the adjacent iliac crest. The insertion is into the lower border of the 12th rib and the transverse processes of the upper four lumbar vertebrae.

Patients with spasm of the QL muscle usually present with low back pain. They have difficulty turning over in bed, increased pain with standing upright. Coughing or sneezing may exacerbate their pain. These patients respond well to trigger point injections and stretching.

16. **(B)** The structures that pass under the inguinal ligament, medial to lateral are: femoral vein, femoral artery, inguinal nerve, femoral nerve, and lateral femoral cutaneous nerve. The following muscles also pass under the inguinal ligament: pectineus, psoas major, iliacus. The inferior epigastric artery passes under the rectus sheath. The obturator nerve passes through the obturator foramen. The sciatic nerve is located posteriorly.

17. **(A)** The flexor reticulum (retinaculum) is fibrous band which is attached medially to the pisiform and the hamate bone. It is attached laterally to the scaphoid and trapezium. The area under the flexor reticulum is known as the carpal tunnel, through which pass flexor tendons of the digits and the median nerve. The radial and ulnar nerves do not pass under the reticulum. The extensor digitorum longus tendon lies on the dorsum of the wrist.

18. **(D)** The boxer's fracture involves the neck of the metacarpal. This is the most common site for fracture when punching a stationary object. The fracture occurs commonly in the fourth and fifth metacarpal bones. A fracture of the scaphoid bone is usually seen after a fall on the outstretched hand. Fracture of the distal radius is also know as Colles fracture and usually occurs after a fall on the outstretched hand.

19. **(B)** The Rexed laminae is a complex of 10 layers of grey matter located in the spinal cord. They are labeled as I to X. Laminae I to VI are in the dorsal horn and VII to IX are in the ventral horn. Lamina X borders the central canal of the spinal cord. Lamina I is also known as the posteromarginal nucleus. The neurons in lamina I receive input mainly from Lissauer tract. They relay pain and temperature sensation. Lamina II is known as substantia gelatinosa. The neurons contain μ- and κ-opioid receptors. C fibers terminate in the substantia gelatinosa. Lamina I and II are found along the entire spinal cord. The neurons in lamina I project to the thalamus. WDR neurons are concentrated in lamina V.

20. **(B)** Wallerian degeneration results after an axonal injury. It starts within 24 hours of the injury and occurs at the distal end of the cut axon. The rate of regeneration is approximately 1 mm/d. Regeneration in the peripheral nervous system is more rapid than the central nervous system. Motor nerve regenerate earlier than sensory nerves.

21. **(B)** Neuropraxia is a nerve damage without any disruption of the myelin sheath. There is an interruption in conduction of nerve impulses. There is a transient loss of motor conduction. Little to no sensory conduction is affected. This is a common sports injury.

22. **(A)** C-fibers are unmyelinated and hence have a slow conduction velocity (2 m/s). All sensory transmission takes place through the dorsal column. Hypophysectomy can be performed for intractable pain.

23. **(C)** A-δ fibers are thin, myelinated fibers, hence have a faster conduction velocity than C fibers. They are high threshold mechanoreceptors. They are associated with sharp pain, temperature, cold, and pressure sensations.

24. **(D)** Fentanyl has a low molecular weight and high lipid solubility; this allows it to be administered by the transdermal route. It interacts primarily with the μ-receptors. It is about 80 times more potent than morphine. The low abuse potential for fentanyl is a property of the transdermal delivery system and not of the opioid itself.

25. **(B)** Clonidine, tizanidine, and dexmedetomidine are α_2-agonists. Antipamazole is an α_2-antagonist. α_2-Agonists have been used in the management of hypertension for many years. Their role has now expanded to chronic pain management and as muscle relaxants. One proposed mechanism of analgesic action of α_2-agonists is by reducing sympathetic outflow by a direct action on the preganglionic outflow at the spinal level.

Clonidine is available in oral, transdermal, and epidural or intrathecal use form. It is used for the treatment of complex regional pain syndromes, cancer pain, headaches, postherpetic neuralgia, and peripheral neuropathy.

Tizanidine has been used for painful conditions involving spasticity. Dexmedetomidine is currently used as sedative in the intensive care unit.

26. (A) Tricyclic antidepressants (TCA) have been known to be effective in managing chronic pain. Unfortunately, their side-effect profile very often limits their clinical use. Some of the major side effects include orthostatic hypotension, anticholinergic effects, weight gain, sedation, cardiac conduction disturbances, sexual dysfunction, and restlessness.

TCAs with lower sedating effects include protriptyline, amoxapine, desipramine, and imipramine. Trazodone is an atypical antidepressant. It inhibits serotonin uptake and blocks serotonin 5-HT$_2$ receptors, α_1-receptor antagonist. Its most common side effects are sedation and orthostatic hypotension. At low doses it is used as an adjunct for insomnia.

27. (C) Methadone is a synthetic opioid derivative which seems to function both as a μ-receptor agonist and an NMDA receptor antagonist. It is equipotent to morphine after parenteral administration. The drug has a tendency to accumulate with repeated administration. It is excreted almost exclusively in the feces and can be given to patients with compromised renal function; however, caution should be used.

One of the two rate-limiting steps in prostaglandin synthesis is the conversion of arachidonic acid to the prostanoid precursor prostaglandin H2(PGH$_2$) by cyclooxygenase (COX). COX-2 is an isozyme of COX and mediates responses to inflammation, infection, and injury.

28. (C) Administration of epidural steroids by interlaminar or transforaminal approach is one of the most common approaches to treating spinal and radicular pain. Steroids decrease inflammation by inhibiting phospholipase A2, thus inhibiting the formation of arachidonic acid, prostaglandins, and leukotrienes.

Steroids may reduce inflammatory edema around the inflamed nerve root and improve microcirculation. They block the conduction of nociceptive C fibers. By restricting the formation of prostaglandins they may decrease sensitization of the dorsal horn neurons.

29. (B) Cold stimulus headache starts with exposure of the head to very cold temperatures as in diving into cold water. An intense focused pain develops in the frontal region when very cold food is ingested. The pain lasts for a short duration of a few minutes. It may be in the frontal or retropharyngeal region. A frontal sinusitis is a persistent frontal headache and does not have an abrupt onset. Conversion headaches are associated with severe behavioral abnormalities. Chronic paroxysmal hemicrania is very similar to a cluster headache in the form that it is similar in intensity and location. The attacks are short and frequent. They respond well to indomethacin.

30. (A) The management of headaches is based on the correct diagnosis. Postdural puncture headaches develop after a dural puncture such as a spinal tap. The pain is usually frontal and occipital. It becomes worse in the upright position and is relieved significantly with lying supine. Some patients develop sixth cranial nerve palsy because of the long intracranial course of the sixth cranial nerve.

The differentiation between tension-type headache (TTH) and migraine without aura is much more difficult. Very often both headaches coexist. TTHs are tightening or pressing in character. They are mild to moderate in intensity and are bilateral. TTH is seldom associated with nausea and in most patients TTH is not greatly exacerbated by physical activity.

Giant-cell (temporal) arteritis affects the extracranial vessels of the head and arms. There is tenderness over the scalp. The temporal or occipital arteries are enlarged and tender. They may have visual symptoms including amaurosis fugax, diplopia, and blindness. Most patients also have symptoms of intermittent claudication with chewing. A temporal artery biopsy is diagnostic.

According to the International Headache Society, headaches are classified into primary and secondary headache disorders. The primary headache disorders consist of:

Migraine with aura
Migraine without aura
Tension-type headache—chronic and episodic
Cluster headache—chronic and episodic

Primary headaches, such as migraine with or without aura, tension-type, and cluster headache constitute about 90% of all headaches. Migraine as defined by the International Headache Society is idiopathic, recurring headache disorder manifesting in attacks lasting 4 to 72 hours.

31. **(D)** The carotid tubercle (Chassaignac tubercle) lies 2.5 cm lateral to the cricoid cartilage. It is a part of the transverse process of the C6 vertebra and can be easily palpated. The carotid tubercle is an important landmark for stellate ganglion blocks.

32. **(B)** The normal cervical spine can rotate between 160° and 180°. Approximately 50% of this occurs at the atlantoaxial joint. The rest of the rotation occurs below that level. Nodding flexion and extension occurs at the atlantooccipital joint. Rotation occurs at the atlantoaxial joint, especially at the atlantoodontoid joint.

33. **(B)** The nucleus pulposus in the cervical disc is present at birth but by the age of 40 years it practically disappears. The adult disc is desiccated and ligamentous. It is mainly composed of fibrocartilage and hyaline cartilage. After the age of 40 years, a herniated cervical disc is never seen because there is no nucleus pulposus.

    A cleft appears in the lateral part of the annulus fibrosus at 9 to 14 years. This cleft gradually dissects toward the midline. By 60 years the annular desiccation is so advanced that a transverse cleft develops from one uncinate process to the other. The disc is bisected.

34. **(D)** The sympathetic supply to the upper extremity is through the grey rami communicantes of C7, C8, and T1 with occasional contributions from C5 and C6. This innervation is through the stellate ganglion. Blocking the stellate ganglion would effectively cause a sympathetic denervation of the upper extremity.

    In some cases the upper extremity maybe supplied by the T2 and T3 grey rami communicantes. These fibers do not pass through the stellate ganglion. These are Kuntz fibers and have been implicated in inadequate relief of sympathetically maintained pain despite a good stellate ganglion block. These fibers can be blocked by a posterior approach.

35. **(D)** Achilles reflex is also referred to as ankle jerk reflex. This reflex tests the S1 and S2 nerve root. The Achilles tendon is tapped while the foot is dorsiflexed.

Reflex	Muscle Contraction	Myotome	Nerve
Patellar	Quadriceps femoris	L2, L3, L4	Femoral
Achilles	Gastroc and soleus	S1, S2	Tibial

The Achilles tendon reflex is diminished when the S1 nerve root is affected.

36. **(A)** Nerve root and corresponding dermatome levels:

Level	Dermatome
L1	Upper thigh and groin
L2	Mid anterior thigh
L3	Medial femoral condyle
L4	Medial malleolus
L5	Dorsum of the foot at metatarsal phalangeal joint
S1	Lateral heel
S2	Popliteal fossa

37. **(A)** The medial branch innervates the facet joint, interspinous ligament and the multifidus muscle. During the stimulation phase of radio frequency of denervation of the medial branch, contraction of the multifidus muscle is often seen.

38. **(B)** The psoas major muscle arises from the anterolateral aspect of the lumbar vertebrae and inserts into the lesser trochanter of the femur. It is a flexor of the hip but does not flex the lumbar spine. Contraction of the psoas major exerts an intense compression on the intervertebral discs.

39. **(B)** The piriformis muscle rotates the extended thigh externally and abducts the flexed thigh. It does not cause flexion of the knee, extension of the thigh, lateral flexion of the thigh. A spasm of the piriformis muscle may present as buttock pain. The piriformis muscle can be tested clinically by asking the subject to abduct the thigh while seated.

40. **(A)** The facet joint capsule has a dual nerve supply. Each facet joint is supplied by the median branch from the dorsal nerve root at the same level and the level above.

41. **(C)** The cervical facet joints are oriented in a coronal plane to allow for extension, flexion, and lateral bending. The thoracic facets are oriented approximately 20° off the coronal plane. The lumbar facet joints are oriented 45° off the saggital plane.

42. **(A)** The lateral femoral cutaneous nerve arises from L2 and L3. It passes below the inguinal ligament, medial to the anterior superior iliac spine. Meralgia paresthetica is caused by neuritis of the nerve, usually by compression of a tight belt or overhanging abdominal fat.

43. **(B)** The lumbar sympathetic chain consists of the preganglionic axons and postganglionic neurons. It lies on the anterolateral border of the vertebral bodies. The aorta is anterior and medial to the chain.

44. **(B)** Postherpetic neuralgia is defined as a syndrome of intractable neuropathic pain persisting for 1 month after the rash following herpes zoster has healed. It has been variably defined as pain persisting beyond 1, 2, or 6 months after the rash. The incidence of postherpetic neuralgia has been estimated from 9% to 14%. Approximately 50% at 60 years age and 75% at age 70 years who develop herpes zoster are likely to develop postherpetic neuralgia.

45. **(D)** Stretching the piriformis muscle by flexing, adducting, and internal rotation of the hip, stretches the piriformis muscle. The sacroiliac joint and hip joint are tested using Patrick test. The gluteus medius is more superficial muscle, laterally and does produce pain with the mentioned maneuver.

CHAPTER 2

Pain Physiology
Questions

DIRECTIONS (Questions 46 through 63): Each of the numbered items or incomplete statements in this section is followed by answers or by completions of the statement. Select the ONE lettered answer or completion that is BEST in each case.

46. Which of the following nerves conduct nociceptive stimuli?

    (A) A-δ fibers and C fibers
    (B) A-δ fibers and A-β fibers
    (C) A-β fibers and C fibers
    (D) B fibers and C fibers
    (E) A-α fibers and A-β fibers

47. Arrange A-δ, A-β, B, C, and A-α nerves according to their conduction velocity (fastest to slowest):

    (A) A-α, A-β, A-δ, B, C
    (B) A-δ, C, B, A-β, A-α
    (C) C, B, A-δ, A-β, A-α
    (D) A-β, A-δ, C, B, A-α
    (E) B, C, A-β, A-α, A-δ

48. The impulse traveling through the C fiber terminates in the Rexed laminae:

    (A) Laminae 1 and 5
    (B) Laminae 1 and 2
    (C) Laminae 1, 2, and 5
    (D) Laminae 2 and 5
    (E) Laminae 3 and 5

49. Some of the naturally occurring chemicals involved in nociceptive input are hydrogen ions, serotonin (5-HT), and bradykinin. What effect do these have on the nociceptors?

    (A) Sensitize the nociceptors
    (B) Activate the nociceptors
    (C) Activate and sensitize the nociceptors
    (D) Block the nociceptors
    (E) Modify the nociceptors

50. Substance P release from the dorsal horn neuronal elements is blocked by

    (A) endogenous opioids
    (B) exogenous opioids
    (C) both type of opioids
    (D) anticonvulsant medications
    (E) local anesthetics

51. Arrange the visceral structures—hollow viscera, solid viscera, serosal membranes—in the order of increasing sensitivity to noxious stimuli:

    (A) Serosal membranes, hollow viscera, solid viscera
    (B) Hollow viscera, solid viscera, serosal membranes
    (C) Solid viscera, hollow viscera, serosal membranes
    (D) Hollow viscera, serosal membranes, solid viscera
    (E) Serosal membranes, solid viscera, hollow viscera

52. Visceral pain is typically felt as

    (A) dull
    (B) sharp
    (C) vague
    (D) all of the above
    (E) A and C only

53. Hollow viscera can be painful during which type of contractions?

    (A) Isotonic
    (B) Isometric
    (C) Sustained
    (D) Isotonic and isometric
    (E) None of the above

54. Certain nociceptors are termed "silent nociceptors." These can be activated ("awakened") by a prolonged noxious stimulus, such as inflammation. These types of receptors were initially identified in which structures?

    (A) Bones
    (B) Brain
    (C) Nails
    (D) Joints
    (E) Nerves

55. Visceral referred pain with hyperalgesia can be explained by which of the following?

    (A) Viscerovisceral convergence
    (B) Viscerosomatic convergence
    (C) Nociceptive perception
    (D) Sympathetic stimulation
    (E) Sympathetic transmission

56. Enkephalins and somatostatin – are these types of neurotransmitters:

    (A) Excitatory
    (B) Inhibitory
    (C) Gastrotransmitters
    (D) Excitatory and inhibitory
    (E) None of the above

57. There are several subtypes of N-methyl-D-aspartate (NMDA) receptors. They are

    (A) NR1, NR2 (A, B, and C)
    (B) NR1, NR2 (A, B, C, and D)
    (C) NR1, NR2 (A, B, and C), and NR3 (A and B)
    (D) NR1, NR2 (A, B, C, and D), and NR3 (A and B)
    (E) NR1, NR2 (A, B, C, and D), NR3 (A and B), and NR4 (A and B)

58. Sodium channels are also important in neurotransmission through the dorsal root ganglion (DRG). How many different types of sodium channels have been identified?

    (A) Four
    (B) Eight
    (C) Seven
    (D) Five
    (E) Nine

59. Ziconotide, found in snail venom, acts primarily on which type of calcium channel?

    (A) N-type
    (B) T-type
    (C) L-type
    (D) P-type
    (E) Q-type

60. Pretreatment with an NMDA antagonist prior to inflammation has been shown to

    (A) enhance central sensitization
    (B) attenuate central sensitization
    (C) have no effect on central sensitization
    (D) enhance peripheral sensitization
    (E) attenuate peripheral sensitization

61. NMDA receptor channels are usually inactive and blocked by zinc and magnesium ions. A depolarization of the cell membrane removes these ions and allows influx of which ions?

    (A) Sodium
    (B) Calcium
    (C) Chloride
    (D) Sodium and calcium
    (E) Sodium and chloride

62. Nociceptive stimuli cause increased activity in the cerebral cortex in

    (A) a focal area around the central gyrus
    (B) widespread areas in the temporal cortex
    (C) a focal area around the posterior cortical areas
    (D) widespread areas in the frontal cortex
    (E) a focal area in the thalamus

63. γ-Aminobutyric acid (GABA) receptors (a type of cellular channel), are these types of ion channels:

    (A) Calcium
    (B) Sodium
    (C) Chloride
    (D) Magnesium
    (E) Potassium

Directions: For Question 64 through 84, ONE or MORE of the numbered options is correct. Choose answer

    (A) if only answer 1, 2, and 3 are correct
    (B) if only 1 and 3 are correct
    (C) if only 2 and 4 are correct
    (D) if only 4 is correct
    (E) if all are correct

64. Nociceptors are present in

    (1) skin
    (2) subcutaneous tissue
    (3) joints
    (4) visceral tissue

65. Substance P is released by the activation of nociceptors and has the following effect(s):

    (1) Vasodilatation
    (2) Vasoconstriction
    (3) Mast cell activation
    (4) Decrease vascular permeability

66. Visceral pain input terminates in the following Rexed lamina(e):

    (1) Lamina 1
    (2) Lamina 2
    (3) Lamina 5
    (4) Lamina 10

67. The visceral pain may be felt as pain in

    (1) the midline
    (2) the unilateral
    (3) the bilateral
    (4) multiple patterns

68. Which of the following induce pain in hollow viscera?

    (1) Cutting
    (2) Ischemia
    (3) Burning
    (4) Distension

69. Viscera are supplied by sympathetic nerves which contribute to pain generation and transmission. They release several chemical substances including the following:

    (1) Norepinephrine
    (2) Histamine
    (3) Serotonin
    (4) Epinephrine

70. Neurotransmitters in the central nervous system (CNS) are classified into which of the following?

    (1) Excitatory
    (2) Inhibitory
    (3) Neuropeptides
    (4) Regulatory

71. These are some of the excitatory neurotransmitters:

    (1) Glutamate
    (2) Glycine
    (3) Aspartate
    (4) GABA

72. NMDA receptor blockade in the spinal cord causes

    (1) inhibition of pain transmission
    (2) modulation of pain transmission
    (3) reduction in pain transmission
    (4) does not have a role in pain transmission

73. The subunit most relevant in nociception is

    (1) NR2A
    (2) NR2B
    (3) NR3A
    (4) NR1

74. Ketamine and Memantine are NMDA receptor

    (1) allosteric regulators
    (2) agonists
    (3) stimulators
    (4) blockers

75. The most important substances found in the descending inhibitory pathways of the CNS include

    (1) acetylcholine
    (2) serotonin
    (3) nitric oxide (NO)
    (4) norepinephrine (NE)

76. There are several types of calcium channels. Which one is the most relevant to pain impulse transmission in the spinal cord?

    (1) L-type
    (2) R-type
    (3) T-type
    (4) N-type

77. N-type calcium channels are highly concentrated in which of the following areas?

    (1) DRG
    (2) Cerebral cortex
    (3) Dorsal horn
    (4) Postsynaptic terminals

78. Windup is a phenomenon that occurs due to constant input of C-fiber activity to the spinal cord. This phenomenon defines

    (1) reduction in excitability of spinal neurons in the DRG
    (2) increase in excitability of spinal neurons in the DRG
    (3) reduction in excitability of spinal neurons in the dorsal horn
    (4) increase in excitability of spinal neurons in the dorsal horn

79. Primary inhibitory neurotransmitters include the following:

    (1) Glycine
    (2) Glutamate
    (3) GABA
    (4) Aspartate

80. Excitatory neuropeptides in the CNS include the following:

    (1) Substance P
    (2) Somatostatin
    (3) Neurokinin A
    (4) Dynorphin

81. Serotonin is released as mediator as a result of tissue injury from which of the following?

    (1) Platelets
    (2) Muscle cells
    (3) Mast cells
    (4) White blood cells

82. Protease-activated receptors (PAR) were detected in which of the following?

    (1) Platelets
    (2) Endothelial cells
    (3) Fibroblasts
    (4) Nervous system

83. Increased nerve growth factor (NGF) levels observed after inflammatory stimuli result from increased synthesis and release of NGF from cells in the affected tissue. Large number of stimuli can alter NGF production including:

    (1) 2IL-1β, IL-4, IL-5
    (2) Tumor necrosis factor α (TNF-α), transforming growth factor β (TGF-β)
    (3) Platelet-derived growth factor
    (4) Epidermal growth factor

84. Endogenous opioid peptides are important in nociceptive perception and modulation. These include which of the following?

    (1) Leucine-enkephalin
    (2) Dynorphin
    (3) Methionine-enkephalin
    (4) Nociceptin

DIRECTIONS (Questions 85 through 90): Each of the statements in this section is either true or false. Choose answer

    (A) **if the statement is TRUE**
    (B) **if the statement is FALSE**

85. Nociceptors are specific receptors within the superficial layers of the skin.

86. Conduction velocity of A-δ fibers is faster than the C fibers.

87. Nociceptive impulse terminates in nociceptive—specific as well as wide dynamic range (WDR) neurons.

88. Hyperalgesia can only occur with somatic nociceptive stimuli and not visceral stimuli.

89. NMDA receptor in the spinal cord dorsal horn is essential for central sensitization, the central facilitation of pain transmission produced by peripheral injury.

90. Neuropeptides are only excitatory in nature.

Answers and Explanations

46. **(A)** Nociceptors transmit impulses mainly through the A-δ and C fibers to the spinal cord. A-β fibers carry impulses generated from low-threshold mechanoceptors. B fibers are mainly preganglionic autonomic (white rami and cranial nerves III, VII, IX, X).

47. **(A)** Conduction velocity is dependent on the size of the nerve fiber as well as myelination. Myelinated nerves conduct the impulse faster than unmyelinated nerves (C) due to jumping from one node to the next node of Ranvier (saltatory conduction).

48. **(C)** Impulses C fibers and their collaterals terminate in the Rexed laminae L1, L2, and L5.

49. **(B)** The sensitization of nociceptors may be caused by prostaglandins and cytokines, whereas activation is caused by substance, such as hydrogen ions, serotonin, and bradykinin.

50. **(C)** Both, endogenous as well as exogenous opioids block the release of substance P in the dorsal horn there by providing analgesia.

51. **(C)** The serosal membranes are the most sensitive and the solid viscera the least sensitive to noxious stimuli.

52. **(E)** The visceral pain is felt as a vague, deep, dull pain as opposed to sharp and well-defined pain. It may mimic other types of pain due to referred pain pattern.

53. **(B)** Viscera can generate painful contraction in an isometric contraction state such as bowel and ureteral obstruction. Isotonic contractions usually are not painful.

54. **(D)** Sleeping or silent nociceptors are population of nociceptors that remain inactive under normal conditions. They are activated because of tissue injury, with consequent release of chemical mediators. They appear to be present in skin, joints, muscle, and visceral tissue.

55. **(B)** The viscerosomatic convergence of signals within the spinal cord at the level of dorsal horn and at supraspinal levels within the brainstem, thalamus, and cortex; explains the phenomenon of referred pain to somatic structures. Viscerovisceral convergence on the other hand has been shown to exist between colon/rectum, bladder, vagina, and uterine cervix, and between heart and gallbladder.

56. **(B)** Dopamine, epinephrine, and norepinephrine are considered to be excitatory neurotransmitters, whereas serotonin, GABA, and dopamine are the other inhibitory neurotransmitters.

57. **(B)** There is accumulating evidence to implicate the importance of NMDA receptors to the induction and maintenance of central sensitization during pain states. However, NMDA receptors may also mediate peripheral sensitization and visceral pain. NMDA receptors are composed of NR1, NR2 (A, B, C, and D), and NR3 (A and B) subunits, which determine the functional properties of native NMDA receptors. Among NMDA receptor subtypes, the NR2B subunit– containing receptors appear particularly important for nociception, thus leading

to the possibility that NR2B-selective antagonists may be useful in the treatment of chronic pain.

58. **(E)** Voltage-gated sodium channels underlie the electrical excitability demonstrated by mammalian nerve and muscle. Nine voltage-gated sodium channels are expressed in complex patterns in mammalian nerve and muscle. Six have been identified in the DRG. Three channels, $Na_v1.7$, $Na_v1.8$, and $Na_v1.9$, are expressed selectively in peripheral damage-sensing neurons. $Na_v1.8$ seems to play a specialized role in pain pathways.

59. **(A)** The nonopioid analgesic ziconotide has been developed as a new treatment for patients with severe chronic pain who are intolerant of and/or refractory to other analgesic therapies. Ziconotide is the synthetic equivalent of a 25-amino-acid polybasic peptide found in the venom of the marine snail *Conus magus*. In rodents, ziconotide acts by binding to neuronal N-type voltage-sensitive calcium channels, thereby blocking neurotransmission from primary nociceptive afferents. Ziconotide produces potent antinociceptive effects in animal models and its efficacy has been demonstrated in human studies.

60. **(B)** Pretreatment with an NMDA antagonist attenuates the central sensitization from inflammation.

61. **(C)** NMDA receptor ion channel has binding sites for zinc, magnesium, and phencyclidine, which are inhibitory. A depolarization causes removal of zinc and magnesium allowing largely calcium and to much lesser extent sodium ions to influx, initiating intracellular activity.

62. **(B)** Noxious stimuli cause widespread activation of cortical area. Increasing stimulus intensity activates increasing number of areas within the cortex. Other areas of the brain are not involved in the interpretation of the noxious stimuli.

63. **(C)** Three major classes of chloride channels have been identified. The first class identified was the ligand-gated chloride channels, including those of the $GABA_A$ and glycine receptors. The ligand-gated chloride channels are common in dorsal horn neurons. The second class, also likely common spinal levels, is the voltage-gated chloride channels. The final chloride channel class is activated by cyclic adenosine monophosphate and may include only the cystic fibrosis transmembrane regulator. Activation of chloride currents usually produces inward movement of chloride to cells that hyperpolarize neurons; facilitation of these hyperpolarizing currents underlies the mechanisms of many depressant drugs. An important exception at spinal levels, however, is that $GABA_A$ receptors on primary afferent terminals gate a chloride channel that allows reflux of chloride with a net effect therefore of depolarizing primary afferent terminals.

64. **(E)** Nociceptors are present in all of the above tissues as well as in periosteum and muscles.

65. **(B)** Substance P activates and degranulates the mast cells, which in turn release histamine and serotonin.

66. **(E)** The visceral afferents usually terminate in the Rexed laminae L1, L2, L5, and L10. These laminae receive input from the nerve fiber types A-δ and C.

67. **(E)** Superficial and deep dorsal horn neurons are involved in pain perception from the abdominal visceral and may present it as vague unilateral, bilateral, and more commonly midline pain. The pattern may change with the course of the disease.

68. **(C)** Hollow viscera are insensitive to normally noxious stimuli that elicit pain in other somatic structures. However certain stimuli like ischemia, necrosis, inflammation, distension, and compression do elicit painful response from a viscus.

69. **(A)** In the viscera, sympathetic nerve terminals, mast cells, and epithelial cells, including enterochromaffin cells in the gastrointestinal tract, release a variety of bioactive substances,

including noradrenaline, histamine, serotonin, adenosine triphosphate (ATP), glutamate, NGF, and tryptase. Resident leukocytes and macrophages attracted to an area of insult collectively contribute products of cyclooxygenase and lipoxygenase, including prostaglandin I_2, prostaglandin E_2 hydroxyeicosatetraenoic acids (HETEs), and hydroperoxyeicosatetraenoic (HPETEs), and a variety of cytokines, reactive oxygen species, and growth factors. Some of these chemicals can directly activate visceral afferent terminals (eg, serotonin, ATP, and glutamate), whereas others probably play only a sensitizing role (eg, prostaglandins, nerve growth factor, and tryptase).

70. **(A)** There are three main classes of neurotransmitters; excitatory, inhibitory, and neuropeptides.

    Tissue injury results in the local release of numerous chemicals which either directly induce pain transduction by activating nociceptors or facilitate pain transduction by increasing the excitability of nociceptors. There are three classes of transmitter compounds; excitatory neurotransmitters, inhibitory neurotransmitters, and neuropeptides, that are found in three anatomical compartments; sensory afferent terminals, local circuit terminals, and descending (or ascending) modulatory circuit terminals.

71. **(B)** Glutamate and aspartate are the main excitatory neurotransmitters, whereas GABA and glycine are inhibitory neurotransmitters.

72. **(B)** NMDA receptor activation causes increased pain transmission whereas its blockade attenuates pain transmission. There are four receptor types for glutamate and aspartate in the somatosensory system. The class of receptors best activated by NMDA is termed the NMDA receptor. The NMDA receptor is usually considered as recruited only by intense and/or prolonged somatosensory stimuli. This characteristic is due to the NMDA receptor's well-known magnesium block that is only relieved by prolonged depolarization of the cell membrane.

73. **(C)** NMDA receptors are critically involved in the induction and maintenance of neuronal hyperexcitability after noxious events. Until

recently, only central NMDA receptors were a primary focus of investigations. With the recognition of peripheral somatic and visceral NMDA receptors, it is now apparent that the role of NMDA receptors in pain is much greater than thought previously. Over the past decade, accumulating evidence has suggested that the *NR2B subunit of NMDA receptor is particularly important for pain perception*. Given the small side-effect profile and good efficacy of NR2B-selective compounds, it is conceivable that NR2B-selective blockade will emerge as a viable strategy for pharmacological treatment of pain.

74. **(D)** Both are clinically used NMDA receptor blockers, causing analgesia. Clinically available compounds that are demonstrated to have NMDA receptor-blocking properties include ketamine, dextromethorphan, and memantine. Dextromethorphan, for example, is effective in the treatment of painful diabetic neuropathy and not effective in postherpetic neuralgia and central pain. NMDA receptor blockers may therefore offer new options in the treatment of pain.

75. **(C)** Nitric oxide is released in response to NMDA receptor activation and is implicated in neuronal plasticity rather than antinociception. Amongst the substances found in the descending inhibitory pathways of the CNS are norepinephrine and serotonin.

76. **(D)** The Ca^{2+} channel can be divided into subtypes according to electrophysiological characteristics, and each subtype has its own gene. The L-type Ca^{2+} channel is the target of a large number of clinically important drugs, especially dihydropyridine, and binding sites of Ca^{2+} antagonists have been clarified.

    N-type calcium channels are primary targets for the calcium channel blockers with analgesic properties. The N-type calcium channel exhibits a number of characteristics that make it an attractive target for therapeutic intervention concerning chronic and neuropathic pain conditions.

77. **(B)** N-type channels are highly concentrated in both DRG cell bodies and also in the synaptic

terminals they make in dorsal horn of the spinal cord (laminae L1 and L2). Commonly they are found in presynaptic terminals. Critically, block of N-type currents inhibits the release of neuropeptides substance P and calcitonin gene-related peptide (CGRP) from sensory neurons.

78. **(D)** Windup refers to the progressive increase in the magnitude of C-fiber evoked responses of dorsal horn neurons produced by repetitive activation of C-fibers. Neuronal events leading to windup also produce some of the classical characteristics of central sensitization including expansion of receptive fields and enhanced responses to C but not A δ-fiber stimulation.

79. **(B)** Primary inhibitory neurotransmitters of the somatosensory system include the amino acids glycine and GABA. Glycine is particularly important at spinal levels, while GABA is the chief inhibitory transmitter at higher levels. Three types of GABA receptors have been identified. $GABA_A$ receptor is linked with a chloride channel and modulated by barbiturates, benzodiazepines, and alcohol. Selective $GABA_A$ agonists include muscimol and selective antagonists include gabazine. The $GABA_B$ receptor has been associated with both a potassium ionophore and G protein-linked complex. Baclofen is a selective $GABA_B$ receptor agonist and phaclofen is a selective antagonist. Finally the newly described $GABA_C$ receptor has also been described as associated with a potassium channel ionophore. Glutamate and aspartate are excitatory neurotransmitters.

80. **(B)** The excitatory neuropeptides in the somatosensory system include substance P and neurokinin A. These peptides are especially concentrated in primary afferent fibers but also present in intrinsic neurons of the spinal dorsal horn and thalamus. The inhibitory neuropeptides at spinal levels include somatostatin, the enkephalins, and possibly dynorphin. These peptides are contained in both intrinsic neurons of the dorsal horn and in the fibers descending to the dorsal horn from various brainstem nuclei.

81. **(B)** Serotonin is one of many mediators that are released from platelets (rats and humans) and mast cells (rats) in injured and inflamed tissues. In situ hybridization, studies have shown that DRG neurons normally express mRNA for 5-HT_{1B}, 5-HT_{1D}, 5-HT_{2A}, 5-HT_{2B}, 5-HT_{3B}, and 5-HT_4 receptors. Many of the excitatory actions of serotonin have been ascribed to the ligand-gated 5-HT_3 receptor, but there is good evidence that serotonin can activate and sensitize nociceptors by actions on G protein–coupled receptors. 5-HT_2 receptors are expressed largely in (calcitonin gene-related peptide) CGRP-containing, small-diameter sensory neurons, and their activation produces thermal hyperalgesia. 5-HT_2 receptors are usually linked to the phospholipase C pathway. Activation of 5-HT_2 receptors depolarizes capsaicin-sensitive DRG neurons by reducing a resting potassium potential, and such an effect could contribute to both excitation and sensitization.

82. **(E)** Four types of G protein–coupled PARs have been identified (PAR1-PAR4). These receptors are activated by a unique mechanism whereby extracellular, soluble, or surface-associated proteases cleave at specific residues in the extracellular N-terminal domain of the G protein to expose a novel N-terminal sequence, which acts as a tethered ligand that activates the receptor by binding to other regions of the protein. These agonist effects can be mimicked by short synthetic peptides based on the sequence of the tethered ligands of the different PARs. PAR1, PAR2, and PAR4 are activated by thrombin produced during the blood-clotting cascade, while PAR3 activation is triggered by tryptase, which is known to be released from mast cells in inflammatory conditions, as well as the blood-clotting factors VIIa and Xa. In this way, PARs are activated as a result of tissue damage and inflammation. Because activation involves an irreversible enzymatic cleavage, restoration of PAR sensitivity requires internalization of the receptors and insertion of new receptor into the plasma membrane. PARs were initially detected in platelets, endothelial cells, and fibroblasts, but are now known to also be expressed in the nervous system. PAR1 and PAR2 are expressed on peripheral sensory neurons. PAR2 is expressed in about 60% of rat DRG neurons, where it is found mainly in the

small to medium-sized neurons, with a significant number coexpressing substance P and CGRP.

83. **(E)** NGF levels increase during inflammation. NGF is a critical mediator of inflammatory pain. NGF clearly has a powerful neuroprotective effect on small-diameter sensory neurons, and NGF levels have been shown to change in a number of models of nerve injury. However, its exact role in the development of neuropathic pain is at present unclear. Blocking NGF bioactivity (either systemically or locally) largely blocks the effects of inflammation on sensory nerve function. Elevated NGF levels have been found in a variety of inflammatory states in humans, including in the bladder of patients with cystitis, and there are increased levels in synovial fluid from patients with arthritis.

84. **(E)** The contribution of endogenous opioid peptides to pain modulation was first suggested by reports that stimulation-produced analgesia in animals and humans is reduced by the narcotic antagonist naloxone. Naloxone also worsens postoperative pain in patients who have not received exogenous opioid therapy, thus establishing the relevance of endogenous opioids to common clinical situations. Peptide transmitters and hormones are derived by the cleavage of larger, usually inactive, precursor. Met- and leu-enkephalin are derived from a common precursor, preproenkephalin, each molecule of which generates multiple copies of met-enkephalin and one of leu-enkephalin. β-Endorphin is cleaved from a larger precursor protein, proopiomelanocortin, which also gives rise to adrenocorticotrophic hormone and several copies of melanocyte-stimulating hormone. Two copies of dynorphin (A and B) and α-neoendorphin are generated from a third endogenous opioid precursor molecule (preprodynorphin).

85. **(B)** Nociceptors are free nerve endings and do not have any specific receptors, but are activated by a tissue injury due to mechanical, thermal, or chemical stimuli.

86. **(A)** "A-δ" fibers are myelinated fibers and conduct the impulses faster (5-20 m/s) than the C fibers, which are unmyelinated (< 2 m/s).

87. **(A)** WDR neurons respond to nociceptive as well as nonnociceptive stimuli transmitted by the peripheral nerves. These types of receptors are located in the dorsal horn of the spinal grey matter.

88. **(B)** Visceral pain is usually felt as referred pain. This type of pain can be "with hyperalgesia" or "without hyperalgesia." Most structures elicit a midline or bilateral pain; however, certain structures such as kidneys and ureters can produce unilateral pain. Referred pain with hyperalgesia is termed "true parietal" pain and usually extends to the muscles, but can extend up to the skin.

89. **(A)** NMDA receptors are involved in the induction and maintenance of certain pathological pain states produced by peripheral nerve injury, possibly by sensitizing dorsal horn neurons. These receptors have been implicated in the phenomenon of windup and related changes such as spinal hyperexcitability that enhance and prolong sensory transmission.

90. **(B)** There are multiple neuropeptides that contribute to signaling of somatosensory information. Some of these could be classified as excitatory compounds and others as inhibitory. Neuropeptides tend to have more gradual onset of effects as well as much more prolonged duration of action once released.

CHAPTER 3

Pain Pathophysiology
Questions

DIRECTIONS (Questions 91 through 138): Each of the numbered items or incomplete statements in this section is followed by answers or by completions of the statement. Select the ONE lettered answer or completion that is BEST in each case.

91. Common causes of acute abdominal pain in adults include

    (A) intussusception in an adolescent patient
    (B) abdominal aortic aneurysm in an adult population, which most likely presents with excruciating abdominal pain
    (C) diabetic ketoacidosis in an elderly patient without a previous history of diabetes
    (D) drug-induced pain from polypharmacy that is rarely a cause of abdominal pain in the elderly
    (E) interstitial cystitis

92. A 35-year-old woman has right arm pain. Which of the following statements regarding her pain is true?

    (A) It is more likely she will have arterial thoracic outlet syndrome than neurogenic thoracic outlet syndrome
    (B) If it began in the ulnar nerve distribution after an injury to the ulnar nerve, she may have complex regional pain syndrome (CRPS) type I
    (C) If she also has pain radiating into her occiput, she may have involvement of the sensory portion of the C1 nerve
    (D) If she has clawing of the small finger, the median nerve is likely involved
    (E) The ulnar nerve is commonly compressed at the cubital tunnel

93. You suspect a patient is having cluster headaches. The most convincing evidence of this type of headache would be if

    (A) the patient is female
    (B) although it is worse on the right side of the head, the symptoms are usually bilateral
    (C) the headaches are occurring at the same time each night
    (D) the patient is having a rebound headache due to excessive use of medication and the most likely underlying recurring headache is a cluster headache
    (E) the patient is urinating frequently and has blurry vision

94. Which of the following statements about migraine headache is true?

    (A) Recent evidence has supported the notion that cortical spreading depression is the mechanism of migraine headache
    (B) Activation of cortical spreading depression has become an interesting target for preventive migraine treatment
    (C) Current evidence shows a clear causal relationship between cardiac right-to-left shunt (RLS) and migraine headaches
    (D) Migraine pathophysiology involves the trigeminovascular system but not central nervous system (CNS) modulation of the pain-producing structures of the cranium
    (E) More than 90% of migraineurs have auras

95. A patient you are seeing recently began experiencing low-back pain. You suspect zygapophysial joint arthropathy as the primary cause of the symptoms. Which of the following can be said about this disease process?

    (A) Predisposing factors include spondylolisthesis and old age; however, degenerative disc pathology is not a risk factor

    (B) The key to diagnosing zygapophysial joint arthropathy is the historic and physical examination

    (C) An accepted method for diagnosing pain arising from the lumbar facet joints is with low-volume intra-articular or medial branch blocks because of the low false-positive rate

    (D) Cadaveric studies of the facet joints in patients with suspected arthropathy have revealed histologic changes

    (E) Its clinical presentation is characterized as a radicular pattern

96. Which of the following statements regarding postmastectomy neuromas is true?

    (A) In general, neuromas are palpable

    (B) Neuromas form with mastectomy but usually not with lumpectomy

    (C) Neuromas are most likely the cause of a painful scar

    (D) Resection should not be considered for an intercostal neuroma

    (E) None of the above

97. You suspect nerve root impingement in the cervical spine. Which of the following physical findings would support this diagnosis?

    (A) You suspect C1 nerve root involvement and the patient has numbness over the occiput

    (B) You suspect C6 nerve root involvement and the patient has loss of the biceps reflex

    (C) You suspect C7 nerve root involvement and the patient has loss of strength in the deltoid

    (D) Carpal tunnel syndrome (CTS) would be excluded by a normal examination of the abductor pollicis brevis (APB)

    (E) You suspect C8 nerve root involvement and the patient has numbness in the lateral aspect of the forearm

98. Which is the following statements regarding neck pain is true?

    (A) Peer reviewed literature suggests that there may be short-term benefit derived from treatment with acupuncture

    (B) Neck pain following an acceleration/deceleration injury most commonly involves the lower cervical spine

    (C) If you suspect an acute cervical disc herniation, it is important to ask about bowel and bladder incontinence because of the risk of cauda equina syndrome

    (D) A patient with neck pain alone may meet the criteria for fibromyalgia

    (E) CTS cannot have associated neck pain

99. Which of the following statements regarding fibromyalgia is true?

    (A) Two central criteria for fibromyalgia are chronic widespread pain (CWP) defined as pain in all four quadrants of the body and the axial skeleton for at least 2 years, and the finding of pain by 25-kg pressure on digital palpation of at least 11 of the 18 defined tender points

    (B) It is generally agreed that abnormal CNS mechanisms are responsible for all of the symptoms of fibromyalgia

    (C) There are both primary and secondary fibromyalgia syndromes

    (D) Fibromyalgia symptoms generally resolve if a rheumatic process is identified and treated appropriately

    (E) Most of fibromyalgia patients are male

100. Which of the following statements regarding endometriosis is true?

(A) The etiology is unclear but it has recently been demonstrated that retrograde menstruation is most likely not the cause

(B) Oral contraceptives tend to exacerbate pain symptoms

(C) The "gold standard" diagnosis of the disease remains magnetic resonance imaging (MRI) of the abdomen

(D) If endometriosis is diagnosed at the time of laparoscopy, laparoscopic surgery should be the first choice of treatment

(E) Endometriosis pain does not follow menstrual cycle

101. A 28-year-old female enters your clinic with upper extremity symptoms. You suspect thoracic outlet syndrome because

(A) she fractured her clavicle and developed symptoms afterward

(B) she has had sensory symptoms along her lateral forearm for some time

(C) radiographs confirm she does not have cervical ribs

(D) she has symptoms consistent with a chronic upper trunk brachial plexopathy

(E) all of the above

102. A 55-year-old homeless woman presents to the emergency room (ER) by ambulance in an unconscious state. The emergency medical technician (EMT) reports discovering the patient while she was experiencing a grand mal seizure. She has no identifying information and is unaccompanied in the ER. An examination of the woman reveals that she has bilateral mastectomies. When the patient wakes up, she reports having severe pain in her ribs and along her spinal column that is getting progressively worse. Which of the following statements is true?

(A) Bisphosphonates not only can treat the bony metastases of breast cancer but can reverse osteonecrosis of the jaw often seen in this type of cancer

(B) A large number of patients with breast cancer have osteolytic metastatic disease involving the bony skeleton

(C) Placebo-controlled trials with oral or intravenous (IV) bisphosphonates have shown that prolonged administration can reduce the frequency of skeleton-related events by 80%

(D) Hypercalcemia is the most frequent symptom of bone metastases

(E) This patient's most significant issue is most likely opiate dependence

103. Which of the following statements is true regarding arthritis?

(A) The biologic precursor to gout is elevated serum glutamic acid levels

(B) In psoriatic arthritis the distal interphalangeal joints are regularly involved

(C) The onset of polyarthritis in rheumatoid arthritis (RA) is usually rapidly progressive and initially affects the small joints of the hands and feet

(D) Inflammatory markers such as the erythrocyte sedimentation rate (ESR) or C-reactive protein (CRP) are abnormal in about 95% of patients with early RA

(E) None of the above

104. A patient enters your office complaining of leg pain after having a sural nerve biopsy. Which of the following statements is true about this type of complex regional pain syndrome (CRPS)?

(A) Increased tremor has been documented in the context of this type of CRPS

(B) This is most likely CRPS type I

(C) This type of CRPS has been described to occur after stroke

(D) The CNS does not appear to be involved in the pathophysiology of CRPS

(E) All of the above

105. Which of the following statements is true regarding pain in the context of human immunodeficiency virus (HIV)/acquired immunodeficiency syndrome (AIDS)?

(A) Distal symmetrical polyneuropathy is the most common peripheral nerve disorder associated with HIV

(B) Headache is the second most common of the AIDS-related pain syndromes

(C) Progressive polyradiculopathy is most commonly associated with herpes virus

(D) Kaposi sarcoma has been shown to cause muscular pain but not bone pain

(E) None of the above

106. Which of the following statements about central pain is correct?

(A) Central pain occurs with stroke and spinal cord injury (SCI) but not with multiple sclerosis

(B) In syringomyelia, central pain is often the first symptom of the disease

(C) The pathophysiology of pain associated with SCI has yet to be completely elucidated, but supraspinal pathways, not spinal pathways, are most likely involved

(D) After injury to the CNS, it is the denervated synaptic sites that serve an inhibitory role preventing the development of central pain

(E) All of the above

107. A 35-year-old female with chronic low-back pain comes to see you in your office for the first time. You immediately notice her unusual affect and behavior. Which of the following statements is true?

(A) Patients with somatization disorder, hypochondriasis, factitious physical disorders, and malingering may have pain complaints as part of their illness

(B) Malingerers, by definition, are not consciously aware of their motivation

(C) Other psychiatric disorders, such as depression, anxiety, and panic attacks, may strongly influence chronic pain without directly causing it; posttraumatic stress disorders do not usually impact a pain complaint

(D) One of the main differences between pain associated with malingering and pain associated with anxiety is that in malingering, complaints or symptoms go beyond what should be expected from a specific disease process

(E) None of the above

108. A patient is referred to you by a dentist friend. This patient is having pain in and around her mouth on one side. Which of the following statements is true?

(A) Primary burning mouth syndrome is a chronic, idiopathic intraoral pain condition that is not accompanied by clinical lesions; some consider it a painful neuropathy

(B) Increasing evidence suggests that very few cases of trigeminal neuralgia that are classified as idiopathic are caused by compression of the trigeminal nerve by an aberrant loop of artery or vein

(C) About 40% of patients with multiple sclerosis develop trigeminal neuralgia

(D) Trigeminal neuralgia can occasionally be present over the occiput

(E) All of the above

109. A patient is referred to you with facial pain. Which of the following statements is true?

(A) The pain of glossopharyngeal neuralgia is very similar to that of trigeminal neuralgia but affects anterior two-thirds of the tongue, tonsils, and pharynx

(B) Giant cell arteritis is a vasculitic condition that can lead to visual loss but has never been reported in a case of stroke

(C) Cervical carotid artery dissection most commonly presents with neck, head, or facial pain

(D) Pure facial pain is rarely associated with sinusitis alone

(E) None of the above

110. A 47-year-old woman comes into the ER complaining of a vague sense of nausea and heart palpitations. She has a history of chronic refractory angina. Which of the following statements regarding chest pain is false?

(A) In acute coronary syndrome men are more likely to present with chest pain, left arm pain, or diaphoresis and women may present with nausea

(B) To consider the diagnosis of cardiac syndrome X, this patient would have to have an abnormal coronary arteriography

(C) Controlled studies suggest that in patients with chronic refractory angina, spinal cord stimulation (SCS) provides symptomatic relief that is equivalent to that provided by surgical or endovascular reperfusion procedures, but with a lower rate of complications and rehospitalization

(D) The mechanism of action of spinal cord stimulation in treating angina is not yet completely defined

(E) None of the above

111. Which of the following statements regarding knee pain is true?

(A) Children and adolescents who present with knee pain are likely to have one of three common conditions: patellar subluxation, tibial apophysitis, or pseudogout

(B) A patient with a history of diabetes who presents with acute onset of pain and swelling of the joint with no antecedent trauma is likely to have a patellofemoral pain syndrome

(C) In pseudogout calcium pyrophosphate crystals are the causative agents

(D) You would not expect to see cystic changes on radiography of a knee with suspected osteoarthritis

(E) All of the above

112. A patient comes into your clinic complaining of right foot pain. Which of the following would be a correct diagnosis?

(A) The most commonly seen neuropathy in diabetes, because the symptoms are unilateral

(B) Plantar fasciitis, because the patient develops the symptoms after prolonged activity

(C) Morton neuroma, because it is located on the heel

(D) Tarsal tunnel syndrome, compression of the posterior tibial nerve as it passes by the medial malleolus

(E) None of the above

113. A 35-year-old woman comes to your clinic complaining of pelvic pain. Which of the following is important to consider during her evaluation?

(A) Endometriosis is the most common cause of pelvic pain in women

(B) Endometriosis most likely does not have an inflammatory component

(C) Endometriosis has been shown to be primarily dependent on blood levels of the hormone progesterone

(D) An inflammatory process would be supported by findings of a decrease of interleukin 8 in testing of peritoneal fluid

(E) All of the above

114. An 85-year-old man comes to your clinic having recovered from "a bad pneumonia" recently. He now complains of chest pain. Which of the following statements is false?

(A) While the parietal pleura does not contain any nociceptive innervation, the visceral pleura does

(B) Viral infection is the most common cause of pleurisy

(C) A description of pain with coughing would be consistent with pleurisy

(D) Pulmonary embolism is a possible cause of these symptoms

(E) None of the above

115. Which of the following statements regarding repetitive strain injuries is true?

- (A) Repetitive strain injury does not include the specific disorder cubital tunnel syndrome
- (B) Repetitive strain injury is a controversial diagnosis partially because there are few studies showing an association between physical risk factors and injury
- (C) Psychosocial factors are more clearly correlated than physical risk factors in repetitive strain injury
- (D) The "unifying hypothesis" of repetitive strain injury states that most often these diseases can be demonstrated to be due to focal injury
- (E) All of the above

116. A 56-year-old woman comes into your clinic complaining of chest pain on the left. She has a history of breast cancer with mastectomy and radiation treatment. She may still have chemotherapy. Which of the following statements is true?

- (A) As treatments for breast cancer have advanced in the past decade, the incidence of this type of pain has plummeted
- (B) The incidence of peripheral neuropathy would be higher with cisplatin than with paclitaxel
- (C) With chemotherapy, there is a higher incidence of motor than sensory neuropathy
- (D) Axillary dissection poses risks to the intercostobrachial nerve and the medial cutaneous nerve of the arm
- (E) All of the above

117. A 52-year-old obese male with a 5-year history of diabetes is complaining of foot pain. Which of the following statements is false?

- (A) If this patient has "large-fiber" nerve dysfunction, it may include weakness
- (B) Blood sugar abnormalities have been shown to correlate with degree of nerve dysfunction

- (C) Neuropathy has been described in the context of diabetes and blood sugar levels less than the criteria for diabetes mellitus as defined by the American Diabetes Association have not been shown to correlate with neuropathy
- (D) Small fiber neuropathy can have autonomic features
- (E) None of the above

118. An 85-year-old woman comes into your clinic with chronic pain over her left breast for more than 1 year. The symptoms began after she broke out in a rash in the same distribution. Which of the following statements is true?

- (A) Zoster reactivation is always accompanied by a rash
- (B) Zoster reactivation may occur two to three times for a healthy individual
- (C) Post herpetic neuralgia (PHN) is pain that persists for more than 120 days
- (D) The incidence of PHN is expected to remain stable in the future
- (E) All of the above

119. A patient comes into your clinic without a referral. He has a long history of chronic pain. He reports having some implantable device but he is unsure what it is. On examination, you find a surgical scar over the left lower quadrant of his abdomen. Over the past several weeks he has been developing worsening lower extremity pain. Your examination reveals spasticity. Which of the following is important to consider?

- (A) If the patient is getting intrathecal morphine, the rate of infusion would not have any impact on his complaint
- (B) If this patient has an intrathecal pump, only intrathecal morphine has been shown to result in granuloma formation
- (C) A microscopic investigation of an intrathecal morphine related granuloma would reveal necrotic tissue without immune cells
- (D) Morphine is a hydrophilic molecule
- (E) All of the above

120. The patient from question 119, relates that over the past decade he has had three back surgeries. This is why he thinks that the intrathecal pump was implanted. He reports that the first back surgery helped him for 6 months but the symptoms returned. The subsequent back surgeries only made his symptoms worse. Which of the following statements regarding this patient's condition is true?

   (A) In failed back surgery syndrome (FBSS), the most common structural cause of symptoms has been shown to be foraminal stenosis

   (B) In FBSS, pure psychogenic pain is somewhat common

   (C) In the context of chronic pain, an improvement of 30% is usually considered satisfactory

   (D) Failed back surgery syndrome, for the most part, implies a specific anatomical derangement

   (E) None of the above

121. Which of the following statements is false regarding pain and pregnancy?

   (A) One of the common causes of pain in early pregnancy includes stretch and hematoma formation in the round ligaments

   (B) Radicular symptoms usually suggest a herniated disc

   (C) Pregnancy is not an absolute contraindication to radiography

   (D) Migraine headaches rarely begin during pregnancy

   (E) All of the above

122. A 10-year-old boy with a diagnosis of sickle cell disease comes into your clinic. Which of the following statements is true regarding his condition?

   (A) A vasoocclusive crisis commonly involves the back, legs, and eyes

   (B) Acute pain in patients with sickle cell disease is caused by ischemic tissue injury resulting from the occlusion of macrovascular beds by sickled erythrocytes during an acute crisis

   (C) When a vasoocclusive crisis lasts longer than 7 days, it is important to search for other causes of bone pain

   (D) Patients with homozygous sickle cell and sickle cell–β-thalassemia have a lower frequency of vasoocclusive pain crises than patients with hemoglobin sickle cell and sickle cell–β-thalassemia genotype

   (E) None of the above

123. You enter a clinic's examination room to do a new evaluation on a patient. You find the patient leaning back on the chair in a deep sleep. Upon waking the patient up, you immediately notice an inappropriate affect and decreased movement of the right arm and leg. Which of the following statements is false?

   (A) Sleep disturbance, which can occur in the context of depression, can cause chronic pain

   (B) The diagnostic criteria of substance abuse includes recurrent substance use in situations where it is physically hazardous

   (C) The diagnostic criteria of substance dependence includes recurrent substance use in situations where it is physically hazardous

   (D) Conversion disorder is voluntary

   (E) None of the above

124. A patient comes into your clinic several years after sustaining a SCI. He complains of pain in multiple areas of his body. Which of the following statements is true regarding this patient's pain?

   (A) Chronic pain is a major complication of SCI with approximately two-thirds of all SCI patients experiencing some type of chronic pain and up to one-third complaining that their pain is severe

   (B) Central pain is the only cause of pain in patients with SCI

   (C) Cervical spine injuries have the highest incidence of central pain of all the spinal cord injuries

   (D) Central pain that occurs at the level of the SCI is because of nerve root damage

   (E) All of the above

125. The patient from the previous question used to be an anatomy and physiology teacher at a local college and is asking about some details about the mechanism of central pain in spinal cord injury (SCI). Which of the following explanations would you not give him?

(A) Prolonged high intensity noxious stimulation activates the *N*-methyl-D-aspartate (NMDA) receptors which induces a cascade that may result in central sensitization

(B) Abnormal sodium channel expression may be involved

(C) Thalamic neurons thought to be involved in the generation of pain undergo changes after SCI

(D) Thalamic neurons in SCI are relay stations for pain signals but not pain generators

(E) All of the above

126. Chronic pancreatitis is the progressive and permanent destruction of the pancreas resulting in exocrine and endocrine insufficiency and, often, chronic disabling pain. Which of the following statements about chronic pancreatitis is incorrect?

(A) Excessive alcohol use plays a significant role in up to 70% of adults with chronic pancreatitis, whereas genetic and structural defects predominate in children

(B) The pain with chronic pancreatitis is commonly described as midepigastric postprandial pain that radiates to the back and that can sometimes be relieved by sitting upright or leaning forward

(C) Autoimmune pancreatitis accounts for up to 5% of cases

(D) Because of its uniform presentation most cases of chronic pancreatitis are diagnosed

(E) None of the above

127. The definition of pain that is endorsed by the International Association for the Study of Pain is "Pain is an unpleasant sensory and emotional experience associated with actual or potential tissue damage, or described in terms of such damage." There are a host of physiologic

mechanisms by which injuries lead to nociceptive responses and ultimately to pain. That being said, not all nociceptive signals are perceived as pain and not every pain sensation originates from nociception. Which of the following statements regarding pain is false?

(A) Mainly two types of pain receptors are activated by nociceptive input. These include low-threshold nociceptors that are connected to fast pain-conducting A-δ fibers, and high-threshold nociceptors that conduct impulses in slow (unmyelinated) C fibers

(B) Many neurotransmitters (ie, glutamate and substance P) are able to modulate postsynaptic responses with further transmission to supraspinal sites (thalamus, anterior cingulated cortex, insular cortex, and somatosensory cortex) via ascending pathways

(C) Prolonged or strong activity of dorsal horn neurons caused by repeated or sustained noxious stimulation may subsequently lead to increased neuronal responsiveness or central sensitization

(D) Windup refers to a mechanism present in the peripheral nervous system in which repetitive noxious stimulation results in a slow temporal summation that is experienced in humans as increased pain

(E) Substance P is an important nociceptive neurotransmitter. It lowers the threshold of synaptic excitability, resulting in the unmasking of normally silent interspinal synapses and the sensitization of second-order spinal neurons

128. The presence of several pain inhibitory and facilitatory centers in the brainstem is well recognized. Which of the following regarding these systems is incorrect?

(A) The dorsolateral funiculus is involved in a pathway for descending pain inhibitory systems

(B) One function of the descending inhibitory pathway is to expand the excitation of the dorsal horn neurons

(C) The activity in descending pathways is not constant but can be modulated, for example, by the level of vigilance or attention and by stress

(D) Certain cognitive styles and personality traits have been associated with amplification of pain and its extension in the absence of tissue damage. These include somatization, catastrophizing, and hypervigilance

(E) All of the above

129. Which of the following statements is incorrect regarding the mechanisms of neuropathic pain?

(A) Injured and neighboring noninjured sensory neurons can develop a change in their excitability sufficient to generate pacemaker-like potentials, which evoke ectopic action potential discharges, a sensory inflow independent of any peripheral stimulus

(B) Central sensitization represents a state of heightened sensitivity of dorsal horn neurons such that their threshold of activation is reduced, and their responsiveness to synaptic inputs is augmented

(C) After peripheral nerve injury C fiber input may arise spontaneously and drive central sensitization

(D) The negative symptoms of neuropathic pain, such as allodynia, essentially reflect loss of sensation owing to axon/neuron loss

(E) All of the above

130. Which of the following statements about prolonged opiate use is false?

(A) A patient who maintains the same dose of opiate over a prolonged period of time is not at risk for developing tolerance

(B) Patients who receive long-term opiate therapy may be at risk of developing a paradoxical opioid induced pain

(C) Pharmacologic induction of pain may occur through activation of the rostral ventromedial medulla

(D) There is evidence that over the long term, opiates suppress pain by upregulation of spinal dynorphin, and enhanced, evoked release of excitatory transmitters from primary afferents

(E) None of the above

131. An anatomy/physiology professor sees you in clinic. You believe he meets criteria for CRPS. He has several questions about the autonomic nervous system. Which of the following would you highlight to him as a significant difference between the peripheral pathways of the autonomic and somatic motor nervous system?

(A) Unlike the somatic motor system which has its motor neurons in the CNS, the motor neurons of the autonomic nervous system (ANS) are located in the periphery

(B) The peripheral efferent pathways of the somatic motor nervous system has two components: a primary presynaptic or preganglionic neuron, and a secondary postsynaptic or postganglionic neuron

(C) The cell bodies of somatic motor nerves forms aggregates in the periphery called ganglia

(D) There are no significant differences

(E) All of the above

132. The professor from question 131 has several more questions about the autonomic nervous system. You would make all of the following statements about the sympathetic and parasympathetic divisions of the autonomic nervous system, EXCEPT

    (A) the parasympathetic preganglionic fibers travel from the CNS to synapse in ganglia located close to their target organs
    (B) while sympathetic nerve fibers are distributed throughout the body, parasympathetic fibers generally only innervate visceral organs
    (C) the preganglionic sympathetic neurons have their cell bodies in the gray matter of the brainstem and their fibers travel with the oculomotor, facial, glossopharyngeal, and vagus nerves
    (D) the efferent portion of the sympathetic division of the ANS includes preganglionic neurons, the two paravertebral (lateral) sympathetic chains, prevertebral and terminal ganglia, and postganglionic neurons
    (E) none of the above

133. A patient with a history of cancer comes to your clinic complaining of neck, shoulder, and arm pain. Which of the following is an important consideration?

    (A) Most tumors that affect the brachial plexus are from skin cancer
    (B) The most common presenting complaint of a tumor affecting the brachial plexus is pain
    (C) Radiation induced plexopathy has not been shown to be dependent on dose of radiation
    (D) Clinically, it is nearly impossible to distinguish between neoplastic and radiation plexopathy
    (E) All of the above

134. A patient with a history of multiple sclerosis comes into your office for an initial consult. She is wheelchair bound and has an intrathecal pump. She skipped the last appointment with her previous pain physician because she "did not like his bed-side manner." She cannot recall exactly, but it probably has been 3 months since she saw a pain physician. Which of the following is an important consideration?

    (A) A withdrawal syndrome from intrathecal baclofen (ITB) may include respiratory depression and hypotonia
    (B) ITB is a calcium channel blocker that acts primarily at the dorsal root ganglion (DRG)
    (C) Withdrawal syndromes from ITB can be fatal
    (D) Symptoms of ITB overdose include pruritus and hyperthermia
    (E) All of the above

135. A hearing impaired patient with severe learning disabilities comes to your office accompanied by his mother. The day prior to seeing you, the patient had a translaminar lumbar epidural steroid injection for low-back pain at a "major medical center" and the physician performing the procedure said it was a perfect injection. The patient is not able to communicate proficiently at his baseline. The mother reports that since the injection was done, the patient appears more comfortable lying down than standing. He is groggy and keeps his eyes closed for most of your interaction, but he has been up most of the night. The patient has a low-grade fever and mild tachycardia. His neck is somewhat stiff but he is otherwise uncooperative. Which of the following is the most appropriate next step of management?

    (A) Place an IV line to prepare the patient for a blood patch
    (B) Explain to the mother that the patient should exhaust conservative therapy for 48 to 72 hours prior to considering a blood patch
    (C) Send the patient to the ER for immediate performance of a lumbar puncture
    (D) Schedule the patient for an MRI of the lumbar spine
    (E) Initiate high-dose narcotic therapy

136. A physician is performing a cervical trans-foraminal epidural steroid injection at the C4-5 level. After the needle is placed in what the practitioner believes is an appropriate position, he removes the stylet and gets return of pulsating red blood. This would be most concerning if

(A) the needle is in the anterior neuroforamen

(B) the needle is in the posterior neuroforamen

(C) no need for concern, as the practitioner is only planning on injecting triamcinolone

(D) the patient is feeling new radicular pain symptoms that are severe in the C5 dermatome

(E) the patient has a significant history of vasovagal responses

137. Which of the following statements is true regarding phantom limb pain and stump pain?

(A) Mastectomy has been documented to lead to phantom sensation in the breast in well more than 90% of cases

(B) Phantom sensations are almost always more vivid in the distal extremity

(C) All amputees that have neuromata have stump pain

(D) Phantom limb sensations usually change with time; the distal part of the limb usually disappears first

(E) None of the above

138. A 35-year-old ex-football player enters your office complaining of shoulder pain. Which of the following statements is true of his condition?

(A) A complaint along the deltoid has been shown to correlate with rotator cuff pathology

(B) A history of a thyroid disorder could suggest dysfunction of the acromioclavicular joint

(C) Acromioclavicular joint pathology usually presents with diffuse shoulder pain

(D) If the pain began before the age of 30, this would most fit the clinical picture of a rotator cuff tear

(E) All of the above

DIRECTIONS: For Question 139 and 140, ONE or MORE of the numbered options is correct. Choose answer

(A) if only answer 1, 2, and 3 are correct

(B) if only 1 and 3 are correct

(C) if only 2 and 4 are correct

(D) if only 4 is correct

(E) if all are correct

139. You suspect nerve root impingement in the lumbar spine. Which of the following physical findings would support this diagnosis?

(1) You suspect L2 nerve root involvement and the patient has weakness of hip flexion and sensory loss on the lateral aspect of the calf

(2) You suspect L4 nerve root involvement and the patient has weakness of leg extension and loss of patellar reflex

(3) You suspect L5 nerve root involvement and the patient cannot dorsiflex his big toe and has a loss of the Achilles reflex

(4) You suspect S1 nerve root involvement and the patient has loss of sensation over the bottom of the foot. Achilles reflex is normal

140. Which of the following structures that play a role in the neurobiology of addiction are properly linked?

(1) Nucleus locus ceruleus—arousal, attention, and anxiety

(2) Anterior cingulate cortex—functional part of limbic system

(3) Amygdala—mediates drug craving

(4) Nucleus accumbens—one of the brain's reward centers

Answers and Explanations

91. **(C)** Diabetic ketoacidosis needs to be ruled out (in addition to myocardial infarction, pneumonia, pyelonephritis, and inflammatory bowel disease) as a cause of abdominal pain. The most common cause of abdominal pain in infants is intussusception. Although abdominal aortic aneurysms, which are a manifestation of atherosclerosis, do occur in an adult population, they usually do not present with specific clinical symptom of abdominal pain. Finally, drug-related abdominal pain is very common in the elderly.

92. **(E)**
    A. The majority of cases of thoracic outlet syndrome are categorized as neurogenic thoracic outlet syndrome.
    B. CRPS type II is when an identifiable neural injury is present.
    C. The first cervical nerve does not have a sensory branch.
    D. Ulnar neuropathy often has clawing of the small finger.

93. **(C)**
    A. Cluster headaches occur predominantly in males.
    B. Cluster headaches occur unilaterally and are accompanied by lacrimation, nasal congestion, conjunctival injection, and ptosis.
       Patients tend to get clusters of headaches occurring the same time daily (often at night).
    C. Patients tend to get cluster headaches the same time daily (often at night).
    D. Patients with rebound headaches are often overmedicating an underlying migraine headache.

    E. Patients with cluster headache do not routinely experience polyuria or changes in visual acuity.

94. **(A)**
    A. The recent discovery of multiple point mutations in familial hemiplegic migraine has led to the suggestion that migraine and its variants may be caused by a paroxysmal disturbance in ion-translocating mechanisms. Mutations associated with familial hemiplegic migraine render the brain more susceptible to prolonged cortical spreading depression caused by either excessive synaptic glutamate release or decreased removal of glutamate and potassium from the synaptic cleft, or persistent sodium influx.
    B. Suppression of cortical spreading depression has become an interesting target for preventive migraine treatment. Prolonged treatment with β-blockers, valproate, topiramate, methysergide, or amitriptyline reduced the number of potassium-evoked cortical spreading depressions and elevated the electrical stimulation threshold for the induction of cortical spreading depression in rats. Recent imaging studies in patients suffering from migraine without aura also points to the presence of silent cortical spreading depression as an underlying mechanism. Repeated waves of cortical spreading depression may have deleterious effects on brain function, and perhaps cause silent ischemic lesions in vulnerable brain regions such as the cerebellum in susceptible individuals.

C. There is an association between RLS and migraine. The relationship between RLS and migraine is further supported by the disappearance and improvement of migraine symptoms after closure of the foramen ovale. Nonetheless, the mechanism as well as the question about causality of this association has to be further elucidated.

D. Migraine pathophysiology has been demonstrated to involve the trigeminovascular system and CNS modulation of the pain-producing structures of the cranium.

95. (D)

A. The onset of lumbar facet joint pain is usually insidious, with predisposing factors including spondylolisthesis, degenerative disc pathology, and old age.

B. The existing literature does not support the use of historic or physical examination findings to diagnose lumbar zygapophysial joint pain.

C. The most accepted method for diagnosing pain arising from the lumbar facet joints is with low-volume intra-articular or medial branch blocks, both of which are associated with high false-positive rates.

D. Histologic studies of the facet joints in patients with suspected arthropathy have revealed pathology.

96. (C)

A. Neuromas can form whenever peripheral nerves are severed or injured. Macro-neuromas consist of a palpable mass of tangled axons unable to regenerate to their target, fibroblasts, and other cells, whereas microneuromas contain small numbers of axons and may not be palpable.

B. Both mastectomy and lumpectomy leave a scar in which neuromas can form. Chronically painful scars can develop after mastectomy and lumpectomy, and abnormal neuronal activity originating in neuromas or entrapped axons within this scar tissue is the likely mechanism of such pain. Neuroma pain may be more common following lumpectomy than mastectomy.

C. Axons entrapped within these scars can cause spontaneous pain and severe mechanosensitivity.

D. Anecdotal reports suggest that resection of intercostal neuromas may alleviate chronic pain after breast cancer surgery.

97. (B)

A. The C1 nerve root has no sensory component.

B. C6 radiculopathy can be accompanied by a loss of bicep reflex.

C. With C7 nerve roots, paresis affects the finger and wrist flexors and extensors. The triceps reflex is also innervated by the C7 nerve root; the deltoid is innervated by C5, C6 nerve roots.

D. Although the median nerve (which is affected in CTS) innervates the APB as well as the opponens pollicis, a normal motor examination does not exclude the possibility of CTS.

98. (A)

A. Peer-reviewed literature suggests that acupuncture is effective in the short-term management of low-back pain, neck pain, and osteoarthritis involving the knee. However, the literature also suggests that short-term treatment with acupuncture does not result in long-term benefits. Data regarding the efficacy of acupuncture for dental pain, colonoscopy pain, and intraoperative analgesia are inconclusive. Studies describing the use of acupuncture during labor suggest that it may be useful during the early stages, but not throughout the course of labor. Finally, the effects of acupuncture on postoperative pain are inconclusive and are dependent on the timing of the intervention and the patient's level of consciousness.

B. Upper cervical pain is most common with involvement of the suboccipital area as well as the C2-3 dermatomes.

C. In cauda equina syndrome, there is acute loss of function of the neurologic elements below the termination of the spinal cord. This occurs at the level of the lumbar spine.

D. In 1990, the American College of Rheumatology (ACR) established criteria for classifying patients with fibromyalgia which consists of tenderness in 11 of 18 standardized tender points. Only six to eight are located in the neck and associated structures.

E. CTS can have associated neck pain.

99. (C)

A. The two operational criteria are chronic widespread pain (CWP) defined as pain in all four quadrants of the body and the axial skeleton for at least 3 months, and the finding of pain by 4-kg pressure on digital palpation of at least 11 of 18 defined tender points.

B. The exact pathogenesis of fibromyalgia has not been cleared up yet, but according to the currently held view a variety of biological, psychological, and social factors play a role in the manifestation of the disorder. Among other things, inflammatory, traumatic, and immunological processes; static problems; endocrine disorders; and depressions, anxiety conditions, and stress factors are thought to trigger the syndrome. A dysfunction of the central affective and/or sensory pain memory may possibly be at work in the different illnesses mentioned above, which then results in fibromyalgia pain.

C. In principle, fibromyalgia can be categorized as primary or secondary fibromyalgia. In primary fibromyalgia, which is much more common than the secondary type, even the most careful work-up will not reveal any definitive organic factor triggering the syndrome. With secondary fibromyalgia, on the other hand, the underlying disease, such as inflammatory rheumatic processes or collagenosis can be diagnosed with relative ease.

D. Symptoms associated with fibromyalgia often do not disappear when the rheumatic processes have subsided, suggesting that some central mechanisms may be responsible for the persistence of generalized pain and hyperalgesia, possibly due to a disorder of the central affective pain memory and/or the memory of sensory pain or else to latent peripheral immunological processes. It is precisely this coexistence of pain and hyperalgesia in secondary fibromyalgia associated with systemic inflammatory rheumatic diseases, which proves that pain and sensitivity to pain cannot be separated strictly in fibromyalgia.

100. (D)

A. Endometriosis is the presence of endometrial glands and stroma outside the endometrial cavity and is a common cause of pelvic pain. The etiology is unknown, although the theory of retrograde menstruation is the prevailing theory.

B. Oral contraceptives, androgenic agents, progestins, and gonadotropin-releasing hormone (GnRH) analogs have all been used successfully in treating the symptoms of endometriosis.

C. The "gold standard" of diagnosis is laparoscopy with direct visualization.

D. If endometriosis is diagnosed at the time of laparoscopy, laparoscopic surgery should be the first choice of treatment, especially in women of reproductive age with an endometrioma.

101. (A)

A. The most frequently fractured bone in the body is the clavicle and the most common cause is a fall or blow on the point of the shoulder. In most instances, clavicular fractures do not involve nearby structures, and their healing is uneventful, except for possibly some residual deformity. Occasionally, however, the blood vessels and the brachial plexus elements situated between the midportion of the clavicle and the first thoracic rib are injured secondarily. This generally occurs in adults, most often following midshaft displaced fractures. This type of neurovascular injury often is referred to as traumatic TOS.

B. The majority of patients report having had sensory disturbances for long periods before that point. The earliest and most common symptoms are intermittent aching or paresthesias along the medial arm and forearm, sometimes extending into the medial hand and fingers. Hand cramping with use sometimes appears later in the course. Although these symptoms, particularly the intermittent aching, may be present for years, they rarely are bothersome enough to cause the patient to seek medical care.

C. Plain cervical spine radiographs are important for diagnosis of thoracic outlet syndrome. Typically, a rudimentary cervical rib or an elongated C7 transverse process is found ipsilateral to the affected limb. Cervical ribs frequently are present bilaterally, and often the one on the contralateral, uninvolved, side is larger. This is inconsequential, however, because the cervical ribs themselves do not compromise the proximal lower trunk axons; instead, it is a radiolucent band extending from the tip of the rudimentary cervical rib to the first thoracic rib that does so. In some patients, cervical ribs are difficult to visualize unless special radiograph views are used.

D. This rare disorder manifests as a very chronic lower trunk brachial plexopathy, most commonly caused by congenital anomalies.

102. **(B)**

A. Bisphosphonates are effective for the management of hypercalcemia of malignancy and bone metastases. This group of drugs has improved the quality of life in many patients with proven efficacy in limiting pain and skeleton-related events. Osteonecrosis of the jaws is a recognized complication of bisphosphonate therapy.

B. In some studies, up to 75% of patients with breast cancer will have metastatic disease. The bony skeleton is frequently involved. On radiologic examination, these metastases are predominantly osteolytic.

C. Placebo-controlled trials with oral or IV bisphosphonates have shown that prolonged administration can reduce the frequency of skeleton-related events by 30% to 40%.

D. Pain is the most frequent symptom of bone metastases and can significantly alter the quality of life of cancer patients. Hypercalcemia classically occurs in 10% to 15% of the cases.

E. This patient likely has a history of breast cancer and now may have diffuse metastases in both her brain and skeletal system. She requires a detailed evaluation.

103. **(B)**

A. The biologic precursor to gout is elevated serum uric acid levels (ie, hyperuricemia).

B. In psoriatic arthritis, the distal interphalangeal joints are regularly involved. The disease can also focus on the larger joints of the lower extremities.

C. The onset of polyarthritis in RA is insidious in about three-quarters of patients and initially affects the small joints of the hands and feet (metacarpophalangeal, proximal interphalangeal and metatarsophalangeal joints) before spreading to the larger joints.

D. Inflammatory markers such as the ESR or CRP are normal in about 60% of patients with early RA.

104. **(A)** This is most likely a case of CRPS type II.

A. CRPS is a painful disorder that develops as a disproportionate consequence of traumas. These disorders are most common in the limbs and are characterized by pain (spontaneous pain, hyperalgesia, allodynia); active and passive movement disorders (including an increased physiological tremor); abnormal regulation of blood flow and sweating; edema of skin and subcutaneous tissues; and trophic changes of skin, organs of the skin, and subcutaneous tissues.

B. CRPS type I (previously known as reflex sympathetic dystrophy) typically develops after minor trauma with no obvious or a small nerve lesion (eg, bone fracture, sprains, bruises, skin lesions, or surgery).

C. CRPS type I can also develop after remote trauma in the visceral domain or even after a CNS lesion (eg, stroke). Important features of CRPS type I are that the severity of symptoms is disproportionate to the severity of trauma and pain has a tendency to spread distally in the affected limb. The symptoms are not confined to the innervation zone of an individual nerve. Thus, all symptoms of CRPS type I may be present irrespective of the type of the preceding lesion.

D. Research is beginning to uncover that the CNS is actively involved in CRPS pathophysiology. Nerve cells, microglia, and astrocytes all may be involved.

105. (A)

A. Distal symmetrical polyneuropathy is the most common peripheral nerve disorder associated with HIV.

B. Headache is the most common of the AIDS-related pain syndromes. Common causes include cerebral toxoplasmosis.

C. Progressive polyradiculopathy is most commonly associated with cytomegalovirus infection. Symptoms include flaccid paralysis and pain with sensory disturbance.

D. Kaposi's sarcoma can cause both muscular and bone pain through infiltration.

106. (B)

A. Central pain affects people with strokes, spinal cord injuries, and multiple sclerosis. It can also occur after neurosurgical procedures on the brain and spine. The mechanism is thought to be because of disruption of spinothalamocortical transmission.

B. Pain may occur with syringomyelia, and it may precede any other sign of the disease by many years.

C. The pathophysiology of SCI has yet to be completely elucidated, but both spinal and supraspinal pathways may be involved.

D. Partial or total interruption of afferent fibers results in the degeneration of presynaptic terminals and an alteration in function and structure. Denervated synaptic sites may be reinnervated by other axons and previously ineffective synapses may become active (unmasking). Excitation spreads to neighboring areas and supersensitivity

occurs, producing an abnormal firing pattern that may depend on stimulation or may occur spontaneously. This sequence of events explains many of the symptoms of central pain, including dysesthesia (abnormal firing pattern), spontaneous shooting pain (paroxysmal burst discharges), evoked pain from nonpainful stimuli, diffusion of the evoked abnormal sensation, and the long-term failure of neurosurgical treatment.

107. (A)

A. Common psychiatric conditions that often feature pain as part of the illness are somatization disorder, hypochondriasis, factitious physical disorders, and malingering.

B. One of the ways to distinguish between these condition is whether there is conscious awareness (or lack of awareness) of both motivation and symptom production. Malingerers have a conscious awareness and motivation for a pain complaint.

C. Other psychiatric disorders may strongly influence chronic pain without directly causing it—depression, anxiety, panic, and posttraumatic stress disorders.

D. Chronic pain complaints often reflect or are influenced by psychiatric factors. Physicians commonly encounter "illness-affirming behaviors" in which patient complaints or symptoms go beyond what should be expected from a specific disease process. This is true of both anxiety and malingering.

108. (A)

A. Primary burning mouth syndrome is a chronic, idiopathic intraoral pain condition that is not accompanied by clinical lesions but some consider it a painful neuropathy. The symptoms are often described as continuous, spontaneous, and often intense burning sensation in the mouth or tongue.

B. Increasing evidence suggests that 80% to 90% of cases that are technically still classified as idiopathic are caused by compression of the trigeminal nerve close to its exit from the brainstem by an aberrant loop of artery or vein.

C. Less than 10% of patients will have symptomatic disease associated with an identifiable cause other than a vascular compressive lesion—usually a benign tumor or cyst—or multiple sclerosis. About 1% to 5% of patients with multiple sclerosis develop trigeminal neuralgia.

D. Trigeminal neuralgia, by definition, has to be in the distribution of the trigeminal nerve (not the distribution occipital nerve). Trigeminal neuralgia is defined as paroxysmal attacks of pain lasting from a fraction of a second to 2 minutes that affect one or more divisions of the trigeminal nerve. Diagnostic criteria for classic trigeminal neuralgia:

- Pain has at least one of these characteristics: intense, sharp, superficial, or stabbing precipitated from trigger areas or by trigger factors.
- Attacks are similar in individual patients.
- No neurological deficit is clinically evident.
- Not attributed to another disorder.

109. (C)

A. The pain of glossopharyngeal neuralgia is very similar to that of trigeminal neuralgia but affects posterior-third of the tongue, tonsils, and pharynx.

B. Giant cell arteritis is a common systemic vasculitis in the elderly. It is commonly associated with visual loss and strokes, so it must be diagnosed and treated aggressively. Temporal artery biopsy is the gold standard in the diagnosis of giant cell arteritis. Steroids are a common mode of treatment.

C. Cervical carotid artery dissection most commonly present with head, facial, or neck pain. Other commonly seen symptoms include Horner syndrome, pulsatile tinnitus, and cranial nerve palsy.

D. Pure facial pain is most often caused by sinusitis and the chewing apparatus, but also a multitude of other causes.

110. (B)

A. There are gender differences in the presentation of acute coronary syndrome. Men are more likely to present with chest pain, left arm pain, or diaphoresis. Nausea is more common in women.

B. Cardiac syndrome X is angina-like chest pain in the presence of a normal coronary arteriography. Although symptoms in cardiac syndrome X are often noncardiac, a sizable proportion of patients have angina pectoris due to transient myocardial ischemia.

C. Despite sophisticated medical and surgical procedures, including percutaneous endovascular methods, a large number of patients suffer from chronic refractory angina pectoris. Improvement of pain relief in this category of patients requires the use of adjuvant therapies, of which spinal cord stimulation (SCS) seems to be the most promising. Controlled studies suggest that in patients with chronic refractory angina, SCS provides symptomatic relief that is equivalent to that provided by surgical or endovascular reperfusion procedures, but with a lower rate of complications and rehospitalization. Similarly, SCS proved cost effective compared to medical as well as surgical or endovascular approaches in a comparable group of patients.

D. Using SCS for the treatment of angina is still met with reluctance by the medical community. Reasons for this disinclination may be related to incomplete understanding of the action mechanism of SCS.

111. (C)

A. Children and adolescents who present with knee pain are likely to have one of three common conditions: patellar subluxation, tibial apophysitis, or patellar tendonitis. Additional diagnoses to consider in children include slipped capital femoral epiphysis and septic arthritis. Pseudogout is more likely present in older adults.

B. Infection of the knee joint may occur in patients of any age but is more common in those whose immune system has been weakened by cancer, diabetes mellitus, alcoholism, acquired immunodeficiency syndrome, or corticosteroid therapy. The patient with septic arthritis reports abrupt onset of pain and swelling of the knee with no antecedent trauma.

C. Acute inflammation, pain, and swelling in the absence of trauma suggest the possibility of a crystal-induced inflammatory arthropathy such as gout or pseudogout. Gout commonly affects the knee. In this arthropathy, sodium urate crystals precipitate in the knee joint and cause an intense inflammatory response. In pseudogout, calcium pyrophosphate crystals are the causative agents. On physical examination, the knee joint is erythematous, warm, tender, and swollen. Even minimal range of motion is exquisitely painful.

D. Osteoarthritis of the knee joint is a common problem after 60 years of age. The patient presents with knee pain that is aggravated by weight-bearing activities and relieved by rest. The patient has no systemic symptoms but usually awakens with morning stiffness that dissipates somewhat with activity. In addition to chronic joint stiffness and pain, the patient may report episodes of acute synovitis. Findings on physical examination include decreased range of motion, crepitus, a mild joint effusion, and palpable osteophytic changes at the knee joint. Radiographs show joint-space narrowing, subchondral bony sclerosis, cystic changes, and hypertrophic osteophyte formation.

112. (D)

A. Distal symmetric polyneuropathy is the most common neuropathy in diabetes (which would affect both legs symmetrically). There are other neuropathic entities that occur in diabetes, such as mononeuropathy, which could affect one foot.

B. The plantar fascia is frequently a site of chronic pain. Patients typically complain of pain that starts with the first step on arising in the morning or after prolonged sitting. Pain onset is usually insidious but also may commence after a traumatic injury. Diagnosis is made by eliciting pain with palpation in the region of origin of the plantar fascia. Pain may be worsened by passive dorsiflexion of the foot.

C. The interdigital spaces of the foot are sites for the occurrence of painful neuromas, a condition termed Morton neuroma. The second and third common digital branches of the medial plantar nerve are the most frequent sites for development of interdigital neuromas.

D. The tarsal tunnel is formed by the medial malleolus and a fibrous ligament, the flexor retinaculum. The posterior tibial nerve passes through the tunnel and can be compressed by any condition that reduces the space of the tunnel. The medial plantar, lateral plantar, and calcaneal branches of the posterior tibial nerve innervate the base of the foot.

113. (A)

A. Endometriosis is the commonest cause of chronic pelvic pain in women. It is characterized by the presence of uterine endometrial tissue outside the uterus, most commonly in the pelvic cavity. The disorder mainly affects women of reproductive age.

B. Endometriosis has been described as a pelvic inflammatory process with altered function of immune cells and increased number of activated macrophages in the peritoneal environment that secrete various local products, such as growth factors and cytokines.

C. Endometriosis is estrogen-dependent, and traditional treatments have aimed to decrease production of estrogens such as estradiol. However, the exact mechanism by which estrogens promote endometriosis is unclear and suppression of estrogens has variable effects.

D. Endometriotic lesions themselves secrete proinflammatory cytokines such as interleukin 8 (IL-8), which recruit macrophages and T cells to the peritoneum and mediate inflammatory responses.

114. (A)

A. The visceral pleura do not contain any nociceptors or pain receptors. The parietal pleura is innervated by somatic nerves that sense pain when the parietal pleura is inflamed. Inflammation that occurs at the periphery of the lung parenchyma can extend into the pleural space and involve the parietal pleura, thereby activating the somatic pain receptors and causing pleuritic pain.

B. Viral infection is one of the most common causes of pleurisy. Viruses that have been linked as causative agents include influenza, parainfluenza, coxsackieviruses, respiratory syncytial virus, mumps, cytomegalovirus, adenovirus, and Epstein-Barr virus. Additionally, pleurisy may be the first manifestation of some less common disorders.

C. Pleuritic pain typically is localized to the area that is inflamed or along predictable referred pain pathways. Patients' descriptions of the pain are consistent in most cases of pleurisy. The classic feature is that forceful breathing movement, such as taking a deep breath, talking, coughing, or sneezing, exacerbates the pain.

D. The differential diagnosis of chest pain in this patient should include myocardial infarction, endocarditis, pulmonary embolism, pneumonia, and pneumothorax. Pulmonary embolism can cause pleurisy.

115. (B)

A. Repetitive strain injury includes specific disorders such as CTS, cubital tunnel syndrome, Guyon canal syndrome, lateral epicondylitis, and tendonitis of the wrist or hand.

B. Ample evidence exists for the association between physical risk factors such as repetitive movements, poor posture, and inadequate strength and the occurrence of repetitive strain injury.

C. The effects of work-related and psychosocial factors are not as clear as those of physical factors, although high workload, stress, and physical or psychological demands, low job security, and little support from colleagues might be important.

D. Several hypotheses for the pathophysiology of repetitive strain injury exist, but none

has been strongly supported by scientific evidence. Despite initial distal presentation, this disorder seems to be a diffuse neuromuscular illness. Mechanical (elastic deformation of connective tissue due to increased pressure within muscles) and physiological (electrochemical and metabolic imbalances) reactions might cause damage to muscle tissue and lead to complaints of strain. Continuous contraction of muscles from long-term static load with insufficient breaks could result in reduced local blood circulation and muscle fatigue. Consequently, pain sensors in the muscles could become hypersensitive, leading to a pain response at low levels of stimulation. Other hypotheses suggest frequent cocontractions in muscles or changes in proprioception as the source of injury. There is no unifying hypothesis.

116. (D)

A. Chronic pain following surgical procedures for breast cancer was once thought to be rare. The results of recent studies, however, suggest that the incidence of chronic pain following breast cancer surgery may be more than 50%. Although most surgical advances are less invasive and have fewer complications, the rapid pace of change in treatment complicates outcome research.

B. Peripheral neuropathy, often painful, is common after paclitaxel, a second-line therapy for metastatic disease, and also occurs with other chemotherapeutic agents. The incidence of peripheral neuropathy is lower with platinum compounds like cisplatin.

C. Sensory neuropathies are more common in chemotherapy than motor neuropathies.

D. Axillary dissection poses risks to the intercostobrachial nerve, from stretch during retraction as well as from frank transection. Many patients will be left with an area of numbness on the upper inner arm, signifying damage to the intercostobrachial nerve, but only a minority of these will be painful. Other nerves at risk for damage from axillary dissection include the medial cutaneous nerve of the arm, which contains fibers from C8 and T1 and arises from the medial cord of the brachial plexus. It can be harmed during section of the tributaries of the axillary vein, leaving patients with sensory loss on the lower medial skin of the upper arm. Pain accompanied by sensory loss in one of these areas provides the basis for a diagnosis of injury to these specific nerves.

117. **(C)**

A. Peripheral nerves are composed of large- and small-diameter nerve fibers. Symptoms associated with large-diameter nerve fiber dysfunction include weakness, numbness, tingling, and loss of balance, while those associated with small-diameter nerve fiber damage include pain, anesthesia to pin and temperature sensation, and autonomic dysfunction (eg, changes in local vasoregulation).

B. Diabetes duration and blood sugar control correlate with the development of neuropathy.

C. Neuropathy with a predilection for small-diameter nerve fibers can appear with impaired glucose tolerance, a prediabetic state that does not meet the criteria for diabetes mellitus as defined by the American Diabetes Association. Although this neuropathy is usually milder than the neuropathy seen in frank diabetes mellitus, impaired glucose tolerance has been associated with severe painful polyneuropathy without another known etiology.

D. As these painful symptoms often result from small-diameter nerve fiber dysfunction, patients may have accompanying abnormalities of autonomic function in the feet (eg, decreased sweating, dry skin, and impaired vasomotor control).

118. **(C)**

A. Reactivation of the varicella-zoster virus can cause dermatomal pain without a rash in a process termed "zoster sine herpete." This cannot be made on the basis of clinical presentation alone and would require evidence of concurrent viral reactivation.

B. Zoster reactivation typically occurs once for an individual. Atypical manifestations that occur in immunocompromised patients include prolonged course, recurrent lesions, and involvement of multiple dermatomes. Diagnostic laboratory tests are recommended when herpes simplex must be ruled out (eg, recurrent rash or sacral lesions) and for patients with atypical lesions.

C. Until recently, these definitions have been arbitrary, but the results of recent research now provide support for the validity of distinguishing between three phases of pain in affected and adjacent dermatomes: (1) herpes zoster acute pain (also termed acute herpetic neuralgia), defined as pain that occurs within 30 days after rash onset; (2) subacute herpetic neuralgia, defined as pain that persists beyond the acute phase but that resolves before the diagnosis of PHN can be made; and (3) PHN, defined as pain that persists 120 days or more after rash onset.

D. It can also be predicted that the number of adults developing herpes zoster in the United States may increase as a consequence of reduced opportunities for subclinical immune boosting resulting from near-universal varicella vaccination of children. Recent data showing an increase in herpes zoster in the United States are consistent with this prediction. An increase in the incidence of herpes zoster could be offset by zoster vaccination, but the extent to which widespread herpes zoster vaccination will occur is presently unknown.

119. **(D)** This patient has evidence of having an intrathecal pump with granuloma formation.

A. There is a strong relationship between higher doses of intrathecal morphine and granuloma formation. The notion that high-dose morphine is causative is not universally accepted. Some authors have suggested that long-term administration of opiates may lead to localized fibrosis and the formation of a granulomatous mass surrounding the catheter tip.

B. There have been cases of granuloma formation reported involving the intrathecal infusion of baclofen. These lesions did not appear to cause any compression of the spinal cord or neurological deficits, resolved when the catheter tip was replaced, and could represent a different disease process.

C. Microscopic pathology of intrathecal morphine related granulomas often reveals necrotic tissue surrounded by macrophages, plasma cells, eosinophils, or lymphocytes. Nearby vessels may be surrounded by mononuclear inflammatory cells consisting predominantly of plasma cells. Gross pathologic examination of catheter tip granulomas related to intrathecal morphine infusions often demonstrates the mass conforming to the distal portion of the catheter.

D. Because of its (morphine) hydrophilic structure, it has a prolonged duration of action and due to the drug's high localization; its analgesic effect is maximized at a lower dose. This results in a lower incidence of systemic side effects, reduces drug dependence, and does not significantly influence motor, sensory, or sympathetic reflexes.

120. (C)

A. In the three studies that looked at the causes of FBSS, the most common structural causes of FBSS are foraminal stenosis (25%-29%), painful disc (20%-22%), pseudarthrosis (14%), neuropathic pain (10%), recurrent disc herniation (7%-12%), iatrogenic instability (5%), facet pain (3%), and sacroiliac joint (SIJ) pain (2%), among some others.

B. Most patients with refractory low-back pain have symptoms of at least one major psychiatric disorder, most commonly depression, substance abuse disorder or anxiety disorder. Pure psychogenic pain (pain disorder, psychological type) is rare in patients with FBSS. All patients have some pain behavior, which may be appropriate or inappropriate.

C. In patients with chronic pain, an improvement in visual analog scale (VAS) score of 1.8 U, equivalent to a change in pain of

about 30%, may be considered a satisfactory result.

D. FBSS is a nonspecific term that implies that the final outcome of surgery did not meet the expectations of both the patient and the surgeon that were established before surgery.

121. (B)

A. True, this process usually begins at 16 to 20 weeks. In early pregnancy it is important to exclude unruptured ectopic pregnancy and ovarian torsion.

B. Radicular symptoms are common during pregnancy; there is a low incidence of herniated disc associated with these complaints.

C. Limited plain radiographs that are considered vital may be okay to perform during pregnancy according to some studies.

D. It is true that if a new onset migraine occurs during pregnancy, one should investigate a secondary cause (including consideration for an MRI).

122. (C)

A. A vasoocclusive crisis most commonly involves the back, legs, knees, arms, chest, and abdomen. The pain generally affects two or more sites. Bone pain tends to be bilateral and symmetric. Recurrent crises in an individual patient usually have the same distribution.

B. Acute pain in patients with sickle cell disease is caused by ischemic tissue injury resulting from the occlusion of microvascular beds by sickled erythrocytes during an acute crisis. Acute bone pain from microvascular occlusion is a common reason for emergency department (ED) visits and hospitalizations in patients with sickle cell disease. Obstruction of blood flow results in regional hypoxemia and acidosis, creating a recurrent pattern of further sickling, tissue injury, and pain. The severe pain is believed to be caused by increased intramedullary pressure, especially within the juxta-articular areas of long bones, secondary to an acute inflammatory response to vascular necrosis of the bone marrow by sickled erythrocytes. The pain may also occur because of involvement of the periosteum or periarticular soft tissue of the joints.

C. When a vasoocclusive crisis lasts longer than 7 days, it is important to search for other causes of bone pain, such as osteomyelitis, avascular necrosis, and compression deformities. When a recurrent bone crisis lasts for weeks, an exchange transfusion may be required to abort the cycle.

D. Patients with homozygous sickle cell and sickle cell–β-thalassemia have a higher frequency of vasoocclusive pain crises than patients with hemoglobin sickle cell and sickle cell–β-thalassemia genotype.

123. (B)

A. Depression produces well documented disturbances to sleep architecture including reduced slow-wave sleep and early onset rapid-eye-movement (REM) sleep. Sleep disturbance has been well documented in fibromyalgia.

B. This is one of the *Diagnostic and Statistical Manual of Mental Disorders* (Fourth Edition) *(DSM-IV)* diagnostic criteria of substance abuse.

C. This is not included as one of the *DSM IV* diagnostic criteria for substance dependence.

D. Conversion disorder is an alteration in voluntary motor or sensory function that suggests a neurologic or general medical condition.

124. (A)

A. Chronic pain is a major complication of SCI with approximately two-thirds of all SCI patients experiencing some type of chronic pain, and up to one-third complaining of that their pain is severe. The prevalence of pain after SCI often increases with time after injury.

B. In addition to central pain, there are multiple types of pain that develop after SCI

including musculoskeletal, visceral, and peripheral neuropathic pain.

C. Central pain has been reported with injury to all levels of the spinal cord. There is conflicting evidence in the literature as to the level of injury that results in greatest frequency or severity of central pain, whether incomplete spinal cord lesions may result in a higher incidence of central pain or whether there is a link between type of injury and the development of central pain.

D. Central neuropathic pain after SCI has been categorized based on the location of the complaint as either at the level of the injury or below the level of the injury. Although it may be difficult to distinguish the two clinically (and both may be present in the same patient), central pain that occurs at the level of injury is because of segmental spinal cord damage, and not because of nerve root damage.

125. (D)

A. Physiologic changes occur to the nociceptive neurons in the dorsal horn following SCI including an increase in abnormal spontaneous and evoked discharges from dorsal horn cell. Noxious stimulation causes primary afferent C-fibers to release excitatory amino acid neurotransmitters in the dorsal horn. Prolonged high intensity noxious stimulation activates the NMDA receptors which induces a cascade that may result in central sensitization.

B. On a molecular level, abnormal sodium channel expression within the dorsal horn (laminae L1-L4) bilaterally has been implicated as a major contributor to hyperexcitability. These pain relay neurons tend to show increase activity with noxious and nonnoxious stimuli thus serving as a pain amplifier.

C. Thalamic neurons appear to undergo changes after SCI in both human and animal models. In the animal model, enhanced neuronal excitability in the VPL has been demonstrated directly and as well as indirectly; enhanced regional blood flow has been found in the rate VPL after SCI suggesting increased neuronal activity.

D. Much like the neurons in the dorsal horn, the thalamic neurons after SCI show increased activity with noxious and nonnoxious stimuli. VPL neurons are spontaneously hyperexcitable following SCI without receiving input from the spinal cord neurons suggesting that the thalamus may act as a pain-signal generator in central pain accompanying SCI.

126. (D)

A. Excessive alcohol use plays a significant role in up to 70% of adults with chronic pancreatitis. Genetic and structural defects predominate in children.

B. Patients may have recurrent episodes of acute pancreatitis, which can progress to chronic abdominal pain. The pain is commonly described as midepigastric postprandial pain that radiates to the back and that can sometimes be relieved by sitting upright or leaning forward. In some patients there is a spontaneous remission of pain by organ failure (pancreatic burnout theory). Patients may also present with steatorrhea, malabsorption, vitamin deficiency (A, D, E, K, and B_{12}), diabetes, or weight loss. Approximately 10% to 20% of patients may have exocrine insufficiency without abdominal pain.

C. Autoimmune pancreatitis accounts for 5% to 6% of chronic pancreatitis and is characterized by autoimmune inflammation, lymphocytic infiltration, fibrosis, and pancreatic dysfunction.

D. Because of its varied presentation and clinical similarity to acute pancreatitis, many cases of chronic pancreatitis are not diagnosed.

127. (D)

A. Mainly two types of pain receptors are activated by nociceptive input. These include low-threshold nociceptors that are connected to fast conducting A-δ pain fibers, and high-threshold nociceptors that conduct impulses in slow (unmyelinated)

C fibers. Within the dorsal horn of the spinal cord, these pain fibers synapse with spinal neurons via synaptic transmission.

B. Many neurotransmitters (ie, glutamate and substance P) are able to modulate the postsynaptic responses with further transmission to supraspinal sites (thalamus, anterior cingulated cortex, insular cortex, and somatosensory cortex) via the ascending pathways.

C. The simplest form of plasticity in nervous systems is that repeated noxious stimulation may lead to habituation (decreased response) or sensitization (increased response). Prolonged or strong activity of dorsal horn neurons caused by repeated or sustained noxious stimulation may subsequently lead to increased neuronal responsiveness or central sensitization. Neuroplasticity and subsequent CNS sensitization include altered function of chemical, electrophysiological, and pharmacological systems. These changes cause exaggerated perception of painful stimuli (hyperalgesia), a perception of innocuous stimuli as painful (allodynia), and may be involved in the generation of referred pain and hyperalgesia across multiple spinal segments. While the exact mechanism by which the spinal cord becomes sensitized or in "hyperexcitable" state currently remains somewhat unknown, some contributing factors have been proposed.

D. *Windup* refers to a central spinal mechanism in which repetitive noxious stimulation results in a slow temporal summation that is experienced in humans as increased pain. In 1965, animal experiments showed for the first time that repetitive C fiber stimulation could result in a progressive increase of electrical discharges from the second-order neuron in the spinal cord. This mechanism of pain amplification in the spinal cord is related to temporal summation of second pain or windup. Second pain, which is more dull and strongly related to chronic pain states, is transmitted through unmyelinated C fibers to dorsal horn nociceptive neurons. During the C fibers transmitted stimuli, NMDA receptors of second-order neurons become activated. It is well-known that NMDA activation induces calcium entry into the dorsal horn neurons. Calcium entry into sensory neurons in the dorsal horn induces activation of nitric oxide (NO) synthase, leading to the synthesis of NO. NO can affect the nociceptor terminals and enhance the release of sensory neuropeptides (in particular, substance P) from presynaptic neurons, therefore contributing to the development of hyperalgesia and maintenance of central sensitization.

E. Substance P is an important nociceptive neurotransmitter. It lowers the threshold of synaptic excitability, resulting in the unmasking of normally silent interspinal synapses and the sensitization of second-order spinal neurons. Furthermore, substance P can extend for long distances in the spinal cord and sensitize dorsal horn neurons at a distance from the initial input locus. This results in an expansion of receptive fields and the activation of wide dynamic neurons by nonnociceptive afferent impulses.

128. (B)

A. The presence of several pain inhibitory and facilitatory centers in the brainstem is well recognized. The dorsolateral funiculus appears to be a preferred pathway for descending pain inhibitory systems.

B. One function of the descending inhibitory pathway is to 'focus' the excitation of the dorsal horn neurons. The effect is to generate a more urgent, localized, and rapid pain signal by suppressing surrounding neuronal activity.

C. Facilitatory pathways leading from the brainstem have also been identified. There is now behavioral evidence that forebrain centers are capable of exerting powerful clinically significant influences on various nuclei of the brainstem, including the nuclei identified as the origin of the descending facilitatory pathway. The activity in descending pathways is not constant but can be modulated, for example, by the level of vigilance

or attention and by stress. This has been referred to as cognitive emotional sensitization. Forebrain products such as cognitions, emotions, attention, and motivation have influence on the clinical pain experience.

D. Certain cognitive styles and personality traits have been associated with the amplification of pain and its extension in the absence of tissue damage. These include somatization, catastrophizing, and hypervigilance. Thus, via descending pathways behavioral and cognitive therapies might also effect synaptic transmission in the spinal cord and thereby have the capacity to prevent or reverse long-term changes of synaptic strength in pain pathways.

129. (D)

A. Injured and neighboring noninjured sensory neurons can develop a change in their excitability sufficient to generate pacemaker-like potentials, which evoke ectopic action potential discharges, a sensory inflow independent of any peripheral stimulus. These changes may manifest at the site of the injury, at the neuroma, and in the DRG. Ectopic input is most prominent in A fibers but also occurs to a more limited extent in cells with unmyelinated axons (ie, C fibers).

B. Central sensitization represents a state of heightened sensitivity of dorsal horn neurons such that their threshold of activation is reduced, and their responsiveness to synaptic inputs is augmented. There are two forms of central sensitization; an activity-dependent form that is rapidly induced within seconds by afferent activity in nociceptors and which produces changes in synaptic efficacy that last for tens of minutes as a result of the phosphorylation and altered trafficking of voltage- and ligand-gated ion channel receptors, and a transcription-dependent form that takes some hours to be induced but outlast the initiating stimulus for prolonged periods.

C. After peripheral nerve injury C fiber input may arise spontaneously and drive central sensitization.

D. Peripheral neuropathic pain, that clinical pain syndrome associated with lesions to the peripheral nervous system, is characterized by positive and negative symptoms. Positive symptoms include spontaneous pain, paresthesia, and dysesthesia, as well as a pain evoked by normally innocuous stimuli (allodynia) and an exaggerated or prolonged pain to noxious stimuli (hyperalgesia/hyperpathia). The negative symptoms essentially reflect loss of sensation due to axon/neuron loss; the positive symptoms reflect abnormal excitability of the nervous system.

130. (D)

A. It is well recognized that the prolonged use of opioids is associated with a requirement for ever-increasing doses in order to maintain pain relief at an acceptable and consistent level. This phenomenon is termed analgesic tolerance. All patients on opiates are at risk to develop tolerance.

B. Tolerance may also be related to a state of hyperalgesia that results from exposure to the opioid itself. Patients who receive long-term opioid therapy sometimes develop unexpected, abnormal pain. Similar paradoxical opioid-induced pain has been confirmed in a number of animal studies, even during the period of continuous opioid delivery. This has been termed opiate-induced hyperalgesia (OIH).

C. A number of recent studies have demonstrated that such pain may be secondary to neuroplastic changes that occur in the brain and spinal cord. One such change may be the activation of descending pain facilitation mechanisms arising from the rostral ventromedial medulla (RVM).

D. Opioids elicit systems-level adaptations resulting in pain due to descending facilitation, upregulation of spinal dynorphin, and enhanced, evoked release of excitatory transmitters from primary afferents. These adaptive changes in response to sustained exposure to opioids indicate the need for the evaluation of the clinical consequences of long-term opioid administration.

131. (A)

A. Unlike the somatic motor system which has its motor neurons in the CNS, the motor neurons of the ANS are located in the periphery.

B. The peripheral efferent pathways of both the sympathetic and parasympathetic nervous system have two components: a primary presynaptic or preganglionic neuron, and a secondary postsynaptic or postganglionic neuron.

C. The cell bodies of the autonomic postganglionic neurons are arranged in aggregates known as ganglia, wherein the synapses between pre- and postganglionic neurons take place. The transmission of signal from the CNS synapses at an autonomic ganglia in the periphery prior to reaching the target organ.

D. There are multiple differences between the two systems. Some of the important points are highlighted above.

132. (C)

A. The parasympathetic preganglionic fibers travel from the CNS to synapse in ganglia located close to their target organs. In most areas, parasympathetic innervation tends to be more precise than sympathetic innervation.

B. Sympathetic fibers are generally distributed throughout the body. Parasympathetic fibers are generally only innervating the visceral organs.

C. The preganglionic parasympathetic neurons have their cell bodies in the gray matter of the brainstem and their fibers travel with the oculomotor, facial, glossopharyngeal, and vagus nerves. The preganglionic fibers from the oculomotor, facial, and glossopharyngeal nerves synapse in the ciliary, sphenopalatine, otic, and submaxillary ganglia, all of which are located in the head. From these ganglia, the postganglionic fibers travel to the target organs (eg, the lacrimal and salivary glands).

D. The efferent portion of the sympathetic division of the ANS consists of preganglionic neurons, the two paravertebral (lateral) sympathetic chains, prevertebral and terminal ganglia, and postganglionic neurons.

133. (B)

A. Most tumors involving the brachial plexus originate from the lung or breast and as a result often invade the lower plexus, particularly the inferior trunk and medial cord.

B. Pain was the most common presenting symptom (75%) in a large study of neoplastic brachial plexopathy and usually was located in the shoulder and axilla. Radicular pain was often distributed along the medial aspect of the arm and forearm into the fourth and fifth fingers. Motor and reflex findings commonly (75%) were in the lower plexus distribution (especially C8-T1). Most remaining patients had signs of more widespread (C5-T1) plexus involvement.

C. Radiotherapy can produce plexus injury by both direct toxic effects on axons and on the vasa nervorum, with secondary microinfarction of nerve. Neurotoxicity is dose-related for greater than 1000 cGy, pathologic changes can be observed in Schwann cells, endoneurial fibroblasts, and vascular and perineural cells. Administration of 3500 Gy has produced injury to anterior and posterior nerve roots in rodents.

134. (C)

A. Overdose of baclofen causes side-effects that range from drowsiness, nausea, headache, muscle weakness, and lightheadedness to somnolence, respiratory depression, seizures, rostral progression of hypotonia, and loss of consciousness progressing to coma. There are a range of symptoms with withdrawal as well; pruritus without rash, diaphoresis, hyperthermia, hypotension, neurological changes, including agitation or confusion, sudden generalized increase in muscle tone, spasticity, and muscle rigidity. With severe withdrawal, rhabdomyolysis and multiple organ failure can occur.

B. Baclofen is a γ-aminobutyric acid (GABA) analogue that has inhibitory effects on spinal cord reflexes and brain. The precise mechanism of action of baclofen as a muscle relaxant and antispasticity agent is not fully understood. Baclofen inhibits both monosynaptic and polysynaptic reflexes at the spinal cord level, possibly by decreasing excitatory neurotransmitter release from primary afferent terminals, although actions at supraspinal sites may also contribute to its clinical effects. Baclofen also causes enhancement of vagal tone and inhibition of mesolimbic and nigrostriatal dopamine neurons (directly or via inhibiting substance P).

C. ITB withdrawal syndrome has been fatal in some cases. Differential diagnoses include malignant hyperthermia, neuroleptic-malignant syndrome, autonomic dysreflexia, sepsis, and meningitis.

D. Refer to explanation A.

135. (C)

A. Although a post–lumbar puncture headache is a possibility, other processes including a CNS infection must be excluded.

B. In general, prior to treating a post–lumbar puncture headache, conservative management should be trialed for at least 48 hours.

C. The most appropriate step.

D. MRI of the lumbar spine does not have a role at this stage.

E. High-dose narcotic therapy does not have a role at this stage.

136. (A)

A. Cervical transforaminal epidural steroid injections are controversial for several reasons. One of the major concerns is the potential involvement of the vertebral artery, which lies in the anterior neuroforamen.

B. See explanation A.

C. Injecting triamcinolone, which is a particulate steroid, could be problematic, especially if the steroid were to enter the vertebral artery circulation.

D. Patients experiencing radicular symptoms in the course of a transforaminal procedure may suggest involvement of a nerve root.

E. If the patient has a history of vasovagal responses, appropriate planning should be made to manage these symptoms should they occur during the procedure.

137. (B)

A. Mastectomy has been reported to lead to phantom sensation in 22% to 64% of women who have had the operation.

B. Phantom sensations are present in the majority of amputees; the sensation is almost always more vivid in the distal extremity. The vast majority of these patients do not have phantom limb pain.

C. Stump pain is perceived to be present in the existing body part in the region of amputation; it is often associated with palpable neuromata at the amputation site—however, all amputees have neuromata and not all amputees have stump pain.

D. Phantom limb sensations "telescope" with time—the proximal part of the limb disappears first.

138. (A)

A. The location of the pain can be helpful for diagnosis. Anterior-superior pain often can be localized to the acromioclavicular joint, whereas lateral deltoid pain is often correlated with rotator cuff pathology. Neck pain and radiating symptoms should be explored because cervical pathology can mimic shoulder pain. Typically, pain that radiates past the elbow to the hand is not related to shoulder pathology. However, it is not uncommon to have pain that radiates into the neck because the trapezius muscle often spasms in patients with underlying chronic shoulder pathology. The presence of both is more likely to be related to cervical pathology. Dull, achy night pain is often associated with rotator cuff tears or severe glenohumeral osteoarthritis

B. The patient's medical history, including joint problems, can help to narrow the differential diagnosis. Autoimmune diseases and inflammatory arthritis can affect the shoulder, resulting in erosions and wear in the glenohumeral joint, whereas diabetes and thyroid disorders can be associated with adhesive capsulitis.

C. Acromioclavicular joint pathology is usually well localized. A history of an injury to the joint (shoulder separation), heavy weight lifting, tenderness to palpation at the acromioclavicular joint, pain with cross-body adduction testing, extreme internal rotation, and forward flexion are consistent with the diagnosis. Radiographs may be difficult to interpret because most patients have acromioclavicular osteoarthritis by the age of 40 to 50 years. A distal clavicle lysis or an elevated distal clavicle supports the diagnosis, whereas the absence of tenderness to palpation at the acromioclavicular joint is inconsistent with the diagnosis.

D. Rotator cuff disorders that affect the function of the rotator cuff include a partial or complete tear, tendinitis or tendinosis, and calcific tendinitis. Initially, it is more important to differentiate this group of disorders from the other groups than it is to identify the specific diagnosis. Typically, the patients are older than 40 years and complain of pain in the lateral aspect of the arm with radiation no farther than the elbow. Weakness, a painful arc of motion, night pain, and a positive impingement sign are components of the history and physical examination that are consistent with this diagnosis. Findings that are inconsistent with this diagnosis include being younger than 30 years, having no weakness, and presenting no impingement signs. Positive radiographs can be helpful to diagnose calcific tendinitis, acromial spur, humeral head cysts, or superior migration of the humeral head, but are typically normal.

139. (C)

1. L2 nerve: weakness of hip flexion (iliopsoas) and sensory loss on anterior groin and thigh. No deep tendon reflex.

2. L4 nerve: weakness of leg extension (quadriceps), ankle dorsiflexion (tibialis

anterior); sensory loss medial calf/foot; loss of patellar reflex.

3. L5 nerve: weakness of dorsiflexion of big toe (EHL) sensory loss lateral aspect of calf and dorsum of foot. No deep tendon reflex.

4. S1 nerve: weakness of toe walking (gastrocnemius); sensory loss on dorsum of foot, loss of Achilles reflex. This is correct because the reflex does not have to be decreased/lost to suspect this nerve root's involvement. The sensory abnormality is enough.

140. **(E)** Addiction is a disease of the CNS. All substances of abuse activate essentially the same neuroanatomic structures. All of the structures listed above are properly linked.

CHAPTER 4

Pharmacology
Questions

DIRECTIONS (Questions 141 through 209): Each of the numbered items or incomplete statements in this section is followed by answers or by completions of the statement. Select the ONE lettered answer or completion that is BEST in each case.

141. Which of the following is true regarding seizures as one of the multiple side effects from the use of opioids?

    (A) Morphine and related opioids can cause seizure activity when moderate doses are given

    (B) Seizure activity is more likely with meperidine, especially in the elderly and with renal dysfunction

    (C) Seizure activity is mediated through stimulation of N-methyl-D-aspartate (NMDA) receptors

    (D) Naloxone is very effective in treating seizures produced by morphine and related drugs including meperidine

    (E) Seizure activity is most likely related with the fact that opioids stimulate the production of γ-aminobutyric acid (GABA)

142. Which of the following is true regarding respiratory depression related to the use of opioids?

    (A) Opioid agonists, partial agonists, and agonist/antagonists produce the same degree of respiratory depression

    (B) Opioids produce a leftward shift of the CO_2 response curve

    (C) Depression of respiration is produced by a decrease in respiratory rate, with a constant minute volume

    (D) Naloxone partially reverses the opioid-induced respiratory depression

    (E) The apneic threshold is decreased

143. The use of which of the following opioids would produce the greatest incidence of delayed respiratory depression?

    (A) 25 μg intravenous (IV) fentanyl (bolus)

    (B) 4 mg IV morphine (bolus)

    (C) 5 μg IV sufentanil (bolus)

    (D) 8 mg epidural, preservative free morphine

    (E) 0.05 mg intrathecal, preservative free morphine

144. Opioids in general reduce the sympathetic output and produce a dose-dependant bradycardia, EXCEPT

    (A) morphine

    (B) fentanyl

    (C) meperidine

    (D) sufentanil

    (E) alfentanil

145. What is the main mechanism by which opioids produce analgesia?

 (A) Coupling of opioid receptors to sodium and potassium ion channels, therefore inhibiting neurotransmitter release (presynaptic) and inhibiting neuronal firing (postsynaptically)

 (B) Coupling of opioid receptor to potassium and calcium channels, inhibiting neurotransmitter release (presynaptic), and inhibiting neuronal firing (postsynaptically)

 (C) Coupling of opioid receptors to sodium and calcium channels, inhibiting neurotransmitter release (presynaptic), and inhibiting neuronal firing (postsynaptically)

 (D) Coupling of opioid receptors to potassium and calcium channels, inhibiting neuronal firing (presynaptically), and inhibiting neurotransmitter release (postsynaptically)

 (E) All the options are true

146. Main mechanics of spinal opioid analgesia is via

 (A) activation of presynaptic opioid receptors

 (B) activation of postsynaptic opioid receptors

 (C) activation of opioid receptors on the midbrain

 (D) activation of opioid receptors on the RVM

 (E) all of the above

147. Opioids act on what type of receptors targets?

 (A) μ-, δ-, κ-, And ORL receptors

 (B) Voltage-dependent sodium channels

 (C) α_{2B}-Adrenoreceptors

 (D) NMDA receptors

 (E) All of the above

148. Which of the following statements is true regarding the use of oxycodone?

 (A) Analgesic efficacy is not comparable with that of morphine

 (B) Typically has been used in combination with nonopioids

 (C) Not available as a long-acting preparation

 (D) Lower bioavailability than that of morphine

 (E) Consistently shows a higher induced rate of hallucinations and itching when compared with morphine

149. One important characteristic of methadone that has to be considered when prescribing it on an outpatient basis:

 (A) Usually there is a low chance for interactions on patients taking multiple medications

 (B) Withdrawal symptoms are as severe as with morphine

 (C) Rarely used in opioid addiction

 (D) Sedation and respiratory depression can outlast the analgesic action

 (E) Allows rapid titration

150. What property of methadone makes it a good option for opioid rotation, when tolerance develops?

 (A) Serotonin agonist

 (B) α_{2B}-Adrenoreceptor agonist

 (C) μ-Agonist

 (D) NMDA agonist

 (E) NMDA antagonist

151. Which one of the following is the only opioid with prolonged activity not achieved by controlled-released formulation?

 (A) Oxycodone

 (B) Fentanyl

 (C) Morphine

 (D) Codeine

 (E) Methadone

152. Which of the following opioids is used in the office-based treatment of addiction?

 (A) Naloxone

 (B) Morphine

 (C) Tramadol

 (D) Buprenorphine

 (E) Meperidine

153. Pharmacologic properties of fentanyl that make it an ideal drug for transdermal and transmucosal administration is

    (A) high lipid solubility, high molecular weight, and high potency
    (B) low lipid solubility, high molecular weight, and high potency
    (C) low lipid solubility, low molecular weight, and low potency
    (D) high lipid solubility, low molecular weight, and high potency
    (E) high lipid solubility, low molecular weight, and low potency

154. Opioids can have drug interactions with

    (A) tricyclic antidepressants (TCAs)
    (B) selective serotonin reuptake inhibitor (SSRIs)
    (C) monoamine oxidase inhibitors (MAOIs)
    (D) metoprolol
    (E) all of the above

155. Which of the following is a long and cumbersome research tool for substance abuse and is very good but not very practical in the setting of a busy pain clinic?

    (A) Screening Tool for Addiction Risk (STAR)
    (B) Severity of Opiate Dependence Questionnaire (SODQ)
    (C) Screening Instrument for Substance Abuse Potential (SISAP)
    (D) Addiction Severity Index (ASI)
    (E) Prescription Drug Use Questionnaire (PDUQ)

156. An opioid specific five-question self-administered tool which can be completed in less than 5 minutes to help predict patients at high-risk for exhibiting aberrant opioid-related behavior is

    (A) Prescription Drug Use Questionnaire (PDUQ)
    (B) Opioid Risk Tool (ORT)
    (C) Screener and Opioid Assessment for Patients with Pain (SOAPP)

    (D) Screening Instrument for Substance Abuse Potential (SISAP)
    (E) Severity of Opiate Dependence Questionnaire (SODQ)

157. The opioid which is largely metabolized by *CYP3A4* is

    (A) morphine
    (B) fentanyl
    (C) methadone
    (D) hydromorphone
    (E) oxymorphone

158. Which of the following is correct regarding patients who are prescribed and taking hydrocodone and found to have different opioid in their urine drug-testing results?

    (A) Norfentanyl, which is expected
    (B) Hydrocodeine, which is expected as a normal metabolite
    (C) Hydromorphone, which is expected as a normal metabolite
    (D) Hydromorphone, which is unexpected and patient is probably taking another opioid
    (E) Hydrocodeine, which is unexpected and patient is probably taking another opioid

159. An opioid-specific instrument which may be useful in predicting opioid misuse and is available as a 5-, 14-, or 24-item questionnaire as well as a revised version designed to be less susceptible to overt deception than the original version is

    (A) Prescription Drug Use Questionnaire (PDUQ)
    (B) Opioid Risk Tool (ORT)
    (C) Screener and Opioid Assessment for Patients with Pain (SOAPP)
    (D) Screening Instrument for Substance Abuse Potential (SISAP)
    (E) Severity of Opiate Dependence Questionnaire (SODQ)

160. A classic example of an opioid partial agonist is

    (A) naltrexone
    (B) butorphanol
    (C) nalbuphine
    (D) buprenorphine
    (E) pentazocine

161. A popular mnemonic for following relevant domains of outcome in pain management for patients on long-term opioid therapy is the so-called 4 A's which include all the following, EXCEPT

    (A) analgesia
    (B) activities of daily living
    (C) adverse events
    (D) affect
    (E) aberrant drug-taking behaviors

162. A popular pain assessment scale which is utilized by preverbal toddler and nonverbal children through age 7 years who may be treated with opioids is

    (A) CRIES
    (B) APPT
    (C) FACES
    (D) FLAC C
    (E) N-PASS

163. The opioid which has some component of metabolism by *CYP1A2* is

    (A) morphine
    (B) fentanyl
    (C) methadone
    (D) hydromorphone
    (E) oxymorphone

164. The opioid which is a metabolite of oxycodone via 3-0-demethylation is

    (A) hydrocodone
    (B) morphine
    (C) codiene
    (D) hydromorphone
    (E) oxymorphone

165. Which of the following two opioids are inherently, pharmacologically, and relatively long-acting?

    (A) Morphine and oxycodone
    (B) Morphine and oxymorphone
    (C) Oxycodone and fentanyl
    (D) Methadone and levorphanol
    (E) Methadone and oxymorphone

166. Oral transmucosal fentanyl citrate (OTFC) is applied against the buccal mucosa. The percentage of the total dose which is absorbed from the gastrointestinal (GI) tract but escapes hepatic and intestinal first-pass elimination is

    (A) 25%
    (B) 33%
    (C) 50%
    (D) 65%
    (E) 75%

167. OTFC is applied against the buccal mucosa. The total apparent bioavailability is

    (A) 25%
    (B) 33%
    (C) 50%
    (D) 65%
    (E) 75%

168. The fentanyl buccal tablet (FBT) utilizes an effervescent drug delivery system and achieves an absolute bioavailability of

    (A) 25%
    (B) 33%
    (C) 50%
    (D) 65%
    (E) 75%

169. After intramuscular administration of fentanyl citrate, the time to onset of analgesia is roughly

    (A) 1 to 3 minutes
    (B) 7 to 15 minutes
    (C) 15 to 30 minutes
    (D) 20 to 40 minutes
    (E) 30 to 50 minutes

170. The oral bioavailability of morphine is roughly

   (A) 10% to 20%
   (B) 25% to 35%
   (C) 35% to 45%
   (D) 40% to 55%
   (E) 50% to 60%

171. In humans, methadone acts as

   (A) an agonist-antagonist
   (B) a pure μ-agonist
   (C) a μ-agonist but also with significant actions at the δ-opioid receptor
   (D) a μ-agonist but also with significant actions at the κ-receptor
   (E) a μ-, δ-, and κ-agonist

172. A tool which documents a quantitative assessment of various opioid-adverse effects is the

   (A) Pain Assessment and Documentation Tool (PADT)
   (B) Translational Analgesic Score (TAS)
   (C) SAFE score
   (D) Numerical Opioid Side Effect (NOSE)
   (E) Severity of Opioid Dependence Questionnaire (SODQ)

173. Which of the following is the best opioid to administer for analgesia in a patient with chronic kidney disease stage V?

   (A) Codeine
   (B) Meperidine
   (C) Morphine
   (D) Fentanyl
   (E) Propoxyphene

174. Which of the following is the most prescribed opioid in the United States, which also undergoes O-demethylation to dihydromorphine and its major metabolites excreted into the urine are dihydrocodeine and nordihydrocodeine?

   (A) Codeine
   (B) Dihydrocodeine
   (C) Hydrocodone
   (D) Hydromorphone
   (E) Morphine

175. Which of the following is essentially responsible for opioid-induced respiratory depression?

   (A) μ-Receptor
   (B) δ-Receptor
   (C) κ-Receptor
   (D) σ-Receptor
   (E) ORL 1 receptor

176. Propoxyphene napsylate has a higher maximum daily dose than propoxyphene hydrochloride because

   (A) propoxyphene napsylate is less potent than propoxyphene hydrochloride
   (B) propoxyphene napsylate is less toxic than propoxyphene hydrochloride
   (C) propoxyphene napsylate is cleared faster than propoxyphene hydrochloride
   (D) the napsylate salt tends to be absorbed more slowly than the hydrochloride
   (E) the napsylate salt makes propoxyphene less active

177. When considering opioid rotation to methadone, which of the following is the most appropriate next step?

   (A) Maintain the equianalgesic dose
   (B) Reduce the dose by 10% to 25%
   (C) Reduce the dose by 25% to 50%
   (D) Reduce the dose by 50% to 75%
   (E) Reduce the dose by 75% to 90%

178. When considering opioid rotation to fentanyl, which of the following is the most appropriate step?

   (A) Maintain the equianalgesic dose
   (B) Reduce the dose by 10% to 25%
   (C) Reduce the dose by 25% to 50%
   (D) Reduce the dose by 50% to 75%
   (E) Reduce the dose by 75% to 90%

179. The equianalgesic conversion ratio of oral oxymorphone to intravenous morphine is

(A) 1 to 1
(B) 1 to 2
(C) 1 to 3
(D) 1 to 4
(E) 1 to 5

180. By approximately what percentage is codeine ineffective as an analgesic in the Caucasian population owing to genetic polymorphisms in *CYP2D6* (the enzyme necessary to O-methylate codeine to morphine)?

(A) 2%
(B) 5%
(C) 10%
(D) 25%
(E) 33%

181. Which of the following is the correct statement regarding the pharmacologic properties of NSAIDs?

(A) They readily cross the blood–brain barrier
(B) Their chemical structure consists of aromatic rings connected to basic functional groups
(C) They act mainly in the periphery
(D) They have a high renal clearance
(E) They are not metabolized by the liver

182. What are the advantages of COX-2 inhibitors versus NSAIDs?

(A) Protective renal effects
(B) Less GI side effects
(C) Protective cardiovascular effects
(D) Inhibits production of thromboxane A2
(E) Increases production of lipooxygenase

183. Which of the following best fits the pharmacologic mechanisms of action of "traditional" NSAIDs?

(A) Inhibition of phospholipase A2
(B) Inhibition of COX-2
(C) Inhibition of lipoxygenase

(D) Inhibition of arachidonic acid
(E) Inhibition of prostaglandin G/H synthase enzymes

184. The main role of prostaglandins in pain is

(A) as important primary pain mediators
(B) sensitization of central nociceptors
(C) sensitization of peripheral nociceptors
(D) facilitation of the production of pain mediators (ie, bradykinin, somatostatin, histamine)
(E) stimulation of κ-receptors on the spinal cord

185. The effects of NSAIDs on the kidneys function or renal function may include

(A) increase in renal blood flow
(B) promotion of salt and water excretion
(C) chronic interstitial nephritis
(D) increased glomerular filtration rate (GFR)
(E) chronic papillary necrosis

186. Platelet dysfunction secondary to the use of NSAIDs is a known effect, in long-term treatment with standard NSAIDs. What laboratory value is most compatible with these effects?

(A) Prolonged prothrombin time (PT)
(B) Prolonged partial thromboplastin time (PTT)
(C) Prolonged activated clotting time (ACT)
(D) Severely prolonged bleeding time
(E) Below the upper limits of normal to mildly prolonged bleeding time

187. The duration of aspirin effect is related to the turnover rate of COX in different target tissues, because aspirin

(A) competitively inhibits the active sites of COX enzymes
(B) nonirreversibly inhibits COX activity
(C) irreversibly inhibits COX activity
(D) noncompetitively inhibits the active sites of COX enzymes
(E) acetylates COX-1

188. The unique sensitivity of platelets to inhibition by low doses of aspirin (as low as 30 mg/d) is related to

    (A) first pass of aspirin through the liver
    (B) presystemic inhibition of platelets in the portal circulation
    (C) irreversible inhibition of COX
    (D) constitutively expression of COX-1 in platelets
    (E) good oral absorption

189. How long before surgery NSAIDs are advised to be stopped?

    (A) 12 hours
    (B) 2 to 3 days
    (C) 7 days
    (D) 10 days
    (E) 14 days

190. Which of the following NSAIDs is as effective as morphine?

    (A) Ketoprofen
    (B) Indomethacin
    (C) Ibuprofen
    (D) Ketorolac
    (E) Diclofenac

191. Rare side effect of NSAIDs is

    (A) GI side effects
    (B) platelet dysfunction
    (C) potentially fatal hepatic necrosis
    (D) renal dysfunction/failure
    (E) all of the above

192. Which of the following is (are) true regarding oxcarbazepine?

    (A) It has more adverse effects than carbamazepine
    (B) It is a sodium channel blocker
    (C) Oxcarbazepine's dose adjustment is unnecessary for renal insufficiency
    (D) Its most frequent adverse effects is weight loss and dizziness
    (E) none of the above

193. Which of the following is a typical adverse effect of pregabalin?

    (A) Constipation
    (B) Dizziness
    (C) Blurred vision
    (D) Dry mouth
    (E) All of the above

194. Which of the following is (are) false regarding gabapentin?

    (A) It is a first-line drug for the treatment of PHN and PDN (painful diabetic neuropathy)
    (B) Its dose should be reduced in renal insufficiency
    (C) It blocks NMDA receptors
    (D) It is thought to inhibit voltage-dependent calcium channels
    (E) It has a chemical structure similar to that of GABA

195. Which of the following is true about zonisamide?

    (A) It is a sulfonamide drug
    (B) It is a sodium channel blocker
    (C) It is 40% to 50% protein bound
    (D) It may potentially lead to renal calculi
    (E) All of the above

196. Which of the following is true about antiepileptic drugs (AED)?

    (A) AEDs have analgesic effect in all subjects with neuropathic pain
    (B) If one AED is ineffective, it is not necessary to try another one
    (C) Newer AEDs have more side effects than older ones
    (D) AEDs could be combined with antidepressants to treat neuropathic pain
    (E) All of the above

197. The antidepressant with the least anticholinergic and least sedating effect is

    (A) trazodone
    (B) desipramine
    (C) imipramine
    (D) doxepin
    (E) amitriptyline

198. Which of the following antidepressant agent selectively inhibits serotonin reuptake with minimal effect on norepinephrine reuptake?

    (A) Duloxetine
    (B) Protriptyline
    (C) Paroxetine
    (D) Amoxapine
    (E) Desipramine

199. The most common adverse effects associated with TCA are (is)

    (A) anticholinergic effects
    (B) seizures
    (C) arrhythmias
    (D) hepatotoxicity
    (E) nephrotoxicity

200. The least common adverse effects associated with TCA are (is)

    (A) dry mouth
    (B) seizure
    (C) urinary retention
    (D) blurred vision
    (E) aconstipation

201. Compared to TCAs, SSRIs

    (A) are more effective in the treatment of pain
    (B) have more side effects
    (C) have less side effects
    (D) have more serious consequence of overdosage
    (E) none of the above

202. Which of the following is false regarding tramadol?

    (A) It has opioid characteristics
    (B) There is a dose limit of 400 mg/d
    (C) It is a centrally acting analgesic
    (D) No effect on norepinepherine or serotonin
    (E) Inhibits the reuptake of norepinephrine and serotonin

203. The benzodiazepine which is used to treat various neuropathic pain syndromes is

    (A) diazepam
    (B) midazolam
    (C) clonazepam
    (D) flunazepam
    (E) lorazepam

204. Which of the following about carisoprodol is true?

    (A) Naloxone may be a useful antidote to its toxicity
    (B) Flumazenil may be a useful antidote to its toxicity
    (C) It is safe to use as a long-term treatment of musculoskeletal disorders
    (D) It is a $GABA_B$ receptor agonist
    (E) It has no abuse potential

205. Which of the following is true regarding tizanidine?

    (A) It is structurally related to clonipine
    (B) It is $GABA_B$ receptor agonist
    (C) It is $GABA_A$ receptor agonist
    (D) Its excretion occurs primarily through the liver
    (E) It is α_2 agonist

206. Which of the following is a false statement about ziconotide?

    (A) It is derived from conus sea snail venom
    (B) It is the synthetic form of cone snail peptide (conotoxin)
    (C) It is effective when given intravenously or orally
    (D) It is N-type calcium channel blocker
    (E) Its common side effects are dizziness, confusion, and headache

207. Which of the following is true regarding capsaicin?

(A) It is a member of the vanilloid family which binds to the TRPV1 receptor

(B) It is commercially available in 0.025% and 0.075% concentrations

(C) It is the active component of chili peppers

(D) It depletes presynaptic substance P

(E) All of the above

208. The following are some of the side effects of lidocaine 5% patches, EXCEPT

(A) methemoglobin

(B) edema

(C) erythema

(D) abnormal sensation

(E) exfoliation

209. Calcitonin may be used as an adjuvant drug for all the following, EXCEPT

(A) phantom limb pain

(B) sympathetically maintained pain

(C) cancer bone pain

(D) postoperative pain

(E) osteoporosis pain

DIRECTIONS: For Question 210 through 251, ONE or MORE of the numbered options is correct. Choose answer

(A) **if only answer 1, 2, and 3 are correct**

(B) **if only 1 and 3 are correct**

(C) **if only 2 and 4 are correct**

(D) **if only 4 is correct**

(E) **if all are correct**

210. Regarding the effects produced by the different subtypes of opioid receptors, which of the following is (are) true?

(1) κ-Receptors produce more respiratory depression than μ-receptors

(2) Opioid receptors mostly affect phosphorylation through G protein coupling

(3) The stimulation of μ_2-receptors to produce analgesia without respiratory depression, has been supported by several studies

(4) Opioid receptors act both presynaptically and postsynaptically

211. The use of pure opioid agonists are preferred in chronic pain patients because of their

(1) low association with addiction

(2) superior analgesic efficacy

(3) low potential for nausea and vomiting

(4) easier titratable nature

212. The systemic administration of opioids exerts its analgesic effects at what level(s)?

(1) Brain cortex

(2) Brainstem and medulla

(3) Dorsal horn of the spinal cord

(4) Sensory neuron (peripheral nervous system)

213. Which of the following condition(s) increase the likelihood of opioid-related toxicity?

(1) Pregnancy

(2) Renal disease

(3) Cardiac heart failure

(4) Cirrhotic liver disease

214. Which of the following is (are) true concerning the use of epidural morphine?

(1) A biphasic respiratory depression pattern can develop, with the initial phase within 30 minutes of the bolus dose and a second phase 2 to 4 hours later

(2) Initial phase within 2 hours of the bolus dose and a second phase 6 to 12 hours later

(3) Patients should be closely monitored for 48 hours after the administration of epidural morphine

(4) Patients should be closely monitored for 24 hours after the administration of epidural morphine

215. Opioids should be used with caution in which of the following scenarios?

   (1) Emphysema
   (2) Kyphoscoliosis
   (3) Chronic obstructive pulmonary disease (COPD)
   (4) Obstructive sleep apnea

216. Indicate what part differs largely among the μ-, δ-, κ-, and ORL (opioid-receptor-like) receptors?

   (1) Transmembrane domains
   (2) Extracellular loops
   (3) Intracellular loops
   (4) N or C terminal tails

217. Opioids modify and relieve the perception of pain without detriment of other sensory mode types. While the pain is still present there is a dissociation of the emotional and sensory aspects of pain, making the patients feel more comfortable. Select the best reason(s) from the following:

   (1) Action of opioids on supraspinal structures, brainstem [ie, PAG (periaqueductal gray) the RVM (rostroventral medulla)], and midbrain
   (2) Action of opioids on peripheral structures via presynaptic receptors
   (3) Enhanced inhibitory activity on descending controls terminating in the dorsal horn of the spinal cord
   (4) Pronounced reduction in activity of OFF cells and decreased activity of ON cells

218. Opioids exert their analgesic effects through

   (1) their central action within the central nervous system (CNS), inhibiting directly the ascending transmission of painful stimuli from the dorsal horn at the spinal cord
   (2) their central action within the CNS activating pain control circuits descending from the midbrain via the RVM to the spinal cord dorsal horn

   (3) their peripheral actions on opioid receptors and the release of endogenous opioid-like substances
   (4) their action on the spinal cord at a presynaptic level only

219. Which of the following is (are) true regarding pharmacologic characteristics of opioids?

   (1) Opioids are the primary pain medication with ceiling effects
   (2) Opioids are the primary pain medication with *no* ceiling effects
   (3) There are sex related differences in opioid-mediated responsiveness
   (4) There are *no* sex related differences in opioid-mediated responsiveness

220. Tramadol has some different characteristics when compared to some other opioids including

   (1) same side effects as morphine
   (2) risk of respiratory depression is lower at equianalgesic doses from that produce with conventional opioids
   (3) less incidence of nausea and vomiting
   (4) low abuse potential

221. Morphine should be used with caution in which situations/conditions?

   (1) Short bowel syndrome
   (2) Mild liver dysfunction
   (3) Vomiting or severe diarrhea
   (4) Renal dysfunction

222. The transdermal fentanyl patch has differences versus sustained-release morphine in patients with cancer and chronic pain:

   (1) It can be used when the oral route can not be used
   (2) It is 80 times as potent as morphine
   (3) It causes less constipation than sustained-release morphine
   (4) Peak plasma concentration occurs in 6 to 12 hours

223. Which of the following is (are) correct regarding the use of meperidine?

(1) The use of meperidine should be limited to 1 to 2 days in the management of acute pain

(2) Normeperidine is a neurotoxic metabolite of meperidine

(3) Meperidine should be avoided in the management of chronic pain

(4) The use of meperidine is recommended in elderly patients

224. Which of the following is (are) true regarding opioids distribution and biotransformation (metabolism)?

(1) Fentanyl is highly protein bound

(2) Fentanyl distributes to fat tissue and redistributes from there into the systemic circulation

(3) Opioids are metabolized by the liver, CNS, kidney, lungs, and placenta

(4) Opioid distribution is independent of protein binding and lipophilicity

225. What is (are) the neuroendocrine effects produced by opioids?

(1) Hypogonadism

(2) Hypothyroidism

(3) Decreased cortisol levels

(4) Decreased pituitary release of prolactin

226. Which of the following drugs may show interactions with NSAIDs/COX-2 inhibitors?

(1) Angiotensin-converting enzyme (ACE) inhibitors

(2) Furosemide

(3) Warfarin

(4) Lithium

227. Which of the following is (are) contraindicated in patients allergic to sulfonamides?

(1) Rofecoxib

(2) Valdecoxib

(3) Meloxicam

(4) Celecoxib

228. Anti-inflammatory agent(s) which may possess advantages when GI side effects are a concern include

(1) ibuprofen

(2) nabumetone

(3) diclofenac

(4) coxibs

229. Which of the following is (are) true for coxibs versus NSAIDs?

(1) Coxibs are associated with less GI side effects

(2) Coxibs have similar renal effects

(3) Coxibs are not associated with platelet dysfunction

(4) Coxibs are associated with increased incidence of nonunion and delayed bone healing

230. Which of the following NSAIDs have higher potency (either analgesic or anti-inflammatory or both) compared to ASA?

(1) Diflunisal

(2) Indomethacin

(3) Ketorolac

(4) Diclofenac

231. Scenarios in which the adjunct use of NSAIDs can be beneficial in postoperative pain:

(1) Use of opioids

(2) No history of induced-opioid side effects

(3) Preexisting ventilatory compromise

(4) History of GI bleeding

232. Options that can be offered to patients with increased risk of GI toxicity:

(1) Diclofenac with enteric coat

(2) NSAIDs combined with GI prophylaxis

(3) NSAIDs combined with antacids

(4) Coxibs

233. Which of the following is (are) NSAID's role in cancer?

    (1) Synergistic effect of NSAIDs and opioids
    (2) Bone and soft tissue pain relief
    (3) Ability to reduce the side effects of opioids
    (4) Visceral pain relief

234. Anti-inflammatory agent(s) which do not interfere with the cardioprotective effects of "low-dose" aspirin include

    (1) naproxen
    (2) ibuprofen
    (3) ketorolac
    (4) celecoxib

235. Which of the following is (are) true regarding carbamazepine?

    (1) It blocks voltage-dependent sodium channels
    (2) Bicuculline antagonizes its antinociceptive effect
    (3) It was first used for trigeminal neuralgia
    (4) All of the above

236. Pregabalin is Food and Drug Administration (FDA) approved for

    (1) diabetic neuropathy
    (2) postherpetic neuralgia (PHN)
    (3) fibromyalgia
    (4) none of the above

237. Which of the following is (are) true regarding gabapentin?

    (1) It has chemical a structure similar to GABA
    (2) It acts directly at GABA-binding site in the CNS
    (3) It inhibits voltage-dependent calcium channels
    (4) It is the drug of choice for fibromyalgia

238. Which of the following is (are) true regarding clonazepam?

    (1) It is a benzodiazepine
    (2) It is effective as anxiolytic and muscle-relaxing agent
    (3) It may be useful for phantom limb pain
    (4) It has short half-life

239. Which of the following is true about lamotrigine?

    (1) It is an anticonvulsive agent
    (2) It is an NSAID
    (3) A rapid titration may result in skin rash
    (4) More than 300 mg/d is always needed for analgesia

240. The antidepressant(s) which is (are) tertiary amine(s) TCA:

    (1) Imipramine
    (2) Nortriptyline
    (3) Doxepin
    (4) Desipramine

241. Which of the following is true about the analgesic properties of TCAs?

    (1) The analgesic effects of TCA are independent of their effects on clinical depression
    (2) Onset of analgesia with TCA ranges from 3 to 7 days
    (3) Analgesia tends to occur at lower doses and plasma levels than that needed for antidepressant effects
    (4) TCA's analgesic property is superior to that of SSRI's

242. Which of the following is (are) true about TCAs?

    (1) They interact significantly with the opioid and benzodiazepine
    (2) They do not have potential for addiction
    (3) They block calcium channels
    (4) They can cause insomnia, restlessness and dry mouth

243. Symptoms of TCA toxicity includes which of the following?

(1) Hyperthermia
(2) Tachycardia
(3) Seizures
(4) Hypertension

244. When prescribing antidepressants for pain

(1) explain to the patient that you are primarily treating the pain not depression
(2) explain to the patient that it will not work immediately
(3) explain to the patient that it may help sleep
(4) none of the above

245. Which of the following is (are) true regarding acetaminophen?

(1) It is an aniline derivative
(2) Induced analgesia is centrally mediated
(3) It has peripheral mechanism of action
(4) It is a drug of choice for relieving mild to moderate musculoskeletal pain

246. Which of the following is (are) true regarding acetaminophen toxicity?

(1) The liver gets the major insult
(2) The heart gets the major insult
(3) *N*-acetylcysteine is beneficial for treatment
(4) Adrenergic agonists are beneficial for treatment

247. Which of the following is (are) true about baclofen?

(1) It is good for muscle rigidity and spasticity
(2) It is used for neuropathic pain

(3) It is $GABA_B$ receptor agonist
(4) It is $GABA_A$ receptor agonist

248. Which of the following is (are) true regarding botulinum toxin A?

(1) The analgesic mechanism of action is well known
(2) It can be administered intrathecally
(3) Botox, Myobloc, and Dysport are available in the United States
(4) Its effect lasts for about 3 to 6 months

249. Which of the following is false regarding cyclobezaprine?

(1) It is structurally similar to anticonvulsive agents
(2) It has cholinergic side effects
(3) It does not require dose adjustment for elderly patients
(4) It can produce sinus tachycardia

250. Which of the following is (are) false about lidocaine 5% topical patch?

(1) Treatment for postherpetic neuralgia
(2) It may not use more than 1 patch per day
(3) It is used 12 hours ON and 12 hours OFF
(4) High plasma levels are normally achieved through the skin

251. Steroids produce analgesia by

(1) anti-inflammatory effects
(2) suppressing ectopic discharge from injured nerves
(3) reducing edema
(4) blocking sodium channels

Answers and Explanations

141. (B) Extremely high doses of morphine and related opioids can produce seizures, presumably by inhibiting the release of GABA (at synaptic level).

Normeperidine a metabolite of meperidine is prone to produce seizures and tends to accumulate in patients with renal dysfunction and in the elderly.

Naloxone may not effectively treat seizures produced by meperidine.

142. (E) Opioids produce a dose-dependant respiratory depression by acting directly on the respiratory centers on the brainstem. Partial agonist and agonist-antagonist opioids are less likely to cause severe respiratory depression, as are the selective K-agonist.

Therapeutic doses of morphine decrease minute ventilation by decreasing respiratory rate (as oppose to tidal volume).

Opioids depress the ventilatory response to carbon dioxide; the carbon dioxide–response curve shows a decrease slope and rightward shift.

The apneic threshold is decreased and also the increase in ventilatory response to hypoxemia is blunted by opioids.

Naloxone can effectively and fully reverse the respiratory depression from opioids.

143. (D) Delayed respiratory depression is likely to occur with larger dose of epidural opioids, particularly morphine which is hydrophilic and therefore subject to spread in the cerebrospinal fluid (CSF), reaching the respiratory center in the brainstem.

Intrathecal doses of morphine produce only a uniphasic pattern of respiratory depression.

144. (C) High doses of any opioid reduce sympathetic output allowing the parasympathetic output to predominate. The heart rate decreases by stimulation of the vagal center, especially with high-doses.

Meperidine because of its similarity to atropine may elevate the heart rate after IV administration.

145. (B) Opioid receptors are coupled to G proteins, able to affect most of the time, protein phosphorylation via a second messenger, thereby altering the conductance of potassium and calcium ion channels. This is believed to be the main mechanisms by which endogenous and exogenous opioids produce analgesia.

The opening of potassium channels—the most well documented—will inhibit the release of neurotransmitters, including substance P and glutamate if the receptors are presynaptic. And will inhibit neuronal firing by hyperpolarization of the cell if the receptors are postsynaptic on the neurons.

146. (A) The different type of opioid receptors contribute in different proportions to the total opioid receptors in the spinal cord. μ-Receptors constitute 70%, δ-receptors 24% and κ-receptors 6%. The main mechanism of spinal opioid analgesia is through presynaptic activation of opioid receptors.

Opioid receptors are synthesized in small diameter DRG cell bodies and transported centrally and peripherally. They are mainly (70%) located presynaptically on small diameter nociceptive primary afferents (C and A-δ fibers).

147. (E) Opioids produce analgesia primarily through interaction with μ-receptors. The activation of κ- and δ-receptors also causes analgesia.

The ORL receptor is a member of the opioid receptors, although ligands do not have the same high affinity for this type of receptors, but effects of high-affinity ligands, such as antinociception, proprioception/hyperalgesia, allodynia and no effect have been reported.

Analysis has shown that some opioid actions are not mediated by opioid receptors, morphine can inhibit voltage-dependant sodium (Na) current, meperidine can block voltage-dependant sodium (Na) channels. Meperidine also has agonist activity at the α_{2B}-adrenoreceptor subtype.

Methadone, meperidine, and tramadol inhibit serotonin and norepinephrin reuptake. High concentrations of opioids, including morphine, fentanyl, codeine, and naloxone directly inhibit NMDA receptor.

148. **(B)** Oxycodone a semisynthetic derivative of thebaine and has analgesic efficacy comparable with that of morphine, with a median oxycodone to morphine dose ratio of 1 to 15.

Oxycodone has been typically used in combination with nonopioids (acetaminophen, aspirin) and a long-acting preparation is available, which has popularized its use in cancer patients.

It has a higher bioavailability than that of morphine (approximately 60%).

There are not consistent observations on reduced rate of hallucinations and itching when compared with morphine.

149. **(D)** Methadone unlike morphine is metabolized through *N*-demethylation by the liver cytochrome P-450 enzyme, which activity can vary widely in different people.

Methadone should be administered with caution in patients receiving multiple medications, specially antivirals and antibiotics.

Methadone's withdrawal symptoms tend to be less severe than morphine's, this and its long duration of action, good oral bioavailability, and high potency made it the maintenance drug or detoxification treatment of opioid addiction.

Methadone has biphasic elimination. A long β-elimination phase (ranges from 30 to 60 hours) producing sedation and respiratory depression can outlast the analgesic action which equates the α-elimination phase (6-8 hours). This biphasic pattern explains why methadone is required once a day for opioid maintenance therapy and every 4 to 8 hours for analgesia.

Rapid titration is not possible, making this drug more useful for stable type of pain.

150. **(E)** When tolerance to opioids, usually after use over long periods of time, opioid rotation, resting period off opioids, and addition of an NMDA antagonist are a number of strategies available.

Opioid rotation, switching from one opioid to another may be helpful because of partial cross tolerance between opioids. Because methadone has NMDA receptor antagonist properties, makes it a good choice.

Methadone is: μ- and δ-antagonist, NMDA inhibitor, inhibitor of serotonin and norepinephrine reuptake.

151. **(E)** Methadone is the only opioid with prolonged activity not achieved by controlled-release formulation.

Oxycodone can be formulated as controlled-release. Codeine half-life is 2 to 4 hours.

152. **(D)** Buprenorphine is a semisynthetic opioid with partial activity at the μ-receptor and very little activity at the κ- and δ-receptors.

It has high affinity but low intrinsic activity at the μ-receptor and has a pharmacologic ceiling owing to its partial agonist activity.

It is available in the United States to be used in the office-based treatment of addiction.

It can be given for withdrawal of heroin or methadone, or used as a maintenance of addicts.

153. **(D)** Fentanyl is a potent mu agonist, with high lipid solubility, low molecular weight and high potency, making it an ideal drug for transdermal and transmucosal administration.

92% of fentanyl delivered transdermally reaches the circulation as unchanged fentanyl.

Transmucosal route at the buccal and sublingual mucosa skips the first pass effect and overall bioavailability is 50%.

154. **(E)** Opioids can have interactions with multiple medications, including all the medications mentioned above.

One of the most remarkable interactions occurs if meperidine and MAOIs are combined, severe respiratory depression or excitation, arrhythmias, delusions, hyperpyrexia, seizures and coma can be seen.

155. **(D)** The Addiction Severity Index (ASI) is especially effective for evaluating the need for substance-abuse treatment. It is a 200-item, hour-long assessment of seven potential problem areas designed to be administered by a trained interviewer.

156. **(B)** The Opioid Risk Tool (ORT) is a five-question self-administered assessment that can be completed in less than 5 minutes and used on a patient's initial visit. Personal and family history of substance abuse; age; history of preadolescent sexual abuse; and the presence of depression, attention-deficit disorder (ADD), obsessive-compulsive disorder (OCD), bipolar disorder, and schizophrenia are assessed. The ORT accurately predicted which patients were at the highest and the lowest risk for exhibiting aberrant, drug-related behaviors associated with abuse or addiction.

157. **(B)**

158. **(D)**

159. **(C)** Screener and Opioid Assessment for Patients with Pain (SOAPP) is a survey tool used to predict opioid abuse and is available as a 5-, 14-, 24-item questionnaire. Although the five-item questionnaire [SOAPP V LO-SF (5Q)] is less sensitive and specific than the longer version, it may suffice for use in primary care settings. The SOAPP-SF is scored by adding up the ratings of each of the five questions. The SQ SOAPP uses a cutoff score of 4 or above (of a possible 20) with a score of more than 4, indicating that the subject may have a potentially increased risk of opioid abuse.

160. **(D)**

161. **(D)**

162. **(D)**

163. **(C)**

164. **(E)**

165. **(D)**

166. **(A)**

167. **(C)**

168. **(D)**

169. **(B)**

170. **(B)**

171. **(B)**

172. **(D)**

173. **(D)**

174. **(C)**

175. **(A)**

176. **(D)**

177. **(E)**

178. **(A)**

179. **(A)**

180. **(C)**

181. **(C)** The NSAIDs are *weak organic acids*, consisting in one or two aromatic rings connected to an acidic functional group. They *do not cross* the blood–brain barrier, are 95% to 99% bound to albumin, are extensively metabolized by the liver and have low renal clearance (< 10%).

NSAIDs act mainly in the periphery, but they may have a central effect. COX-2 induction within the spinal cord may play an important role in central sensitization. The acute antihyperalgesic action of NSAIDs has been show to be mediated by the inhibition of constitutive spinal COX-2, which has been found to be upregulated in response to inflammation and other stressors.

182. (B) Coxibs do not have any advantages in terms of renal effects.

COX-2 inhibitors are associated with less GI toxicity than standard NSAIDs but they are more expensive.

There is a possible increased risk of myocardial infarction (MI) and thrombotic stroke events associated with the continuosly long-term use of coxibs. Those concerns led to rofecoxib and valdecoxib being withdrawn from the market in the year 2004 and 2005, respectively.

Regular NSAIDs inhibit the synthesis of TXA2 by inhibiting COX-1, which is spared with the use of COX-2 inhibitors.

183. (E) NSAIDs inhibits the prostaglandin G/H synthase enzymes, colloquially known as the COX, therefore inhibiting the synthesis of prostaglandin E, prostacyclin, and thromboxane. NSAIDs inhibit the production of not only COX-2 but also COX-1.

Steroids inhibit phospholipase A2.

184. (C) Prostaglandins are not important primary pain mediators, they do cause hyperalgesia by sensitizing peripheral nociceptors (to mechanical an chemical stimulation) to the effects of pain mediators, such as bradykinin, somatostatin, and histamine, producing hyperalgesia. They do so by lowering the threshold of the polymodal nociceptors of C fibers.

NSAIDs act mainly in the periphery, but they may have a central effect. COX-2 induction within the spinal cord may play an important role in central sensitization. The acute antihyperalgesic action of NSAIDs has been shown to be mediated by the inhibition of constitutive spinal COX-2, which has been found to be upregulated in response to inflammation and other stressors.

185. (C) In the kidney, prostaglandins help to maintain GFR and blood flow.

They also contribute to the modulation of renin release, excretion of water, and tubular ion transport. In patients with normal renal function NSAID-induced renal dysfunction is extremely rare.

Risk factors for NSAID-induced renal dysfunction are:

- Prolonged and excessive NSAID use
- Older patients
- Chronic renal dysfunction
- Congestive heart failure
- Ascites
- Hypovolemia
- Treatment with nephrotoxic drugs (aminoglycosides and vancomycin)

In these scenarios NSAIDs may decrease rapidly the GFR, release of renin, which can progress to renal failure. Sodium, water retention, hyperkalemia, hypertension, acute papillary necrosis, chronic interstitial nephritis, and nephrotic syndrome can also occur.

Coxibs (COX-2 inhibitors) have similar renal effects and it should be closely monitored, as is required for conventional NSAIDs.

186. (E) Platelets are very susceptible to COX inhibition, which also inhibits the endogenous procoagulant thromboxane. Long-term use of standard NSAIDs produces a consistently prolonged bleeding time, but the prolongation is mild and values tend to remain below the upper limits of normal.

187. (C) Aspirin covalently acetylates COX-1 and COX-2, *irreversibly* inhibiting COX activity. This makes the duration of aspirin's effects related to the turnover rate of COX in different target tissues.

NSAIDs competitively inhibit the active site of COX enzymes which relates its duration more directly to the time course of drug disposition.

188. (B) The unique sensitivity of platelets to inhibition by low doses of aspirin, as low as 30 mg/d is related to their presystemic inhibition in the portal circulation before aspirin is deacetylated to salicylate on first pass through the liver.

Aspirin irreversibly inhibits COX activity, making the aspirin's effect related to the turnover rate of COX in different target tissues. Enzyme turnover is most notable in platelets because they are anucleated with a marked limited capacity for protein synthesis. Therefore the inhibition of platelet COX-1 (COX-2 is expressed only in megakaryocytes) last for the lifetime of the platelet, 8 to 12 days (10 days average) after therapy has been stopped.

In general NSAIDs are well absorbed orally, but that is not the reason for high platelet sensitivity to ASA.

189. **(B)** The antiplatelet effect of NSAIDs is rapidly reversible, 24 hours cessation is probably sufficient, although 2 to 3 days cessation is advised.

Aspirin because of its irreversible antiplatelet effect should be stopped 10 days before elective surgery.

190. **(D)** Ketorolac is one of the few NSAIDs that the FDA approved for parenteral use. It is highly efficacious, with efficacy close to that of morphine and other opioids for simple outpatient procedures to major operations.

Ketorolac's side effects, like other NSAIDs include GI bleeding, other bleeding problems, and reversible renal dysfunction (Possibly related with use of high doses or failure to recognize its contraindications).

Nonunion, deleterious effects in bone osteogenesis during bone repair are some other side effects, more likely to occur if ketorolac was administered after surgery, compared with no use of NSAIDs. Decreased posterior spine fusion rates have been demonstrated in rat models, with the long-term use of indomethacin, but even the short-term administration of NSAIDs may possibly significantly affect spinal fusion. These findings have not been confirmed in humans, but many surgeons prefer to avoid the use of NSAIDs in the postoperative period of bone fusion, especially in the spine. COX-2 inhibitors can have similar effects, which is unlikely with short-term perioperative use in humans. No human studies to date document that coxibs have these negative effects in bone healing.

191. **(C)** All are well-known and not uncommon side effects of NSAIDs. Borderline increases of one or more liver tests, may occur in up to 15% of patients taking NSAIDs, approximately 1% of patients taking NSAIDs have shown notable increases in alanine aminotransferase (ALT) or aspartate aminotransferase (AST) (X3 or more the upper limit of normal). These findings may

progress, remain unchanged, or be transient with continuing therapy. Rare cases of severe hepatic reactions, including jaundice and fatal fulminant hepatitis, liver necrosis, and hepatic failure (some with fatal outcome), have been reported with NSAIDs.

192. **(B)** Oxcarbazepine [10, 11-dihydro-10-oxo-5H-debenz (b, f) azepine-5-carboxanide] is an analogue of carbamazepine with a keto group at the 10 carbon position. It is roughly 50% protein bound in the plasma. The dose should be at least cut by half if the patient has significant renal insufficiency.

The most frequent adverse effects experienced include dizziness and vertigo, weight gain and edema, GI symptoms, fatigue, and allergic-type reactions. Cross-allergy to carbamazepine occurs in about 25% of patients and may be severe.

193. **(E)**

194. **(C)** A structural analogue of GABA is considered by many practitioners to be a first-line drug for treatment of PHN and PDN because of its tolerability and efficacy. Dose should be reduced in renal dysfunction. Dose increases are usually made every 3 to 4 days.

195. **(E)**

196. **(D)**

197. **(B)** Anticholinergic side effects are generally very significant for TCAs.

198. **(C)** Antidepressants which selectively inhibit serotonin with minimal effects on norepinephrine reuptake are referred to as SSRIs (eg, paroxetine). Protriptyline, desipramine, and amoxapine are secondary amine TCAs. Duloxetine inhibits both norepinephrine and serotonin (SNRIs).

199. **(A)** Side effects of antidepressants include anticholinergic effects, antihistaminergic effects, α_1-aderenergic receptor bloackade, and cardiac effects. Individual may possess significant side effects in one specific area (eg, doxepin is a strong antihistaminergic agent). As a generalization,

the most common adverse effects associated with TCAs are anticholinergic in nature.

200. **(B)**

201. **(C)**

202. **(D)** Tramadol hydrochloride is a centrally acting analgesic which is thought to provide analgesia via at least two mechanisms: some analgesia may be derived from the relatively weak interaction of tramadol with the μ-opioid receptor. The second and major mechanism, which is thought to account for at least 70% of tramadol′s analgesic activity, is via inhibiting the reuptake of norepinephrine and serotonin.

203. **(C)** Clonazepam is a benzodiazepine—which binds to the $GABA_B$ receptor (other benzodiazepines bind to the $GABA_A$ receptor) and has been utilized to treat various neuropathic pain syndrome and lower extremity muscle conditions.

204. **(B)** Carisoprodol may be useful for the short-term treatment of acute musculoskeletal disorders, especially in combination with acetaminophen, aspirin, or NSAIDs. Carisoprodol is primarily metabolized in the liver to several metabolites, including meprobamate. This metabolic conversion, although relatively small, has been postulated to be the reason that carisoprodol may have abuse potential. The formation of meprobamate from carisoprodol is by *N*-dealkylation via *CYP2C19*. Poor metabolizers of mephenytoin have a diminished ability to metabolize carisoprodol and therefore may be at increased risk of developing concentration-dependent side effects (eg, drowsiness, hypotension, CNS depression) at "usual" adult doses.

Although the precise mechanisms of action of carisoprodol (as well as meprobamate) are uncertain, one theory is that they act as indirect agonists at the $GABA_A$ receptor, yielding CNS chloride ion channel conduction effects similar to benzodiazepines. Therefore, flumazenil may be a potentially useful antidote to carisoprodol toxicity.

205. **(E)** Tizanidine is an imidazoline derivative that is structurally related to clonidine. Its action is primarily derived from agonism at the α_2-adrenoreceptor.

Metabolism of tizanidine occurs primarily in the liver through oxidative processes, and metabolites of the parent compound have no known pharmacologic activity. Excretion of tizanidine and its metabolites occurs primarily via the kidneys (53%-66%).

206. **(C)**

207. **(E)**

208. **(A)**

209. **(D)**

210. **(C)** The previously proposed classification of μ-receptors into μ_1 and μ_2 subtypes, with the rationale that selective μ_1-agonist could produce analgesia without the undesirable effects of respiratory depression has not been proven. Gene experiments have demonstrated that μ-receptors mediate all morphine activities including analgesia, tolerance, dependence, and respiratory depression.

Opioid receptors are coupled to G proteins and they act mostly through phosphorylations via a second messenger.

Opioids act pre- and postsynaptically. Presynaptically, inhibit the release of neurotransmitters including substance P and glutamate. Postsynaptically inhibit neurons by hyperpolarization, through the opening of potassium channels.

211. **(C)** When choosing between partial agonists (ie, buprenorphine) and mixed agonist-antagonists (ie, pentazocine, nalorphine) versus pure agonists, pure opioid agonists are preferred, especially in chronic pain patients, because of their superior efficacy and easier titratable nature.

212. **(E)** Analgesic effects of systemic administration of opioids result from receptor opioid activity at different sites, including:

1. The sensory neuron in the peripheral nervous system.
2. The dorsal horn of the spinal cord (inhibition of transmission of nociceptive information).

3. The brainstem medulla (potentiates descending inhibitory pathways that modulate ascending pain signals).

4. The cortex of the brain (decreases the perception and emotional response to pain).

213. **(C)** The liver metabolizes opioids by dealkylation, glucuronidation, hydrolysis, and oxidation, any hepatic disease can increase the accumulation of toxic metabolites, that is, morphine-6-glucuronide, normeperidine (CNS toxicity), norpropoxyphene (cardiac toxicity).

Kidneys account for 90% of opioid excretion. Therefore any hepatic or renal disease increases the likelihood of opioid-related toxicity.

214. **(C)** The use of hydrophilic opioids like morphine in the epidural space produces a biphasic respiratory depression pattern. One portion of the initial bolus is absorbed systemically, accounting for the initial phase, which usually occurs within 2 hours of the bolus dose. The second phase occurs 6 to 12 hours later owing to the slow rostral spread of the remaining drug as it reaches the brainstem.

215. **(E)** Opioids should be used with caution in any situation with decrease respiratory reserve, that is, emphysema, obesity, scoliosis. Opioids that release histamine (ie, morphine) may precipitate bronchospasm, especially in asthma.

216. **(C)** The opioid receptors, μ-, δ-, κ-, ORL receptors are highly similar, their genes have been cloned in many species, including humans.

The molecular structure of these G protein–coupled receptors (GPCRs) comprises 7 hydrophobic transmembrane domains interconnected by short loops, an intracellular C-terminal tail and an extracellular N-terminal domain.

The *transmembrane* domains and intracellular loops have amino acid sequences that are *65% identical or similar*, whereas the amino (N), carboxy (HOOC) terminal and the extracellular loops are very different.

217. **(B)** When noxious stimuli are produced, they are transmitted to higher centers through spinal routes arriving at the parabrachial area, central gray, and the amygdala. The pathways which project to these supraspinal sites and the sites themselves contribute mostly to the emotional aspects of pain, whereas those which project to the thalamus and somatosensory cortex produce the sensory aspects of pain.

Opioids suppress both pathways but the dissociation of the emotional and sensory aspects of pain is most likely produced by brain mechanisms.

Opioids can also prevent the supraspinal activation by noxious stimuli through increased activity in inhibitory descending controls terminating in the dorsal horn of the spinal cord.

The action of opioids on peripheral structures does not abolish the emotional aspects of pain.

There is a hypothesis describing two major populations of RVM output neurons, ON cells and OFF cells. ON cells activity coincides with spinal reflexes and OFF cell activity is associated with the suppression of those reflexes. Morphine produces a pronounced reduction in the activity of ON cells.

218. **(A)** Opioids exert their analgesic effects through central and peripheral mechanisms. Although it was believed that opioids act exclusively within the CNS, there are opioid receptors outside the CNS able to produce analgesic effects in the periphery. The opioid receptors are synthesized in the dorsal root ganglia (DRG) and transported toward the peripheral sensory nerve endings. These peripheral actions are enhanced under inflammatory conditions. Immune cells may release endogenous opioid-like substances, which act on opioid receptors located on the primary sensory neuron.

Centrally, the opioids inhibit directly the ascending transmission of painful stimuli arising from the spinal cord (dorsal horn) and activate circuits that descend from the midbrain via the RVM to the dorsal horn.

219. **(B)** Opioids are a primary pain medication that has no ceiling effect , and there is no "mild" opioids, because they can be titrated to produce equianalgesic effects. Although some opioids have been considered "mild" because of

dose-related side effects or because commercial preparations are combined with adjuvant drugs (ie, aspirin or acetaminophen) limiting its dosing.

There is evidence indicating that morphine has greater potency but slower speed of onset and offset in women.

Opioids acting in μ- and κ-receptors constrict the pupil by exciting the Edinger Westphal nucleus (parasympathetic). Long-term opioid use can produce tolerance to miotic effects of opioids.

220.   **(C)** Tramadol has a different profile from that of conventional opioids. It is very effective in the treatment of severe pain, with fewer side effects than morphine.

The risk of respiratory depression is lower at equianalgesic doses; the risk of fatal respiratory depression is minimal at appropriate oral dosing, and limited essentially to patients with severe renal failure.

Tramadol has a low abuse potential, however, nausea and vomiting occur at the same rate as with other opioids.

221.   **(D)** Morphine is metabolized by the liver to morphine-6-glucuronide which is more potent than morphine itself and has a longer half-life, resulting in additional analgesia. Morphine is also metabolized to morphine-3-glucuronide which causes adverse effects and is inactive according to others.

Renal dysfunction can produce accumulation of morphine-6-glucuronide, with subsequent opioid effects, including respiratory depression, so morphine should be used with care in renal dysfunction.

Patients with liver failure can tolerate morphine (even in hepatic precoma), because glucuronidation is rarely impaired.

Short bowel syndrome and vomiting and diarrhea limit the efficacy of controlled-release morphine, which relies in slow absorption from the GI tract.

222.   **(A)** Fentanyl is 80 times as potent as morphine. Transdermal fentanyl is extremely useful as a treatment in chronic pain especially in cancer patients. It causes less constipation than sustained-release morphine. Ninety-two percent of fentanyl delivered transdermally reaches systemic circulation as unchanged fentanyl.

Peak plasma concentration after application is 12 to 24 hours and a residual depot remains in subcutaneous tissues for about 24 hours after removal of the patch, therefore care needs to be taken with the use of transdermal system.

223.   **(A)** Normeperidine is a neurotoxic metabolite of meperidine; its accumulation is more likely in patients with poor renal function, especially in the elderly. The use of meperidine should be limited to 1 to 2 days for acute pain and should be avoided in chronic pain management.

224.   **(A)** Opioid distribution is a function of lipophilicity and plasma protein binding. Fentanyl is both lipophilic and highly protein bound. Fentanyl also distributes to fat tissue and redistributes slowly from there into the systemic circulation.

The opioids are mainly metabolized in the liver and to a minor extent in CNS, kidneys, lung, and placenta.

225.   **(B)** Investigations have showed that endogenous and exogenous opioids can bind to opioid receptors primarily in the hypothalamus but also in the pituitary gland and testes, decreasing the release of gonadotropin-releasing hormone (GnRH), luteinizing hormone–follicle-stimulating hormone (LH–FSH), and testosterone-testicular interstitial fluid, respectively. Clinically this will manifest as hypogonadism, including: loss of libido, impotence, infertility (males and females), depression, anxiety, loss of muscle strength, fatigue, amenorrhea, irregular menses, galactorrhea, osteoporosis, and fractures.

Opioids have also been found to decrease cortisol levels and cortisol responses, but they do not modify thyroid function.

Opioids also have been shown to increase pituitary release of prolactin in preclinical studies and one study also documented decreased growth hormone (GH), without clear clinical significance.

226.   **(E)** NSAIDs may diminish the antihyperptensive effects of ACE inhibitors (ACEIs) and the

natriuretic effect of furosemide and thiazides in some patients.

Anticoagulant therapy with warfarin should be monitored, especially in the first few days of changing therapy, because all the currently available COX-2 inhibitors may increase serum warfarin levels.

Lithium levels may also increase with celecoxib, valdecoxib, and rofecoxib.

227. **(C)** All sulfonamides can be regarded to one of the two main biochemical categories, arylamines or nonarylamines. The sulfonamide allergicity is thought to be related to the formation of hydroxylamine a metabolite of the nonarylamine group. Celecoxib and valdecoxib belong to the former group and are contraindicated in patients allergic to sulfonamides.

228. **(C)** Nabumetone (nonacidic prodrug metabolized to a structural analogue of naproxen) is minimally toxic to the GI tract, and it is the choice when GI side effects are a special concern.

Coxibs are also a good choice if there is any history of GI symptoms. Coxibs are associated with less GI toxicity than standard NSAIDs, since they do not inhibit the constitutive COX-1 and therefore the production of the cytoprotective PGI_2 in the stomach mucosa.

229. **(A)** Coxibs show less GI side effects, and have similar renal effects to those of standard NSAIDs.

COX-2 is not present in platetelets, and up-to-date under most conditions, coxibs are not associated with platelet dysfunction.

There is no documentation in humans that the coxibs impairs bone remodeling and delay fracture healing.

230. **(E)** The potency of NSAIDs in general is similar or equipotent to ASA, except for diflunisal, indomethacin, ketorolac, and diclofenac.

Diflunisal is a difluorophenyl derivative of salicylic acid, more potent than aspirin in anti-inflammatory tests in animals. It is used primarily as analgesic in osteoarthritis and musculoskeletal sprains, where is 3 to 4 times more potent than ASA. It also produces fewer and less intense GI and antiplatelet effects than ASA.

Indomethacin is 10 to 40 times more potent inhibitor of COX than ASA, but intolerance limits its dosing to short-term. It also may have a direct, COX-independent vasoconstrictor effect. Some studies have suggested the possibility of increased risk of MI and stroke, but controlled trials have not been performed.

Ketorolac is a potent analgesic, poor anti-inflammatory. Has been used as a short term alternative (less than 5 days) to opioids, for moderate to severe pain.

Diclofenac is more potent than ASA; its potency against COX-2 is substantially greater than that of indomethacin, naproxen, or several other NSAIDs.

Naproxen is more potent in vitro.

231. **(B)** A multimodal approach (the combination of different, appropriate pain treatments) seems to be the best approach in terms of synergy and reducing the side effects of each.

The opioid sparing effects of NSAIDs use in postoperative pain, has been confirmed in multiple controlled trials. This can be of particular benefit when the opioids side effects are especially undesirable, including preexisting ventilatory compromise, strong history of opioid induced side effects and the very young.

232. **(C)** Coxibs are a good choice in patients with a history of GI symptoms or sensitivity to NSAIDs, because they are associated with less GI side effects than standard NSAIDs. Although they are more expensive and they carry the concern of increase cardiovascular risk (increased thrombotic events: MI, stroke), with continuous and prolonged used.

Standard NSAIDs combined with GI prophylaxis seems to be equally effective in terms of efficacy and freedom from GI toxicity. The GI prophylaxis can consist of: parietal cell inhibitors (acid inhibitors, ie, omeprazole), prostaglandin analogues (misoprostol), and H blockers (ie, ranitidine, cimetidine).

Diclofenac is available in combination with misoprostol, retaining the efficacy of diclofenac while reducing the frequency of GI toxicity; it is cost effective relative to coxibs despite the cost of added misoprostol.

Diclofenac with enteric coat does not offer a marked less GI toxicity.

233. **(E)** The combination of opioid/nonopioid (ie, NSAIDs) for mild to moderate cancer pain is synergistic and has the ability to reduce the side effects of each drug.

NSAIDs in advanced cancer, are particularly useful for bone pain (distension of the periosteum by metastases, for soft tissue pain (distension or compression of tissues), and for visceral pain (irritation of the pleura or peritoneum).

ASA and other salicylates are contraindicated in children and young adults (younger than 20 years) with fever associated with viral illness, owing to the association with Reye syndrome.

Acetaminophen: nonacidic, crosses the blood–brain barrier, acts mainly in the CNS, peripheral, and anti inflammatory effects are weak.

234. **(D)** Unlike ibuprofen, naproxen, and ketorolac, celecoxib does not interfere with the inhibition of platelet COX-1 activity and function by aspirin.

235. **(E)**

236. **(A)** The drug was approved by the European Union in 2004. Pregabalin received US FDA approval for use in treating epilepsy, diabetic neuropathy pain, and pain in June 2005, and appeared on the US market in 2005. In June 2007 the FDA approved it as a treatment for fibromyalgia. It was the first drug to be approved for this indication and remained the only one, until duloxetine gained FDA approval for the treatment of fibromyalgia in 2008.

237. **(B)** GBP has a chemical structure similar to GABA. It seems not to act directly at the GABA-binding site in the CNS, however. The mechanism of action is still unclear. It may enhance the release or activity of GABA and seems to inhibit voltage-dependent sodium channels.

238. **(A)** Case report evidence suggests that clonazepam may have a useful effect in treatment of the shooting pain associated with phantom limb pain. Somnolence is a predominant side effect, and with this drug's long half-life, daytime sedation may complicate use. As it belongs to the benzodiazepine group of drugs, anxiolysis and muscle relaxation may also be produced by its use, and this combination of properties may, in some patients, be useful.

239. **(B)** Case report evidence suggests that lamotrigine may reduce the symptoms of complex regional pain syndrome (type 1), with the sudomotor changes seen in this condition being alleviated along with pain and allodynia. Perhaps the major side effect limiting rapid titration to a therapeutic dose is skin rash.

Higher doses may be used, but, if no effect is observed at 300 mg/d, further increases are unlikely to produce analgesia. In view of the relatively long half-life of lamotrigine, once-daily dosing may be appropriate.

240. **(B)** The TCAs can be divided into tertiary amines and their demethylated secondary amine derivatives.

Tertiary amine TCAs
Amitriptyline
Imipramine
Tripramine
Clomipramine
Doxapin
Secondary amine TCAs
Nortriptyline
Desipramine
Protriptyline
Amoxapine

241. **(E)**

242. **(C)**

243. **(A)**

244. **(A)**

245. **(E)**

246. **(B)** The liver receives the major insult from acetaminophen toxicity, with the predominant lesion

being acute centrilobular hepatic necrosis. It is suggested the use of the glutathione precursor of N-acetylcysteine for the treatment of acetaminophen intoxication in efforts to maintain hepatic reduced glutathione concentrations and adrenergic agonists may lower hepatic glutathione significantly.

247. **(A)** Baclofen is the ρ-chlorophenyl derivative of GABA. Baclofen is a $GABA_B$ agonist that has been used for muscle spasms and spasticity, neuropathic pain, and so on. Baclofen may enhance the effectiveness of antiepileptic drugs in certain neuropathic pain states. Side effects include sedation, weakness, and confusion. Abrupt cessation may cause a withdrawal syndrome, such as hallucinations, anxiety, tachycardia, or seizures.

248. **(D)** The two clinically available botulinum toxins in the United States are botulinum toxin type A and botulinum toxin type B. A different formulation of botulinum toxin A is used in Europe as well as a version used in China but are currently not available in the United States. Effects seem to last for roughly 3 to 6 months after injection, at which point a repeat injection generally reproduces the effect.

Although it is generally accepted that botulinum toxins may lead to diminished pain in patients with painful muscle spasms or cervical dystonia by diminishing muscle tone, it is also felt that botulinum toxin may itself possess analgesic properties. The mechanism of botulinum toxin–induced analgesia are unknown.

The most evident mechanism of botulinum toxin-induced analgesia is via reduction of muscle spasm by cholinergic chemodenervation at motor end plates and by inhibition of gamma motor endings in muscle spindles.

Future uses of botulinum toxins for analgesia may lead to redesign toxins for intrathecal use.

249. **(A)** Cyclobenzaprine is structurally similar to TCAs and, as such, demonstrates significant anticholinergic side effects. It exhibits a side-effect profile similar to that of the TCAs, including lethargy and agitation, although it usually does not appear to produce significant dysrhythmias beyond sinus tachycardia. Elderly patients seem to tolerate cyclobenzaprine less well and may develop hallucinations as well as significant anticholinergic side effects, such as sedation. The use of significant lower dosing schedules in elderly patients may be prudent.

250. **(C)**

251. **(A)**

CHAPTER 5

Diagnosis of Pain States
Questions

DIRECTIONS (Questions 252 through 318): Each of the numbered items or incomplete statements in this section is followed by answers or by completions of the statement. Select the ONE lettered answer or completion that is BEST in each case.

252. A 59-year-old female comes to your office complaining of moderately severe low back pain and right buttock pain which is exacerbated with prolonged sitting. On physical examination there is sciatic notch tenderness and the pain is exacerbated with flexion, adduction, and internal rotation of the right hip. Which of the following is the most likely diagnosis?

    (A) L5-S1 facet syndrome
    (B) Piriformis syndrome
    (C) Sacroiliac (SI) joint syndrome
    (D) Sciatica
    (E) L3 radiculopathy

253. A 77-year-old female comes to your office complaining of 6 months of severe right buttock pain radiating into the right lower leg. The pain is also present at night and not uncommonly interferes with sleep. The pain is severe with sitting or lying on her back or right side, however, quickly dissipates with normal erect posture. Which of the following is the most likely diagnosis?

    (A) Snapping bottom
    (B) Sciatica
    (C) Radiculopathy
    (D) Piriformis syndrome
    (E) Weaver's bottom

254. A 53-year-old male comes to your office complaining of foot pain (predominantly in the heel—but also with diffuse plantar symptoms) which also occurs at night and can be exacerbated by prolonged standing or walking. It is associated with weakness of the phalanges (impairing the pushing off phase of walking) as well as sensory loss and paresthesia. After a complete history and physical examination are completed, which of the following is the next most appropriate step?

    (A) Magnetic resonance imaging (MRI) of the ankle
    (B) MRI of the lumbar spine
    (C) Initiate anti-inflammatory medications
    (D) Trial of arch support
    (E) Electrodiagnostic testing

255. A 53-year-old male comes to your office complaining of foot pain (predominantly in the heel—but also with diffuse plantar symptoms) which also occurs at night and can be exacerbated by prolonged standing or walking. It is associated with weakness of the phalanges (impairing the pushing off phase of walking) as well as sensory loss and paresthesia. Which of the following is the most likely diagnosis?

    (A) Morton neuroma
    (B) Peripheral neuropathies
    (C) Medial plantar nerve entrapment
    (D) Tarsal tunnel syndrome
    (E) March fracture

256. A 47-year-old female comes to your office complaining of an aching forearm with discomfort and numbness in the thumb and index finger, and weakness in the hand. A positive Tinel sign is present in the forearm. Which of the following is the most likely diagnosis?

(A) Anterior interosseous nerve syndrome
(B) Posterior interosseous nerve syndrome
(C) Ulnar nerve entrapment
(D) Pronator syndrome
(E) Radial nerve entrapment

257. Complex regional pain syndrome type II (CRPS II) differs from CRPS I because in CRPS II there is

(A) allodynia
(B) movement disorder
(C) sudomotor and vasomotor changes
(D) evidence of major nerve damage
(E) severe swelling

258. Which of the following range is the temperature most appropriate to use as a stimulus when evaluating warm temperature sensation?

(A) 25°C to 30°C
(B) 30°C to 35°C
(C) 35°C to 40°C
(D) 40°C to 45°C
(E) 45°C to 50°C

259. Which of the following range is the temperature most appropriate to use as a stimulus when evaluating cold temperature sensation?

(A) −5°C to 0°C
(B) 0°C to 5°C
(C) 5°C to 10°C
(D) 10°C to 15°C
(E) 15°C to 20°C

260. Which of the following may potentially facilitate or perpetuate myofascial trigger points in some patients?

(A) Low creatine kinase
(B) Low aldolase
(C) Low cholesterol

(D) Low vitamin D
(E) Low vitamin B_{12} or folate

261. A 39-year-old male with persistent coughing attributed to upper respiratory infection (URI) comes to your office complaining of moderate anterior chest wall pain—it is only on the left side—predominantly over the second and third costal cartilages. Bulbous swellings and point tenderness are present at these sites. Which of the following is the most appropriate diagnosis for this patient?

(A) Intercostal neuralgia
(B) Tietze syndrome
(C) Acute myocardial infarction
(D) Pneumonia
(E) Pleurisy

262. A 66-year-old woman who did not have a history of trauma comes to your office complaining of acute, severe, constant medial right knee pain for 6 weeks. MRI imaging demonstrated extensive narrow edema of the medial femoral condyle with significant soft tissue edema around the superficial and deep compartment of the medial collateral ligament (MCL) but without MCL disruption. Which of the following is the most likely diagnosis?

(A) Stress fracture
(B) MCL tear
(C) Medial meniscal tear
(D) Spontaneous osteonecrosis of the knee (SONK)
(E) Medical femoral condyle contusion

263. A 49-year-old male comes to your office after climbing several mountain passes in the Pyrenees on a bicycle with thigh complaints. He relates to you that he developed a painful sensation on the lateral aspect of his right thigh, which lasted for about a week. This was followed by numbness and paresthesia in the same location. Physical examination revealed sensory loss in the same location. Which of the following is the most likely diagnosis?

(A) Tensor fascia lata syndrome
(B) Meralgia paresthetica

(C) Iliotibial band syndrome

(D) Greater trochanteric bursitis

(E) Lumbar radiculopathy

264. A 43-year-old male runner comes to your office complaining of a dull ache in the anterior aspect of the lower legs bilaterally which occurs about 10 minutes into his running routine each time he runs and dissipates with rest. The patient states that he needs to stop running because of this ache and also notes dysesthesia in the first web space of both feet. Which of the following is the most likely diagnosis?

(A) Shin splints

(B) Stress fractures

(C) Chronic osteomyelitis

(D) Periostitis

(E) Chronic exertional anterior compartment syndrome of the lower leg

265. A 32-year-old construction worker felt a sharp pain in his back radiating down to the heel of his right foot after lifting a large, metal girder. Two days later he noticed numbness in the sole of his right foot and fifth toe. Physical examination is notable for a decreased ability to walk on his toes, a positive straight leg raising test on the right, and a markedly diminished ankle jerk reflex. Which of the following is the most likely diagnosis?

(A) L4-5 herniated disc

(B) Discogenic low back pain

(C) L5-S1 herniated disc

(D) Spinal stenosis

(E) Piriformis syndrome

266. An 80-year-old man presents with a 2-year history of low back pain radiating down from both legs to his ankles. He also notes numbness in his left foot and slight weakness. The pain is increased with walking and relieved within seconds of cessation of activity. Leaning forward eases his pain and lying supine relieves it. Which of the following is the most likely diagnosis?

(A) Herniated nucleus pulposus

(B) Facet arthropathy

(C) Muscle spasm

(D) Arachnoiditis

(E) Spinal stenosis

267. A 31-year-old woman presents to your office with marked pain and swelling in her ankle 6 weeks after an open reduction internal fixation with casting. On examination, the ankle is warm and erythematous. Lightly touching the ankle with a cotton swab evokes severe, lancinating pain. You suspect CRPS I. Which of the following tests will confirm your diagnosis?

(A) Lumbar sympathetic block

(B) Phentolamine infusion test

(C) Triple phase isotope bone scan

(D) Erythrocyte sedimentation rate

(E) None of the above

268. A 46-year-old man complains of worsening back and new onset leg pain and paresthesia 10 weeks after an L4-S1 posterior spinal fusion. One week after the surgery, the patient reported 85% pain relief. Which radiologic test would be most appropriate for detecting the cause of failed back surgery syndrome (FBSS) in this patient?

(A) Computed tomographic (CT) scan with contrast

(B) Myelography

(C) Epidural mapping via the injection of contrast under fluoroscopy through a catheter inserted through the caudal canal

(D) T2-weighted MRI with contrast

(E) Further radiologic study is not indicated at this point

269. Which of the following is false regarding discogenic low back pain?

    (A) Sitting bent forward subjects the intervertebral disc to a greater amount of pressure than lying down, standing or sitting with one's back straight

    (B) It is often diagnosed by using provocative discography

    (C) Because of their caudad position in the spine, the lower lumbar discs are most prone to degenerative disc disease (DDD)

    (D) Studies have shown a genetic predisposition to DDD

    (E) Intradiscal steroids are an effective means for treating DDD

270. Which of the following statements concerning central pain is true?

    (A) Spinal cord injury is the leading cause of central pain in the United States

    (B) Lesions involving spinothalamocortical pathways are necessary and sufficient to cause central pain

    (C) Central pain is a common sequelae following neurosurgic procedures

    (D) Motor cortex stimulation is an effective means to treat central pain

    (E) The most typical presentation of central pain is a spontaneous, burning sensation on the entire body contralateral to the lesion site

271. Which of the following is not commonly used to diagnose the level of nerve root involvement in radicular pain?

    (A) MRI

    (B) CT scan

    (C) Selective nerve root block

    (D) Electromyography (EMG)/nerve conduction studies (NCS)

    (E) Epidural injections with local anesthetic and steroids

272. Which of the following conditions is not generally associated with a painful neuropathy?

    (A) Chronic renal failure

    (B) Celiac disease

    (C) AIDS

    (D) Fabry disease

    (E) Amyloidosis

273. A previously healthy 31-year-old woman presents to her internist with generalized muscle pain, most prominent in her right thigh. The pain travels down the back of her leg to the bottom of her foot. She also notes progressive numbness and weakness in her arms and legs. Walking is difficult and a loss of fine motor control makes routine tasks like eating a challenge. A review of her medical record reveals an URI 3 weeks earlier. Which of the following is the most likely diagnosis?

    (A) Multiple sclerosis

    (B) Guillain-Barré syndrome

    (C) Chronic fatigue syndrome

    (D) Acute lumbar and cervical radiculopathies

    (E) Diabetic neuropathy

274. Which of the following statements is true regarding SI joint pain?

    (A) The SI joint is a diarthrodial synovial joint designed primarily for stability

    (B) Patrick's and Gaenslen's tests are definitive diagnostic tests for SI joint pain

    (C) CT scanning is the most sensitive means for diagnosing SI joint pain

    (D) Lifting heavy objects is the one of the most common causes of SI joint injury

    (E) When diagnostic blocks fail, surgery can usually provide long-term pain relief

275. Which of the following statements regarding headaches is false?

    (A) The International Headache Society's diagnostic criteria for cervicogenic headaches includes unilaterality of symptoms and relief of pain by diagnostic anesthetic blocks

    (B) Migraine with aura is more common than migraine without aura

(C) In chronic tension-type headache, the average headache frequency is equal to or greater than 15 days per month

(D) Cluster headaches are more prevalent in men than in women

(E) Tricyclic antidepressants are a mainstay of treatment for both migraine and tension-type headaches

276. Which of the following statements regarding postamputation pain is correct?

(A) Vascular conditions are the leading cause of both lower and upper extremity amputations

(B) There is no relationship between persistent stump pain and phantom limb pain in amputees

(C) The intensity of pain and the length of the phantom increases with time

(D) Phantom breast pain is a common cause of postmastectomy pain

(E) Phantom pain was first described in the American Civil War

277. Which of the following statements regarding the assessment of pain in pediatric patients is true?

(A) Palmar sweating and reduced transcutaneous oxygen concentrations are indicative of pain

(B) In a hospitalized 2-year-old child, crying and increased vitals signs are likely to indicate chronic pain

(C) The FACES scale and Charleston Pain Pictures provide accurate assessments of pain in preschool children

(D) The COMFORT scale and facial action coding system (FACS) are pain instruments used in young children that are based predominantly on facial actions

(E) Visual analogue and numerical rating scales are inappropriate pain indices for most adolescents

278. Which of the following statements is not correct regarding herpes varicella zoster?

(A) The most common presentation of acute herpes zoster (AHZ) is pain and a vesicular rash in the midthoracic dermatomes

(B) The polymerase chain reaction (PCR) is the most common means to diagnose AHZ

(C) The incidence of both AHZ and postherpetic neuralgia increases with age

(D) There is no generally accepted time period from the onset of AHZ to when a diagnosis of postherpetic neuralgia is made

(E) AHZ involving the lumbosacral dermatomes may be misdiagnosed as a herniated disc

279. Which of the following statements regarding electrophysiologic testing is true?

(A) Nerve conduction velocities are more likely to decrease in conditions such as alcoholic and diabetic neuropathy that are characterized by Wallerian degeneration than in demyelinating neuropathies such as Guillain-Barré

(B) EMG can provide information about the type, extent and timing of injuries to motor units and individual muscle fibers

(C) The H reflex can aid in the evaluation of brachial plexus injuries

(D) The F response is used to diagnose pure sensory neuropathies

(E) EMG can readily identify processes causing muscle denervation (neuropathies), but is incapable of identifying myopathies

280. Which of the following statements is true about quantitative sensory testing (QST)?

    (A) QST can be used to pinpoint which nerve is injured and where along its path the lesion lies

    (B) Thermal sensation is used to measure the integrity of large, myelinated nerve fibers

    (C) A beta function can be evaluated using either a tuning fork or von Frey hair

    (D) QST can be used to evaluate the function of all different types of nerve fibers

    (E) An advantage of QST is that it can accurately assess function in uncooperative or incapacitated patients

281. A 38-year-old construction worker presents to you with complaints of right lower extremity pain for the last 8 months. Pain radiates from the lower back to the outer aspect of the right leg and goes down to the dorsum of the right foot. The patient reports a problem with walking and on examination reveals an antalgic gait and inability to do heel-walking on right, though toe-walking is not affected. Strength is 5/5 in all muscle groups except dorsi-flexion of the right ankle which is 4/5 and strength testing for extensor hallucis longus reveals 4/5 strength. Deep tendon reflexes are 2+ at both knees and both ankles. Sensory testing reveals mildly reduced sensation to light touch and pinprick on the dorsum of the right foot when compared to the left foot. This patient most likely has

    (A) right piriformis syndrome
    (B) right L4 radiculopathy
    (C) right L5 radiculopathy
    (D) right S1 radiculopathy
    (E) facet arthritis

282. A 46-year-old female with past medical history of depression, anxiety, irritable bowl syndrome, and asthma is referred to you for evaluation of her lower back pain. History reveals onset of generalized pain that started after she was involved in a car accident 4 years ago. Physical examination reveals nonfocal neurologic examination. Musculoskeletal examination reveals multiple areas of hypersensitivity. The patient reports marked pain with moderate digital pressure at base of skull, her neck, front of her chest, her elbows as well as her lower back, and bilateral lower extremities. The patients MRI scan of the lumbar spine reveals preserved disc height, no facet arthritis and minimal disc bulge at L4-5 without any spinal or foraminal stenosis. This patient most likely has

    (A) fibromyalgia syndrome
    (B) discogenic pain
    (C) myofascial pain disorder
    (D) somatoform disorder
    (E) opioid hyperalgesia

283. A 25-year-old, healthy female volleyball player has developed severe pain in right hand. This pain started while playing volleyball and after a reported wrist sprain. One month after the initial injury and despite conservative care with nonsteroidal anti-inflammatory drugs (NSAIDs), muscle relaxants, and hand splint to avoid any movement related pain, the patient complains of even worse burning pain. Pain is worse with light touch, even blowing air or rubbing of clothes trigger unbearable pain. The patient also reports her right hand to be cold and often wet because of localized sweating. On examination the patient has a markedly swollen, red-appearing hand. Patient is unable to make a fist with her fingers and measurement of temperature reveals a 7°C lower temperature compared to opposite extremity. Which of the following is the most likely diagnosis?

    (A) CRPS I (RSD)
    (B) CRPS II (causalgia)
    (C) Peripheral vascular disease
    (D) Deep venous thrombosis of upper extremity
    (E) Median neuralgia

284. A 38-year-old man developed complete T4 spinal cord injury after a motorcycle accident. Two months after the injury the patient continues to complain of severe radiating pain to the front of chest just above nipple line. The pain is worse with light touching and improves with movement restriction and use of morphine on as needed basis. This patient most likely has

(A) central dysesthesia syndrome
(B) syringomyelia
(C) transitional zone pain
(D) myofascial pain
(E) autonomic dysreflexia

285. After a car accident 5 days ago, a 42-year-old engineer reports severe neck and midback pain. The patient was rear ended while stopped at a traffic light by a pickup truck. The patient reports severe pain in neck that radiates down to both shoulders and upper arm as well as to the midback region. The pain is a severe stabbing and aching sensation that is markedly exaggerated by movement of neck. Examination reveals otherwise intact neurologic system, 5/5 strength, and intact deep tendon reflexes without any sensory deficit. Imaging studies are essentially normal except for straightening of cervical lordosis. The patient most likely has

(A) bilateral C5 radiculopathy
(B) myofascial pain
(C) fibromyalgia
(D) thoracic outlet syndrome
(E) malingering

286. A 64-year-old female with a history of coronary artery disease, peripheral vascular disease, and type 1 diabetes mellitus, controlled with insulin, presents to your pain clinic with gradually worsening bilateral leg and feet pain. The patient reports a history of a fall approximately 5 years ago which resulted in severe back and leg pain. That pain resolved, however, the patient started developing numbness and tingling in both legs and feet. On examination the patient reveals otherwise normal appearing legs and feet, patient does have a nonhealing ulcer on her right great toe. Neurologic testing reveals bilateral 5/5 muscle strength and 2+ patellar and ankle reflexes. Sensory testing reveals intact proprioception but reduced sensation to light touch and

pinprick. The patient also reported marked sensitivity to light touch. This patient most likely has

(A) CRPS I
(B) peripheral vascular disease
(C) diabetic polyneuropathy
(D) lumbar spondylosis
(E) central pain

287. A 32-year-old female develops severe stabbing, "like an ice pick," pain at the base of tongue after an infratemporal neurosurgic procedure. Pain comes in paroxysms and last a few seconds and is triggered by swallowing, yawning, and coughing. This patient most likely has

(A) trigeminal neuralgia
(B) geniculate neuralgia
(C) glossopharyngeal neuralgia
(D) migraine with atypical aura
(E) cluster headache

288. A 38-year-old patient care technician while lifting a 400 lb patient heard a pop in his back. The patient developed severe back pain with radiation to the right leg. Patient described the pain as stabbing back pain with electrical sensations down the back of the right leg all the way to the sole of the right foot. On examination the patient appeared very uncomfortable, sitting in a wheel chair. Straight leg raise and cross straight leg raise test was positive. Muscle strength was 5/5 in all muscle groups except plantar flexion at right ankle which was 4/5. Deep tendon reflexes were intact at the patella bilaterally; however, the reflex at the right ankle is diminished compared to the left ankle. The patient most likely has a herniated disc at

(A) L4-L5 resulting in L4 nerve root compression
(B) L4-L5 resulting in L5 nerve root compression
(C) L5-S1 resulting in L5 nerve root compression
(D) L5-S1 resulting in S1 nerve root compression
(E) L1-L2 resulting in compression of cauda equina

289. A 48-year-old patient after a gunshot wound to the upper chest develops a partial cord transection involving the right spinothalamic tract at T2 level. This patient is most likely to develop loss of pain and temperature sensation:

    (A) At the level of the transection
    (B) Below and on right side from the level of transection
    (C) Below and on left side from the level of transection
    (D) Patient is not likely to develop central dysesthetic pain
    (E) Below and bilateral lower extremity

290. A 38-year-old police officer reports continuous neck pain lasting past 6 months. The patient recalls lifting and carrying heavy boxes while moving his house and reports some neck pain at that time. Pain has gradually worsened over the past 6 months and now patient reports heaviness and occasional weakness in his right hand. The patient often feels numbness in right index finger as well. On examination, the patient has 5/5 strength in all muscle groups except mild weakness in flexors of the right elbow. Light-touch sensation is intact in all dermatomes, however, the patient reports increased sensation to light touch in the radial aspect of the right forearm. Deep tendon reflexes are intact bilaterally except for right brachioradialis reflex which is 1$^+$ compared to left. This patient most likely has

    (A) right C5 radiculopathy
    (B) right C6 radiculopathy
    (C) right C7 radiculopathy
    (D) right C8 radiculopathy
    (E) cervical facet arthritis with referred pain

291. A 42-year-old man underwent a celiac plexus block procedure with 20 mL of 50% alcohol. All of the following listed conditions are complications of this intervention EXCEPT

    (A) genitofemoral neuralgia
    (B) hypertension
    (C) diarrhea

    (D) paralysis
    (E) infection

292. A two-needle lumbar sympathetic plexus block at L2 and L3 when performed appropriately may help in the diagnosis of

    (A) sympathetically mediated pain
    (B) lumbar discogenic pain
    (C) lumbar radiculopathy
    (D) diabetic neuropathy
    (E) facet arthritis

293. A patient who received 1 cc of 0.25% bupivacaine after negative aspiration following a cervical selective nerve root injection became agitated and then developed generalized tonic-clonic movements. Which of the following is the most likely explanation?

    (A) High spinal anesthetic from accidental intrathecal injection
    (B) Anxiety attack from pain during injection
    (C) Vertebral artery injection of local anesthetic
    (D) Injection into spinal cord
    (E) Hypoxia

294. Medial branch nerve blocks may aid in the diagnosis of

    (A) facet arthritis
    (B) sympathetically mediated pain
    (C) spinal nerve irritation
    (D) sciatica
    (E) myofascial pain

295. Which of the following is the most likely side effect of a SI joint injection?

    (A) Perforation of bladder
    (B) Left lower extremity weakness
    (C) Stroke
    (D) High spinal resulting in cardiorespiratory depression
    (E) Injury to pudendal nerve

296. The potential complications of the vertebroplasty procedure include all EXCEPT

   (A) spinal cord compression
   (B) venous embolism
   (C) pedicle fracture
   (D) cement leak in soft tissue
   (E) bowl perforation

297. A 70-year-old man reports severe cramps and "charley horse" sensation in both legs when walking more than one block. Resting usually helps in relieving pain. On examination patient reveals an intact neurologic examination without any sensory or motor deficit. Lower extremity examination reveals normal appearance, and no vascular insufficiency. Ankle brachial index performed 1 month ago is unremarkable. Which of the following is the most likely diagnosis?

   (A) Neurogenic claudication
   (B) Vascular claudication
   (C) Diabetic peripheral neuropathy
   (D) Amyloid neuropathy
   (E) Fibromyalgia

298. A 32-year-old healthy female presents with a 2-month history of gradually worsening right lower extremity pain. The pain is sharp shooting in character and radiates down the right leg all the way to the right foot. On examination, patient has 5/5 muscle strength in all muscle groups except plantar flexors of the right ankle. The patient is unable to stand on her toes. There is no sensory deficit. Flexion, adduction, and internal rotation of the right hip results in reproduction of the symptoms. MRI of lumbar spine is normal with no evidence of herniated discs. This patient most likely has

   (A) right S1 radiculopathy
   (B) piriformis syndrome

   (C) SI arthritis
   (D) somatization disorder
   (E) discogenic pain

299. A 25-year-old construction worker, 8 months after a fall from a ladder, is unable to walk without assistance. However, worker compensations lawyers have provided video evidence of the patient being able to walk and also able to run with his dog. Which of the following is the most likely diagnosis?

   (A) Hypochondriasis
   (B) Factitious disorder
   (C) Malingering
   (D) Conversion disorder
   (E) Somatization disorder

300. A 43-year-old gentleman has developed left groin pain 6 months after an inguinal hernia repair. The patient reports pain to be severe stabbing pain in the left groin radiating down to the left testicle. On examination, the patient has a well-healed incision and marked cutaneous allodynia and hyperalgesia. This patient most likely has

   (A) ilioinguinal neuralgia
   (B) mesh infection
   (C) recurrent hernia
   (D) wound dehiscence
   (E) incarceration

301. Which of the following is the most common complication from the celiac plexus block?

   (A) Hypotension
   (B) Seizure
   (C) Diarrhea
   (D) Hematoma
   (E) Subarachnoid injection

302. A patient with history of three lumbar spinal fusions from an injury while working in a halfway home who is responsive to MS Contin (sustained-release morphine) 30 mg, three times a day and Norco (hydrocodone 5 mg with acetaminophen 325 mg) eight tablets per day with adequate analgesia and improved functionality, but limited activity secondary to side effects, receives an intrathecal opioid pump trial after been cleared by his psychologist. After confirmation of appropriate placement of the catheter under fluoroscopy, he is put on 0.5 mg/d of intrathecal morphine and gradually escalated up to 10 mg/d because of inadequate analgesia. Twelve hours after the procedure, he complains of nausea, headache, and sensation of "skin peeling off his body." Which of the following is the best course of action in this case?

    (A) Increase the intrathecal morphine until pain relief and resolution of symptoms
    (B) CT scan of his spine to confirm correct placement of the catheter
    (C) Removal of the catheter and institution of oral opioids
    (D) Urine toxicology
    (E) Consultation with a spine surgeon

303. Migraine headaches are directly related to

    (A) estrogen increase
    (B) estrogen decrease
    (C) progesterone increase
    (D) progesterone decrease
    (E) none of the above

304. A 50-year-old female comes in complaining of sudden onset pain in bilateral lower extremities and loss of bladder function. Her physical examination reveals motor weakness in her left lower extremity 3/5 compared to the right along with diminished sensation to light touch, pinprick, and temperature along L5 and S1 dermatomes on the right compared to the left. Rest of her physical, musculoskeletal, and neurologic examination is normal. Lumbosacral x-rays done by her primary care physician demonstrate anterolisthesis of L5 on S1. Which of the following is the most appropriate immediate action?

    (A) Consult the spine surgeon
    (B) Intravenous Opioids
    (C) Physical therapy
    (D) Reassurance and return to home with a follow-up visit in 2 weeks if symptoms persist
    (E) A course of oral steroids

305. The approaches to celiac plexus block are all EXCEPT

    (A) retrocrural
    (B) transcrural
    (C) transaortic
    (D) intercrural
    (E) lateral

306. A 25-year-old male presents to you with left-sided neck pain with radiation along lateral aspect of the left arm, forearm, and thumb, index, and middle finger. He has associated tingling and numbness. On neurologic examination, the sensation to pinprick is diminished in the above mentioned distribution and brachioradialis jerk is lost on the left compared to intact 2^+ on the right. The MRI of C-spine is compatible with an acute cervical disc herniation. Which of the following is the most appropriate initial treatment?

    (A) A course of oral opioids, oral steroids, and spine surgical consultation
    (B) A series of cervical epidural steroid injections under fluoroscopy
    (C) Physical therapy
    (D) Spinal cord stimulation (SCS)
    (E) Referral to pain psychologist for coping strategies

307. Hoffmann sign is indicative of

    (A) upper motor neuron lesion (UMNL)
    (B) lower motor neuron lesion (LMNL)
    (C) radiculopathy
    (D) instability of cervical spine
    (E) malingering

308. A 65-year-old male comes in complaining of pain in between the third and the fourth toes. The pain can be reproduced by palpation of the pulp between metatarsal heads. There is some relief of pain following localized administration of local anesthetic. Which of the following is the most likely diagnosis?

(A) Plantar fascitis
(B) Metatarsalgia
(C) Tarsal tunnel syndrome
(D) Morton neuroma
(E) Painful calcaneal spur

309. Which of the following is the most common nerve missed with the interscalene brachial plexus nerve block?

(A) Ulnar
(B) Radial
(C) Musculocutaneous
(D) Median
(E) Axillary

310. A 23-year-old gymnast while performing a double loop hears a popping sound in her left knee. Her knee immediately swells up and is very painful. On physical examination, tenderness on palpation and effusion is demonstrated. McMurray test is positive. Which of the following is the most likely diagnosis?

(A) Baker cyst
(B) Anterior cruciate ligament tear
(C) Posterior cruciate ligament tear
(D) Torn medial meniscus
(E) Pes anserine bursitis

311. A 35-year-old female is rear ended at 45 mph resulting in acute neck pain that was diagnosed to be of musculoskeletal nature in the emergency room. On the next day, her symptoms progress to right upper extremity pain and weakness, both of which are exacerbated with ipsilateral flexion of her neck and reaching overhead. She has no neurologic deficits and MRI of her neck shows no obvious pathology. There is obliteration of the radial pulse with arm extension and abduction. Which of the following is the most likely diagnosis?

(A) Brachial plexitis
(B) Cervical degenerative disc disease
(C) Whiplash injury
(D) Pancoast tumor
(E) Thoracic outlet syndrome

312. The following is true about the H reflex EXCEPT

(A) in clinical practice H reflex is limited to calf muscles
(B) it is recorded in gastrocnemius and soleus muscles by stimulating the posterior tibial nerve in the popliteal fossa
(C) because of the distance the impulse travels, the latency of the H wave is shorter than the F wave
(D) the H reflex recorded from the soleus muscle is primarily mediated by the S1 nerve root
(E) H reflex is normal in L5 radiculopathy whereas is prolonged in S1 radiculopathy

313. The arteria radicularis magna, also known as artery of Adamkiewicz arises from aorta, at the following spinal levels:

(A) L4-5
(B) T9-12
(C) T5-8
(D) T11-12
(E) T5-9

314. A 56-year-old male who is an avid golfer comes in with left elbow pain not relieved after anti-inflammatory medication trial, warm compress, and physical therapy. He has not been able to play 18 holes recently and this is making him quite depressed. On examination, passive flexion or extension against resistance of his left wrist causes pain. Which of the following is the most probable diagnosis in this patient?

(A) Posterior interosseous nerve entrapment
(B) Medial epicondylitis
(C) Lateral epicondylitis
(D) de Quervain disease
(E) Brachioradialis tendonitis

315. All of these cervical pathologies are seen in patients with rheumatoid arthritis EXCEPT

    (A) subaxial subluxation
    (B) cranial settling
    (C) posterior-longitudinal ligament thickening
    (D) atlantoaxial subluxation
    (E) instability of cervical-zygapophyseal joints

316. While undergoing lumbar sympathetic block for CRPS, patient complains of sudden onset of sharp ipsilateral groin and genital pain on injection of the contrast agent. Which of the following is the most likely cause of this symptom?

    (A) Trauma to L2 nerve root
    (B) Trauma to genitofemoral nerve
    (C) Psoas spasm
    (D) Epidural injection
    (E) Successful lumbar sympathetic block

317. Which of the following is the most common inherited neuropathy?

    (A) Familial amyloid polyneuropathy
    (B) Fabry disease
    (C) Porphyric neuropathy
    (D) Charcot-Marie-Tooth disease
    (E) Diabetic polyneuropathy

318. A 52-year-old man comes to your office complaining of $1\frac{1}{2}$ years of "burning" pain in the metatarsal areas of his left foot. Which of the following is the most likely diagnosis?

    (A) Posterior tibial neuritis
    (B) Plantar fasciitis
    (C) Morton neuroma
    (D) Tarsal tunnel syndrome
    (E) Hallux rigidus

DIRECTIONS: For Question 319 through 331, ONE or MORE of the numbered options is correct. Choose answer

    (A) if only answer 1, 2, and 3 are correct
    (B) if only 1 and 3 are correct
    (C) if only 2 and 4 are correct
    (D) if only 4 is correct
    (E) if all are correct

319. In MRI of the lumbar spine T2-weighted images

    (1) are generally more time-consuming to obtain
    (2) are ideal to image the anatomic detail of end-plate reactive changes
    (3) exhibit increased sensitivity to higher water content and thus, may be useful in imaging infectious processes or inflammation
    (4) can be used in place of gadolinium-DTPA (diethylenetriamine penta-acetic acid) contrast in imaging of post-operative patients to differentiate scarring from intervertebral disc issues

320. In EMG and NCS, the H reflex

    (1) is the electrical equivalent of a muscle stretch reflex elicited by tendon tap
    (2) is mostly present in the soleus muscle but at times also can be elicited in the forearm flexor muscles
    (3) may be delayed or absent in S1 radiculopathy
    (4) latencies are length-dependent and should be adjusted for patient's height

321. A previously healthy 83-year-old male presents to your office complaining of acute abdominal pain but without obvious etiology. Medical conditions which should be investigated include

    (1) pneumonia
    (2) inflammatory bowel disease
    (3) pyelonephritis
    (4) inferior wall myocardial infarction

322. Patients diagnosed with cubital tunnel syndrome may have

    (1) pain and numbness in the ulnar border of the forearm and hand
    (2) clawing of the small finger

(3) Wartenberg sign

(4) a deep aching sensation in the mid forearm

323. A 53-year-old male comes to your office complaining of foot pain (predominantly in the heel—but also with diffuse plantar symptoms) which also occurs at night and can be exacerbated by prolonged standing or walking. It is associated with weakness of the phalanges (impairing the pushing off phase of walking) as well as sensory loss and paresthesia. After a complete history and physical examination are completed, the differential diagnosis may include

(1) plantar fasciitis

(2) peripheral neuropathies

(3) posterior tibial nerve entrapment

(4) tarsal tunnel syndrome

324. The diagnostic criteria for CRPS I—as accepted in 1994 by the International Association for the Study of Pain (IASP)—includes which of the following?

(1) The presence of an initiating noxious event, or a cause of immobilization

(2) Continuing pain, allodynia, or hyperalgesia with which the pain is disproportionate to any inciting event

(3) Evidence at some time of edema, changes in skin blood flow, or abnormal sudomotor activity in the region of pain

(4) This diagnosis is excluded by the existence of conditions that would otherwise account for the degree of pain and dysfunction

325. The paroxysmal hemicranias are rare benign headache disorders that may typically be associated with

(1) conjunctival injection

(2) rhinorrhea

(3) ptosis

(4) eyelid edema

326. Which of the following statement(s) is (are) true?

(1) The most common cause of thoracic radiculopathy is diabetes mellitus

(2) The most common levels affected by herniated disc at cervical level are C4-5, C5-6, and C6-7

(3) L4-5 disc is more commonly herniates than L5-S1

(4) The nerve roots involved most commonly in thoracic outlet syndromes are C8 and T1

327. The characteristics of conus medullaris syndrome include

(1) asymmetric paraplegia

(2) symmetric paraplegia

(3) bladder function preservation

(4) upper motor neuron lesion signs

328. Which of the following statement(s) is (are) true for central pain of spinal cord origin?

(1) Most common etiology is of traumatic origin

(2) Most common type of pain in these patients is spontaneous steady, burning, or dysesthetic pain affecting approximately 96% of patients

(3) Bowel and bladder dysfunction can be seen in these patients

(4) Most patients will develop cord central pain within 1 to 6 months of causative lesion although some may present more than 5 years out

329. A positive Froment sign indicates which of the following?

(1) Weakness of first dorsal interosseous

(2) Weakness of flexor pollicis brevis

(3) Weakness of adductor pollicis

(4) Weakness of hypothenar muscles

330. The potential for drug-induced painful neuropathies exist with which of the following agents?

(1) Amiodarone

(2) Metronidazole

(3) Pyridoxine

(4) Vincristine

331. Spinal cord stimulation (SCS) has been used for the treatment of

(1) failed back surgery syndrome

(2) CRPS

(3) angina

(4) peripheral vascular disease

Answers and Explanations

252. **(B)** The piriformis syndrome was originally described by six common characteristics (1) trauma; (2) pain in the muscle with sciatica and difficulty in walking; (3) worsening with squatting or lifting; (4) a sausage-like mass within the muscle; (5) positive Lasègue sign; and (6) gluteal atrophy. The female to male ratio is 6 to 1.

There are many approaches to evaluate piriformis syndrome. One method is in the sitting position which involves the examiner stretching the piriformis muscle by passively moving the hip into internal rotation reproducing buttock pain which is relieved by the examiner passively moving the hip into external rotation. The patient then actively rotates the hip against the resistance which reproduces buttock pain. Furthermore, there is generally point tenderness on palpation of the belly of the piriformis muscle. There tends to be prolongation of the H-reflex with flexion, adduction, and internal rotation.

253. **(E)** In classic weaver's bottom (ischiogluteal bursitis)—the patients invariably get pain sitting which goes away upon standing or lying on their contralateral side. However, the pain promptly returns upon resuming a seated position. Typically, the patient can consistently point to the spot where it hurts with their finger and state "it hurts right here." On physical examination, tenderness is evoked with palpation over the ischiogluteal bursa.

254. **(E)** Imaging studies are most appropriate with bony point tenderness or when the differential diagnosis is likely calcaneal stress, fracture Paget disease, tumors, calcaneal apophysitis (Sever disease in adolescents), or calcaneal stress fracture. The most appropriate diagnostic evaluation for suspected tarsal tunnel syndrome is electrodiagnostic evaluation.

255. **(D)** The tarsal tunnel located behind and inferior to the medial malleolus. It is bounded on the lateral aspect by the tibia and medially by the flexor retinaculum (laciniate ligament). Its contents include the tibial nerve, posterior tibial tendons, flexor digitorum longus tendon, flexor hallucis longus tendon, tibial artery, and tibial vein. Within the tarsal tunnel or immediately distal to it, the tibial nerve divides into the medial and lateral plantar nerves. The calcaneal branch originates variably above or below the flexor retinaculum to supply the heel and calcaneal skin. The tarsal tunnel syndrome most commonly arises from trauma (eg, fractures, ankle dislocations) and is characterized by foot pain and paresthesia, as well as potentially by sensory loss and Tinel sign at the ankle. The pain may be similar to carpal tunnel syndrome in that it often occurs at night. Furthermore, it may be exacerbated by prolonged standing or walking. A march fracture is a stress fracture of the metatarsal bone. The second and third metatarsals are the most common sites. Patients complain of increased intensity of pain with activity or exercise. The pain is localized to the site of the fracture.

256. **(D)** Pronator syndrome may result from compression of the median nerve proximal to the branching of the anterior interosseous nerve. Patients with pronator syndrome generally complain of an aching discomfort of the forearm, numbness in the thumb and index finger, and weakness in the hand. On physical examination there may be tenderness over the proximal part of the pronator teres muscle that is exacerbated by pronation of the forearm against resistance. Resisted pronation may also result in paresthesia in the distribution of the median nerve. A positive Tinel sign is often present at the proximal edge of the pronator muscle. If the entrapment is under the bicipital aponeurosis this may result in weakness of the pronator muscle and depending on the degree of compression, weakness of other muscles (eg, long flexor muscles of the fingers and thumb, abductor pollicis brevis).

257. **(D)** CRPS I and CRPS II are clinically indistinguishable. The only difference is that in CRPS II there is evidence of major nerve damage.

258. **(D)** The temperature range to test warm temperature sensation is 40°C to 45°C—usually done via a glass or metal tube with hot (40°C-45°C) water. Temperatures higher than 45°C are generally perceived as painful.

259. **(C)** The temperature range to test cold temperature sensation is 5°C to 10°C—which may be done with a thermophore. Temperatures lower than 5°C are generally perceived as painful.

260. **(E)** Low levels of vitamin B_{12} and/or folate may be associated with increased trigger points in many patients who suffer from myofascial pain syndrome. Multiple coexisting systemic conditions may also be associated with myofascial pain syndrome and should be investigated in patients with severe painful myofascial trigger points.

261. **(B)** Tietze syndrome (costochondritis) should only be diagnosed after other diagnoses are ruled out. It is most frequently unilateral involving the second and third costal cartilages and is characterized by mild to moderately severe anterior chest wall pain. The pain is typically localized in the region of the costal cartilages but may occasionally radiate to the arm and shoulder. Tietze syndrome occurs more commonly under the age of 40 years. On physical examination, tenderness to palpation

as well as bulbous swelling over the costochondral junctions may be found.

262. **(D)** Spontaneous osteonecrosis of the knee (SONK) is an entity whose precise pathogenesis remains unclear. The pain may be present at rest and is generally well-localized without trauma or associated incited event. It is classically defined as unilateral and spontaneous with predilection for the medial femoral condyle. It occurs typically in the elderly population (> age 60) and is three times more common in women than men. Initial radiographs tend to be normal.

263. **(B)** Meralgia paresthetica is a painful mononeuropathy of the lateral femoral cutaneous nerve (LFCN). Although it may be idiopathic in nature it is commonly caused by focal entrapment of the LFCN as it passes through the inguinal ligament. Although there have been numerous reported associated conditions, some of these include weight change (eg, obesity, pregnancy), possibly external compression (eg, seat belts, tight clothing), perioperative factors/trauma, retroperitoneal tumors, and strenuous walking/cycling (the iliopsoas muscle and tensor fascia lata are heavily involved in walking and/or cycling movement).

264. **(E)** Chronic exertional compartment syndrome of the anterior tibial compartment may occur in runners, soccer players, and racers and may present with a fullness in the anterior compartment, exacerbation of pain on passive dorsiflexion of the great toe, weakness of the extensor hallucis longus muscle, and decreased sensation in the first web space. Symptoms are usually bilateral 75% to 95% of the time.

265. **(C)** Symptoms from an L5-S1 herniated disc are typically experienced in the distribution of the S1 nerve root. These symptoms may include pain or sensory changes in the calf, lateral border of the foot, heel, sole, and sometimes fourth and fifth toes. On physical examination, the patient may have diminished strength in the gastrocnemius, soleus, and the peroneus longus and brevis muscles. An L4-5 herniated disc most frequently results in L5

symptoms, which include diminished sensation in the lateral leg, dorsum of the foot, and the first two toes. Spinal stenosis is narrowing of the spinal canal that occurs with aging. Patients may present with decreased strength and loss of sensation, but with central stenosis it is usually nondermatomal. Piriformis syndrome is an uncommon cause of buttock pain and/or sciatica that is caused by sciatic nerve compression by the piriformis muscle. Although sciatica is often present, pain from piriformis syndrome is nonadicular, and hence straight leg raising tests should not be positive. Discogenic pain is pain that results from internal disc disruption. The neurologic examination should be nonfocal when pain results solely from internal disc derangement.

266. **(E)** As we age, our spinal canal starts to narrow. This narrowing is a result of many different processes including disc bulging from a progressive loss of disc height and elasticity, hypertrophy of the facet joints and ligamentum flavum and osteophyte formation. Technically, the term "spinal stenosis" can refer to central canal stenosis, lateral recess stenosis, or foraminal stenosis. The typical presentation of someone with spinal stenosis is an elderly person with low back and leg pain brought on by walking, especially on stairs or hills. Frequently, the pain is bilateral. In contrast to vascular claudication, patients with neurogenic or pseudoclaudication often find that the cessation of walking brings immediate pain relief. Like spinal stenosis, facet arthropathy is more common in the elderly, but the pain does not typically radiate into the lower leg and is usually not associated with loss of sensation.

267. **(E)** In the early 1990s, a panel of experts reached a consensus that the terms "reflex sympathetic dystrophy" and "causalgia" had lost their utility as clinical diagnoses and suggested a new nomenclature be adopted. The new terms designated for these conditions are "CRPS types I and II". According to the new diagnostic criteria, CRPS need not be maintained by sympathetic mechanisms. A three-phase isotope bone scan is often positive in CRPS, but a normal bone scan does not exclude the diagnosis.

Erythrocyte sedimentation rate is a nonspecific test that is positive in many painful conditions including infection, inflammatory arthritides and inflammatory myopathies. As a syndrome, CRPS is diagnosed by history and physical examination. For CRPS I, the diagnostic criteria include (1) an initiating noxious event; (2) spontaneous pain and/or allodynia occur outside the territory of a single peripheral nerve, and are disproportionate to the inciting event; (3) there is or has been evidence of edema, cutaneous perfusion abnormalities, or abnormal sudomotor activity, in the region of pain since the inciting event; and (4) the diagnosis is excluded by the existence of any condition that would otherwise account for the degree of pain and dysfunction.

268. **(D)** The type and timing of pain after spine surgery provide important clues as to the possible diagnosis. For example, no change in a patient's pain pattern after surgery may indicate that either the wrong surgery was done or the procedure was technically unsuccessful. In this case, the patient experienced initial pain relief, which was followed by worsening back pain and new-onset leg pain several weeks later. Possible causes of this scenario include epidural fibrosis, arachnoiditis, discitis, battered root syndrome with perineural scarring, or an early recurrent disc herniation. Pseudoarthrosis, juxtafusional discogenic pain, and lumbar instability can also be causes of FBSS, but in these cases the recurrence of pain typically occurs much later. For detecting disc pathology, MRI is more sensitive than CT or myelography. It is also more sensitive than CT for identifying contrast enhancement. For the possible etiologies that fit this patient's pain history (ie, arachnoiditis, epidural fibrosis, and discitis), contrast enhancement with gadolinium will greatly enhance the sensitivity of MRI. Epidural mapping via the injection of radiopaque contrast under fluoroscopy through a catheter inserted through the caudal canal is sometimes used to determine the location of epidural scar tissue in FBSS patients, often as a precursor to epidural lysis of adhesions (ie, Racz procedure) or epiduroscopy. However, this procedure provides very little additional information. In the

patient with implanted hardware, foreign ferromagnetic metal objects give rise to local distortion of the magnetic field, which can greatly degrade MRI results. When implants are made of non-superparamagnetic materials like titanium, MRI distortion is less but the anatomy may still be obscured. Since this patient did not have hardware implanted, this should not deter the use of MRI. Generally, T2-weighted images are more sensitive for detecting pathology, whereas T1-weighted images are better for discerning anatomy. The use of MRI to follow a stable, pathologic condition of the lumbar spine is controversial. The use of MRI to evaluate a patient with chronic low back pain who has recently undergone spine surgery and presents with new symptoms is justified.

269. **(E)** Sitting bent forward subjects the lumbar intervertebral discs to greater stress than standing, sitting with one's back straight, or lying down. This helps explain why patients with discogenic low back pain often present with sitting intolerance. Although controversial, discography, with or without CT scanning, is still commonly used to diagnose discogenic pain. Patients at high risk for false-positive discography include those with psychopathology and previous back surgery. The lower lumbar discs are more likely to develop degenerative changes, and hence become pain generators, than more cephalad discs because of the increased load they bear. Recent studies have shown a genetic predisposition for both degenerative disc disease and sciatica. Several prospective studies have been conducted evaluating intradiscal steroids in patients with discogenic low back pain, and none have found them to be efficacious.

270. **(D)** Owing to its high incidence, stroke is the leading cause of central pain in the industrialized world. The chance of developing central pain following spinal cord injury is higher than after stroke (30%-50% vs 8%), but the overall number of stroke patients with central pain is higher. Syringomyelia is the disorder with the highest incidence of central pain (60%-80%). According to neurosurgical studies conducted by V. Cassinari and C.A. Pagni in the 1960s,

injury to spinothalamocortical pathways is necessary but not sufficient to cause central pain. The reason why some patients develop central pain but others with identical injuries do not is unknown. Central pain may occur after neurosurgical procedures and intracranial bleeds, but these are unusual occurrences. There are now several prospective studies showing motor cortex stimulation to be an effective treatment for central pain. There is no typical presentation for central pain. While spontaneous pain is almost universal, allodynia also affects a majority of central pain patients. The time lag between the injury and onset of pain, and the location of central pain are extremely variable.

271. **(E)** MRI is usually the first test used to evaluate new-onset radicular pain. CT scan is less sensitive than MRI for detecting disc pathology, but is used in patients with pacemakers, spinal hardware (owing to the poor resolution of MRI in patients with ferromagnetic metal objects) and when MRI is not available. Selective nerve blocks are sometimes used to diagnose nerve root pathology prior to surgery, but there is little evidence as to whether or not this improves outcomes. Although the terms are sometimes used interchangeably, selective nerve blocks are not the same as transforaminal epidural injections. Since transforaminal epidural injections typically result in injectate spread to contiguous spinal levels, they cannot be considered diagnostic. In addition to providing information about the site of nerve root lesions, EMG/NCS can help determine whether or not the lesion is axonal or demyelinating; whether it is focal, multifocal or diffuse; and the age, severity, and prognosis of the lesion. QST is a subjective test used to evaluate large and small fiber neuronal dysfunction. It may be helpful in clarifying mechanisms of pain, diagnoses, and guiding treatment. It is not used to diagnose nerve root pathology.

272. **(A)** Chronic renal failure is associated with large, myelinated fiber loss that is rarely painful. Celiac disease is a chronic inflammatory enteropathy resulting from sensitivity to gluten. Neurologic complications are estimated

to occur in approximately 10% of patients with peripheral neuropathy and ataxia being the most common. The neuropathy is usually sensory, although infrequently motor weakness may develop. There is some evidence that the neurologic symptoms associated with celiac disease may be ameliorated by a gluten-free diet. Peripheral neuropathies are reported to affect up to 35% of AIDS patients, being more common in later stages of the disease. The most common neuropathy in AIDS patients is a distal sensory polyneuropathy caused by the human immunodeficiency virus (HIV). Other causes of neuropathy in AIDS patients include toxic neuropathies from medications, co-infection with cytomegalovirus (CMV) and other organisms, and vitamin B_{12} deficiency. Fabry disease is an X-linked, lysosomal storage disease that involves the accumulation of galactosylglucosylceramide because of deficiency of α-galactosidase A. It usually presents in adulthood; if symptoms occur in childhood they usually take the form of a painful neuropathy. Amyloidosis may result in a painful peripheral or autonomic neuropathy secondary to deposition of amyloid in nervous tissue. In one study, 35% of patients with amyloidosis were found to have peripheral neuropathy.

273. **(B)** The patient's symptoms are most consistent with Guillain-Barré (GB) acute inflammatory demyelinating polyneuropathy. Patients with GB syndrome generally present with diffuse muscular or radicular pain followed by sensorimotor dysfunction. Most, but not all (72%) patients with GB syndrome experience pain during the course of their illness. GB syndrome affects 1 to 1.5 people per 100,000 and shows no age or gender preference. About 60% to 70% of cases are preceded by an URI or gastrointestinal (GI) illness 1 to 3 weeks before symptoms begin. Cerebrospinal fluid (CSF) analysis reveals normal pressures, increased protein and no cells. The pathology of GB syndrome is demyelination, with most patients fully recovering. Multiple sclerosis is a demyelinating disease that typically presents in early adult life. The most common presenting symptom of multiple sclerosis is ocular complaints, which affects most patients at some time during the course of their illness. Spinal cord lesions can produce a myriad of sensorimotor problems including weakness, spasticity, hyperreflexia, bladder dysfunction, sensory loss, and diminished temperature sensation and proprioception. Central dysesthetic pain affects approximately 20% of multiple sclerosis patients. The diagnosis of multiple sclerosis is usually supported by MRI, with or without CSF analysis. Although muscle pain and weakness may be present in chronic fatigue syndrome (CFS), the hallmark of this disorder is disabling physical and mental fatigue present for more than 6 months. There is no firm data causally linking viral infection to CFS despite frequent reported associations. The most common presentation of acute radiculopathy is pain or sensory changes in a lower extremity. The most common form of diabetic neuropathy is distal, symmetrical polyneuropathy. It is predominantly a sensory disturbance, occurring in a stocking-glove distribution. Because the feet are innervated by the longest nerves in the body, they are usually the first part of the body to be affected. Other types of neuropathy that may be present in diabetics include lower extremity proximal motor neuropathy, truncal neuropathy, cranial mononeuropathy, and autonomic neuropathy. The cause of diabetic neuropathy is most likely related to metabolic and ischemic nerve injury.

274. **(A)** The SI joints are large, paired, diarthrodial synovial joints whose primary functions are stability and dissipating truncal loads. The joints are also involved in limiting *x*-axis rotation and in women, parturition. There are literally dozens of provocative tests that have been advocated as screening tools for SI joint pain, but several studies have shown that these tests lack both specificity and high sensitivity. On a similar note, CT scanning may show SI joint pathology in over 30% of asymptomatic control patients, and be negative in over 40% of patients with SI pain. The most reliable method for diagnosing SI joint pain is through diagnostic local anesthetic blocks. The mechanism of SI joint injury has been described as a combination of axial loading and sudden rotation. Common causes of SI joint pain include motor

vehicle accidents, falls, athletic injuries, spondyloarthropathies, and pregnancy. SI joint injections with corticosteroids have been shown in some but not all studies to provide short-term pain relief. SI joint pain is usually not amenable to surgical correction.

275.   **(B)** In population-based studies, migraine without aura is about twice as frequent as migraine with aura. Major criteria for the diagnosis of cervicogenic headache include signs and symptoms of neck involvement such as the precipitation of head pain by neck movement or external pressure over the upper cervical or occipital region, restricted range of motion in the neck, unilaterality of head pain with or without shoulder or arm pain, and confirmatory evidence by diagnostic anesthetic blocks. Chronic tension-type headache differs from episodic tension-type headache in that the average headache frequency is equal to or greater than 15 days per month or 180 days per year. A shift from peripheral to central mechanisms is believed to play a role in the evolution of episodic to chronic tension-type headache. Cluster headaches typically present as a series of intense unilateral headaches occurring over a period of 2 weeks to 3 months. They are associated with unilateral autonomic features such as nasal congestion, rhinorrhea, miosis, or lacrimation. The attacks are usually brief, lasting between 15 and 180 minutes, and occur in the orbital, supraorbital and/or temporal regions. Unlike migraine headaches, tension-type headaches, temporal arteritis, and cervicogenic headaches, cluster headaches are more frequent in men, with an average male to female ratio of 5 to 1. Tricyclic antidepressants have been shown in numerous clinical trials to be effective in the prevention of both migraine and tension-type headaches.

276.   **(D)** Phantom breast pain occurs in roughly 20% of mastectomy patients, and phantom sensations in close to half. Originally thought to be rare, phantom limb pain is now recognized to occur in between 60% and 80% of limb amputees. Phantom limb pain must be distinguished from phantom sensations, which occur in over 90% of patients. Vascular conditions account for over 80% of limb amputations in the United States. However, trauma is responsible for approximately 75% of upper extremity amputations. Most researchers have found a statistically significant association between phantom limb pain and persistent stump pain. Although earlier studies found a correlation between preamputation pain and phantom limb pain, more recent studies have not confirmed this relationship. It is widely held that phantom pain diminishes with time and eventually fades away. Though described, phantom pain associated with congenital absence of a limb is rare. Phantom pain is generally worse in the distal part of a limb. Most phantoms shrink with time, with the most distal aspect of a limb being the last to disappear. This is known as "telescoping," and occurs in approximately half of all limb amputees. Archaeological records demonstrate that purposeful amputations have been practiced since Neolithic times. The concept of "phantom pain" has been recognized for hundreds, if not thousands, of years. In the 16th century, the French military surgeon Ambrose Paré outlined clear distinctions between phantom limb pain, phantom sensation, and stump pain. The term "phantom pain" was coined by Weir Mitchell in the American Civil War. A few years earlier, Mitchell used the word "causalgia" to describe the characteristic autonomic changes found in the extremities of soldiers who suffered major nerve damage.

277.   **(A)** Palmar sweating and reduced transcutaneous oxygen concentration are indicative of, though not specific for, acute pain. In a young child, crying and increased vital signs (eg. heart rate, respiratory rate, and blood pressure) are associated with distress, which includes but is not limited to pain. Other factors that may cause these signs include separation anxiety, hunger, and fear. Unlike acute pain, chronic pain is usually not associated with elevated vital signs. The FACES scale and Charleston Pain Pictures are designed to provide assessments of pain in school aged, not preschool children. The FACS and COMFORT scale are used to assess pain in infants and young children. The FACS is a comprehensive coding

system based on a wide range of facial actions. The COMFORT scale is an eight-item scale designed to measure distress (including pain) that includes alertness, calmness, respiratory response, physical movement, blood pressure, muscle tone, and facial tension. Pain scales used in adults such as verbal pain scores, numerical rating scales, and visual analogue scales provide accurate assessments of pain in most adolescents.

278. **(B)** The most common way to diagnose AHZ is clinically. In a small percentage of patients, AHZ may occur without a rash, a condition known as "zoster sine herpete" (zoster without rash). The PCR is often used to aid in the diagnosis of this condition. In descending order, the most common sites for AHZ are the midthoracic dermatomes, the ophthalmic division of the trigeminal nerve, and the cervical region. The incidence of both AHZ and postherpetic neuralgia increases with age. Other risk factors for AHZ include HIV infection and transplant surgery, which is likely because of the resultant immunosuppression. There is no standard time period after which persistent pain from AHZ is diagnoses as postherpetic neuralgia. Postherpetic neuralgia has been variably defined as the persistence of sensory symptoms 1 month, 6 weeks, 2 months, 3 months, and 6 months after herpes zoster. AHZ affects the lumbosacral dermatomes in between 5% and 15% of patients. Lumbosacral AHZ may be misdiagnosed as a herniated disc.

279. **(B)** EMG provides a wealth of information about the integrity, function, and innervation of motor units and (using special techniques) individual muscle fibers. Serial EMG examinations permit monitoring of recovery or disease progression. A normal EMG indicates the absence of motor unit involvement. In neuropathies characterized by Wallerian degeneration, nerve conduction velocities range from low normal to mildly slow. In contrast, demyelinating neuropathies of the acute and chronic inflammatory types produce segmental demyelination, which markedly slows conduction velocities. The H wave is the electrical representation of the tendon reflex circuit. In adults, it is only obtainable

in the lower reflexes. It is most prominent during stimulation of the tibial nerve, being particularly helpful in the diagnosis of S1 radiculopathy and predominantly sensory polyneuropathies. The F wave is a late response that is evoked by supramaximal stimulation of a motor nerve. It occurs when a small percentage of the stimulated motor neurons "rebound." The initial response to stimulation of a motor nerve is the M wave. Unlike H waves, F waves are not true reflexes.

280. **(C)** Large, myelinated nerves are more vulnerable to injury than small neurons. The function of large, myelinated A-β function can be measured using both vibratory thresholds and von Frey filaments. QST is used to evaluate the function of individual nerve fibers. It is not useful in determining which nerve is injured and where along its path the injury lies. Both cold and hot thermal sensations are used to measure the function of small myelinated (A-δ) and unmyelinated C fibers. QST cannot be used to assess B (preganglionic autonomic) and A-γ (muscle spindle efferent) function. A downside of QST is that its accuracy is dependent on the cooperation and reliability of the patient.

281. **(C)** Lumbar radiculopathy most often results from disc herniation. Depending on the level of herniated discs radiculopathy may affect specific nerve roots. Disc herniation at L4-5 and L5-S1 is most likely caused by mobility of the segment. A herniated disc may compromise the nerve root at the same level if displaced laterally in the recess or in the foramen (L4-5 disc affecting L4 nerve root), or it may effect the traversing nerve root to the level below (L4-5 disc affecting L5 nerve root). L5 radiculopathy results in pain, sensory, and motor changes in L5 dermatomal distribution. Pain is usually described as shooting or occasionally aching and burning sensation on the outside of leg radiating to the dorsum of foot. Sensory testing may also reveal a decrease in light-touch and pinprick sensation in the same distribution. L5 radiculopathy also may result in weakness in the extensor hallucis longus and thus heel walking. Deep tendon reflexes may be spared in the lower extremity.

282. **(A)** Fibromyalgia syndrome is a common pain condition, estimated to occur in 2.4% of the general population. The syndrome is characterized by widespread musculoskeletal pain, sleep disturbance, psychologic distress, and comorbidity with other pain syndromes [eg, irritable bowel syndrome (IBS), interstitial cystitis, and the female urethral syndrome], which have considerable impact on the everyday life of patients. Fibromyalgia syndrome occurs predominantly in women and demonstrates familial aggregation. Since 1990, the diagnosis of fibromyalgia syndrome has been based on criteria of the American College of Rheumatology (ACR). A key dimension of the ACR criteria is the concept of tender points, 18 specific points on the body surface at which digital palpation elicits pain (11/18 "positive" tender points fulfills an fibromyalgia criteria).

It is not uncommon for patients to have other pain pathologies in addition to fibromyalgia. However a complete clinical picture should be viewed before consideration of treatment options especially if it involves interventional procedures. Patient describes above most likely has fibromyalgia as evidenced by the presence of tender points. A negative physical examination except for tender points and hypersensitivity argues against other listed options.

283. **(A)** Following is the diagnostic criteria for CRPS I:

1. The presence of an initiating noxious event or a cause of immobilization.
2. Continuing pain, allodynia, or hyperalgesia with which the pain is disproportionate to any inciting event.
3. Evidence at some time of edema, changes in skin blood flow, or abnormal sudomotor activity in the region of the pain.
4. This diagnosis is excluded by the existence of condition that otherwise would account for the degree of pain and dysfunction.

The patient in the question meets all the criteria for diagnosis of CRPS I (RSD). CRPS II (causalgia) by definition has a known injury to a major nerve. Vascular etiology though possible after trauma, is unlikely to give symptoms of allodynia as well as sudomotor changes. Median neuralgia would result in a similar clinical pain picture but only hand discomfort would be expected to be confined only to the distribution of median nerve.

284. **(C)** Spinal cord injury may result in various types of pain. To provide the most effective treatment—understanding the mechanism of pain is very important. Taxonomy of spinal cord injury pain may be divided into neuropathic or nociceptive pain. The patient in question appears to have most likely nerve root impingement at T4-5, level of his spinal cord injury, resulting in severe T4 neuralgic pain radiating towards the front of chest wall.

285. **(B)** Myofascial pain may result after a sudden acceleration-deceleration insult. Neck muscles may reflexly go into spasm. It may also result in straightening of cervical lordosis secondary to spasm of posterior supporting neck muscles. Myofascial pain from cervical neck muscle may radiate between shoulder blades as well into the upper extremity. Negative imaging studies are essential to rule out traumatic disc herniation or fracture. Treatment includes nonsteroidals, muscle relaxants, and physical therapy. In a small percentage of patients, if pain doesn't resolve trigger point injections or cervical medial branch blocks may provide help with continuing physical therapy.

286. **(C)** In type 1 diabetes mellitus, distal polyneuropathy typically occurs after many years of chronic prolonged hyperglycemia. Conversely, in type 2, it may present after only a few years of poor glycemic control. Occasionally, in type 2, diabetic neuropathy is found at the time of diagnosis (or even predating diagnosis).

Diabetic neuropathy can manifest with a wide variety of sensory, motor, and autonomic symptoms. Sensory symptoms may be negative or positive, diffuse or focal. Negative sensory symptoms include numbness; "deadness"; feeling of wearing gloves or walking on stilts; loss of balance, especially with the eyes closed; and painless injuries. Positive symptoms include burning, pricking pain, electric shocklike feelings, tightness, and hypersensitivity to touch.

Motor symptoms can cause distal, proximal, or focal weakness. Autonomic symptoms may be sudomotor, pupillary, cardiovascular, urinary, GI, and sexual.

A generally accepted classification of diabetic neuropathies divides them broadly into symmetric and asymmetric neuropathies. Symmetric polyneuropathies involve multiple nerves diffusely and symmetrically and are the most common form. The patient in question appears to have symmetrical small and large fiber neuropathy resulting in pain in both legs and feet, and decreased light-touch sensation as well as allodynia.

287. **(C)** Glossopharyngeal neuralgia is a disorder characterized by intense pain in the tonsils, middle ear, and back of the tongue. The pain can be intermittent or relatively persistent. Swallowing, chewing, talking, sneezing, or eating spicy foods may trigger the disorder. It is often the result of compression of the 9th nerve (glossopharyngeal) or 10th nerve (vagus), but in some cases, no cause is evident.

Skull base surgery or surgeries in the infratemporal region may result in damage or irritation of glossopharyngeal nerve. Conservative treatment includes using anticonvulsants. In refractory cases glossopharyngeal nerve block may be helpful. Radiofrequency lesioning or neurolytic treatment should be reserved for resistant cases or ones associated with head and neck cancer. Surgical decompression should be reserved for nonresponders and resistant cases.

288. **(D)** Lumbar radiculopathy most often results from disc herniation. Depending on the level and "direction" of herniated discs a resultant radiculopathy may affect specific nerve roots. Disc herniation at L5-S1 is most likely a result of mobility of the segment. A herniated disc may compromise the nerve root at the same level if displaced laterally in the recess or in the foramen (L5-S1 disc affecting L5 nerve root), or it may affect the traversing nerve root to the level below (L5-S1 disc affecting S1 nerve root). S1 radiculopathy results in pain, sensory, and motor changes in S1 dermatomal distribution. Pain is usually described as shooting or occasionally as an aching and burning sensation on the back of thigh radiating to the plantar aspect (sole) of foot. Sensory testing may also reveal a decrease in light-touch and pinprick sensation in the same distribution. S1 radiculopathy also may result in weakness in Plantar flexion and thus toe walking. Most often with significant S1 nerve root compression, ankle reflex is diminished. Examination also may reveal positive straight leg raise and cross straight leg raise test (reproduction of radiating pain in lower extremity by raising the opposite extremity).

289. **(C)** The spinal cord is organized into a series of tracts or neuropathways that carry motor (descending) and sensory (ascending) information. These tracts are organized anatomically within the spinal cord. The corticospinal tracts are descending motor pathways located anteriorly within the spinal cord. Axons extend from the cerebral cortex in the brain as far as the corresponding segment, where they form synapses with motor neurons in the anterior (ventral) horn. They decussate (cross over) in the medulla prior to entering the spinal cord.

The dorsal columns are ascending sensory tracts that transmit light-touch, proprioception, and vibration information to the sensory cortex. They do not decussate until they reach the medulla. The lateral spinothalamic tracts transmit pain and temperature sensation. These tracts usually decussate within three segments of their origin as they ascend. The anterior spinothalamic tract transmits light touch. Autonomic function traverses within the anterior anteromedial tract. Sympathetic nervous system fibers exit the spinal cord between C7 and L1, while parasympathetic system pathways exit between S2 and S4.

Injury to the corticospinal tract or dorsal columns, respectively, results in ipsilateral paralysis or loss of sensation of light touch, proprioception, and vibration. Unlike injuries of the other tracts, injury to the lateral spinothalamic tract causes contralateral loss of pain and temperature sensation two to three segments below the level of injury. Because the anterior spinothalamic tract also transmits light-touch information, injury to the dorsal columns may result in complete loss of vibration sensation and proprioception but only partial loss of light-touch sensation. Anterior cord injury causes paralysis and incomplete loss of light-touch sensation.

290. **(B)** Patients with a C6 radiculopathy should have pain in the neck, shoulder, lateral arm, radial forearm, dorsum of hand, and tips of thumb, index, and long finger. Distribution of pain is less extensive and more proximal, whereas paresthesias predominate distally. In some individuals, a C6 lesion will manifest as a depressed or absent biceps reflex; in others, an abnormal brachioradialis or wrist extensor reflex can be found. Elbow flexion will be weak, and the patient will be unable to supinate the forearm against resistance with the elbow held in extension. Conservative treatment includes physical therapy, traction, and analgesics. If pain persists, cervical epidural steroid injection may provide relief from pain and aid in physical therapy. However, if symptoms persist or weakness/numbness doesn't improve surgical decompression with or without anterior fusion may be considered.

291. **(B)** Celiac plexus block is both a diagnostic and therapeutic tool to help in managing upper abdominal pain arising from viscera. Pancreatic cancer is the leading diagnosis for neurolytic celiac plexus block; other conditions may include visceral pain arising from malignancies of liver or GI tract.

      The procedure is performed either under fluoroscopic guidance or CT scan, though blind approaches have also been described. Both single transaortic as well bilateral needle approaches have been described. The fluoroscopic image in question demonstrates a single needle transaortic celiac plexus block. Complications include diarrhea, hypotension, genitofemoral neuralgia, infection, bleeding, damage to surrounding structures and rarely paralysis. All complications mentioned above may occur except hypertension.

292. **(A)** A proper diagnostic test requires a preblock patient evaluation (with special attention to the ipsilateral lower extremity pain, temperature,

and condition), a local anesthetic injection using appropriate volume to avoid spread to adjacent nerves and a postblock evaluation of subjective improvement in pain score as well an objective increase in the temperature of the involved extremity is crucial. Significant improvement in pain scores with increase in temperature of the involved extremity points toward a positive diagnosis of sympathetically mediated pain.

      Discography is performed for diagnosis of lumbar discogenic pain. Whereas diabetic neuropathy may result in sympathetically mediated pain, it is a mixed somatic polyneuropathy and diagnosis is a clinical one. Lumbar selective nerve root block and facet joint injections may aid in the diagnosis of lumbar radiculopathy and facet arthritis resulting in pain.

293. **(C)** Cervical selective nerve root injection may be indicated for diagnosis and treatment of cervical radiculopathy. Complication other than infection, bleeding, and nerve damage, include intravascular uptake into vertebral artery or radicular arteries resulting in seizure, stroke, or paraplegia. Intraspinal spread into epidural or intrathecal spread is also possible resulting in high spinal anesthetic. Damage to spinal cord has also been reported with injection into the spinal cord. Considering the life-threatening complications, cervical selective nerve root block should only be performed by physicians well versed in this technique.

294. **(A)** Medial branches of the dorsal ramus provide innervations to the respective facet joint as well to the joint below. A diagnostic medial branch block with local anesthetic performed at appropriate levels (eg, L3 and L4 for L4-5 facet joint) may provide diagnostic and prognostic information to help with pain associated with facet arthritis.

      If pain is considerably albeit transiently improved after diagnostic medial branch blocks, a radiofrequency ablative procedure may be considered to provide longer lasting pain relief.

295. **(B)** SI joint injection is performed for both diagnostic and therapeutic reasons in patient complaining of SI joint pain. After a therapeutic

injection with 5 to 10 mL of local anesthetic; it is possible that the local anesthetic may spill inferiorly and anteriorly and anesthetize sciatic nerve resulting in leg weakness. Patients may be warned about this, if observed afterward, and should be accompanied by a reasonable adult to avoid any falls and resultant injuries.

296. **(E)** Vertebroplasty is an advanced procedure that is performed to stabilize recently fractured vertebral bodies resulting in excruciating back pain. Performed properly and by trained physicians, vertebroplasty is a safe procedure. However, complications, though rare, are possible and uncompromising. These may include infection; bleeding; pulmonary embolus; damage to pedicles, spinal cord, or surrounding structures; allergic reactions to injectate; and cement leak into soft tissue or in spinal canal resulting in spinal cord compression.

297. **(A)** Spinal stenosis may result from narrowing of the spinal canal secondary to hypertrophy of ligamentum flavum, articular processes and anteriorly from degenerative bulging discs. Stenosis may result in a classical presentation of neurogenic claudication with pain in lower legs or feelings of "charley horse" that come with walking an unpredictable distance and is relieved by resting or sitting down. In contrast to vascular claudication, the patient may report some back pain as well. In addition, pain is not predictably elicited after a certain walking distance because it is relative extension of the lumbar segments that results in worsening stenosis and neurogenic claudication rather than ischemia. Pain is relieved in neurogenic claudication by assuming a flexion posture (bending forward).

Treatment includes posture education, education and improvement of body mechanics, and physical therapy. Epidural steroid injection series may provide pain relief in some patients. If pain or significant limitation in activity persists a decompressive laminectomy may be considered.

298. **(B)** The piriformis is a sausage-shaped muscle which originates from the anterior surface of the lateral sacrum and attaches to the greater trochanter. In most individuals the sciatic nerve lies anterior to the muscle belly. Spasm of the muscle may result in irritation of the sciatic nerve and resultant sciatica. The patient may report localized tenderness in the lower part of the buttock. In addition, if patients have irritation of sciatic nerve, they may also report symptoms suggestive of sciatica which may easily be confused with lumbar radiculopathy. However, flexion, adduction, and internal rotation of the thigh results in tightening of piriformis muscle which may reproduce pain symptoms. MRI should be carefully evaluated to rule out any radicular component.

Treatments include muscle relaxants and physical therapy to break muscle spasm. If pain persists or if the patient is unable to continue with physical therapy, piriformis muscle injection may aid in treatment.

299. **(C)** There can be physical and psychologic symptoms of malingering and factitious disorder. In these conditions the patient willfully produces or feigns symptoms of illness or injury. In the factitious disorder the goal of the behavior is the patient's need to be in sick role—a need not understood by the patient. Placing blood into urine and pretending to have posttraumatic stress disorder are examples. There is no apparent external goal such as to obtain money or drugs. It is always a psychiatric illness. This contrast with malingering, in which there is a clearly defined external goal. Malingering is not a psychiatric illness.

Diagnosis of hypochondriasis require at least 6 month of preoccupation with the fear or belief that one has a serious disease, based on the interpretation of physical signs or sensations as evidence of illness. Somatization disorder is characterized by an extensive history of multiple somatic symptoms that are psychologic in nature. In addition to many physical complaints or a belief that one is sickly, the criteria require at least 13 symptoms from a list of 41. The symptom list includes 6 GI symptoms, 7 pain symptoms, 4 cardiopulmonary symptoms, 12 conversion/pseudoneurologic symptoms, 4 sexual symptoms, and 4 female reproductive symptoms. Conversion disorders are patients presenting with physical symptoms without any anatomic or pathophysiologic basis (pseudoneurologic symptoms; pseudoparalysis, pseudoseizure etc).

300. **(A)** Ilioinguinal neuralgia may develop after any surgery in inguinal area resulting in damage to the ilioinguinal nerve. Pain may start immediately after the surgery or may start after a reasonable period of healing has passed. Wound infection, recurrent hernia, and mesh infection should be ruled out to avoid any correctable causes of ilioinguinal pain. Pain is usually described as sharp, electrical sensation or sometimes as constant burning sensations in the groin area with occasional radiation into the testicles. Pain is exacerbated by light touch or rubbing of clothes. Treatment includes anticonvulsants and other adjuvant medications. If pain persists, local anesthetic diagnostic and therapeutic block as well as other treatment approaches may be warranted. Radiofrequency ablation, peripheral nerve stimulation, neurectomy, and repeat surgery should be reserved for resistant cases.

301. **(A)**

A. Hypotension from sympathetic blockade is the most common complication. It is important to optimally prehydrate these patients prior to the onset of the block.

B. Seizure results from intravascular injection of large volume of local anesthetic stressing the need to confirm negative aspiration prior to injecting the solution.

C. Diarrhea ensues as a result of sympathetic blockade and unopposed parasympathetic tone.

D. Retroperitoneal hematoma is a rare complication of celiac plexus block.

E. Subarachnoid injection is the most serious and very rare complication celiac block.

302. **(D)**

A. Increase in the intrathecal morphine dose is warranted in some situations when a patient demonstrates signs and symptoms consistent with withdrawal or has inadequate analgesia. In that case it is important to carefully evaluate the equianalgesic dose accounting for change in route or incomplete cross tolerance with change of drugs. In this case, considering the oral to intrathecal conversion is 300 to 1, the patient has been escalated to 10 mg of intrathecal morphine a day; it seems unlikely that his symptoms would be because of opioid withdrawal provided his catheter is in the correct position as had been confirmed under fluoroscopy in this case.

B. CT scan can be done to confirm the correct placement of the catheter if necessary; however it is highly unlikely that the catheter would move in a short time in a sedentary postsurgical patient.

C. Removal of catheter followed by reimplantation is a possibility if indeed catheter is determined to be malpositioned. It seems rather premature to pursue such option at this time.

D. Urine toxicology seems like a more viable option considering this patient's association with a half way home and the time of onset of his symptoms approximately 12 hours after the hospitalization. Also, the symptoms experienced although nonspecific, point toward possible withdrawal from a substance of abuse. It is reasonable to order a urine/serum toxicology screen as an initial step at this point while instituting conservative treatment with nonopioid analgesics and antinausea preparations.

E. Spine surgeon consultation does not seem necessary at this point since the symptoms experienced are not truly suggestive of spinal hematoma, infection, or neurologic deficits warranting acute surgical intervention.

303. **(B)** The mechanism by which ovarian hormones influence migraines remain to be determined, but an abrupt decrease in serum estrogen concentrations before the onset of an attack appears to be a critical factor. Sometimes the use of percutaneous estrogen gel applied just before and through the menstrual cycle may reduce the frequency of headaches. However, in some other cases use of low-dose estrogen oral contraceptive formulation are

associated with a haphazard occurrence of attacks during the cycle, probably because of fluctuating estrogen levels. Therefore, it seems prudent to have the treatment strategies aimed toward preventing either a decrease or substantial fluctuation in the levels of estrogen.

304. (A)

A. Considering the acute onset of bladder dysfunction and neurologic deficits on physical examination along with the anterolisthesis of L5 on S1, urgent evaluation by a spine surgeon seems to be the best immediate option of all. This patient needs further workup and possibly even urgent intervention by the spine surgeon at this time.

B. While intravenous opioids can be used to control acute pain, they by no means should be considered adequate in managing this situation that demands urgent surgical attention.

C. Physical therapy may be considered in future for this patient for physical rehabilitation once surgical evaluation and/or intervention has been completed. Physical therapy for acute pain management is inappropriate for this case considering the risk of neurologic deficits that may ensue from further movement of an unstable spine.

D. This condition could be a surgical emergency and so this patient should be actively managed in an in-patient setting.

E. Oral steroids may sometimes be beneficial in such setting to decrease the pain and inflammation associated with acute spine pain, but the surgical evaluation should take precedence over all conservative treatment options that may delay resolution of the spinal pathology.

305. (E) Celiac plexus or ganglia, these terms often used interchangeably, are a dense network of pre- and postganglionic fibers. The three splanchnic nerves; greater, lesser, and least synapse at the celiac ganglia.

A. Retrocrural approach is the most commonly utilized by anesthesiologists and considered the most traditional. The landmarks include iliac crests, 12th rib, dorsal midline, vertebral bodies (T12-L2), and lateral border of the paraspinal (sacrospinalis) muscles.

B. Transcrural approach involves placement of needle tips anterior and caudal to the diaphragmatic crura. Advocates of this approach believe that this approach maximizes spread of injected solutions anterior to the aorta where the celiac plexus is most concentrated and this minimizes the somatic nerve block.

C. Transaortic approach to celiac plexus has been described under both fluoroscopic and CT guidance. It is considered safe by many because of the use of single fine needle compared to two-needle posterior approach. This approach has three distinct advantages over the classic two-needle approach. First, it avoids the risk of neurologic complications related to posterior retrocrural spread of drugs. Secondly, the aorta provides a definitive landmark for needle placement when radiographic guidance is not available and thirdly, much smaller volumes of local anesthetic and neurolytic solutions are required to achieve efficacy equal to or greater than that of classic retrocrural approach.

D. Intercrural approach is a term that can technically be applied to transaortic approach since the needle tips are placed in front of the diaphragmatic crura in this approach, but more commonly this term is used to refer to the classic anterior approach to celiac plexus under CT or ultrasound guidance.

E. Lateral approach has not been described in literature.

306. (A)

A. The trial of oral opioids, steroids, and urgent consultation with a spine surgeon are the most appropriate initial steps in management of what seems to be a case of acute radiculopathy secondary to acute disc herniation. Because these substantial neurologic deficits may be reversed with appropriate and timely decompression, the surgical evaluation and course of steroids are top priorities here.

B. Cervical epidural steroid injections can be considered to decrease the inflammation, but does not qualify to be "most appropriate initial treatment."

C. Physical therapy can be instituted further down the road for rehabilitation.

D. SCS may be beneficial to decrease neuropathic pain of chronic nature, but it has no role in an acute setting of this nature.

E. Pain psychologist can prove to be very useful in patients suffering from chronic pain, but again has little role in acute pain management in this setting.

307. (A) Hoffmann sign is indicative of UMNL. In fact, it is the upper extremity equivalent of Babinski reflex. The examiner holds the patient's middle finger and briskly flicks the distal phalanx. A positive sign is noted if the interphalageal joint of thumb of the same hand flexes.

308. (D)

A. Plantar fascitis is an inflammation of the tendons and the fascia of the foot as they insert into the calcaneal periosteum. It is typically seen in the people who stand on hardwood floors for a prolonged period of time. Pain is elicited with plantar compression over the anterior calcaneus and also may radiate along plantar fascia.

B. Metatarsalgia is characterized by pain in the plantar surface of the metatarsal heads caused by prolonged weight-bearing. It can also be replicated with manual compression over the metatarsal heads. Pain is most commonly increased in combined pronation and eversion.

C. The etiology and diagnosis of tarsal tunnel syndrome is somewhat controversial. This syndrome involves compression or inflammation of the posterior tibial nerve that provides sensory innervation to medial aspect of the calcaneus, motor supply to small lateral musculature of the foot and to the medial and lateral plantar branches. The symptoms are usually vague with activity related problems. Pain along with

paresthesia, cramping, and burning is seen in the distribution. Palpation reveals sensitivity in the area. EMG testing can be utilized in diagnosis of tarsal tunnel syndrome but is controversial.

D. Morton neuroma (interdigital neuroma) is the compression of the interdigital nerves in between the metatarsal heads and deep transverse metatarsal ligaments. The third interspace between third and fourth metatarsal is most frequently involved, it is believed to be so because lateral plantar nerve sends a branch to the medial plantar nerve to form a larger third common digital nerve making it less mobile. The condition is usually unilateral and affects females more commonly than men, usually in their 50s. The most common symptom is plantar pain that is increased by walking or by palpation between the third and fourth metatarsal heads.

E. Painful calcaneal spur is often seen in morbidly obese people or those who stand or walk excessively. Pain is increased in the morning or after a prolonged rest and similar to plantar fascitis except that it is more predominant in the posterior aspect of the plantar calcaneus.

309. (A) Interscalene block of brachial plexus is especially effective for surgery of the shoulder or upper arm, as the roots of the brachial plexus are most easily blocked with this technique. Ulnar nerve is most frequently spared since it is derived from the eighth cervical nerve and the block is placed at a more cephalic site with this approach. This block is ideal for reduction of a dislocated shoulder or any other type of surgery on shoulder or upper arm.

310. (D)

A. A baker (popliteal) cyst represents ballooning of the synovium-lined joint capsule, usually on the posteromedial aspect of the knee. It is usually a secondary manifestation of underlying condition that causes chronic inflammation of the knee, such as meniscal tear, knee synovitis or intra-articular loose body. The diagnosis of the popliteal cyst can be made by direct palpation of the mass. Arthrography or an MRI can verify the diagnosis and demonstrate its communication with the joint cavity. The cyst usually resolves with correction of the underlying pathology.

B. Anterior cruciate ligament is the most commonly injured knee ligament in athletes. Injury to this ligament will result in a bloody knee effusion that is very indicative of this particular kind of injury. Three tests used to diagnose anterior cruciate ligament injury are anterior drawer test, Lachman test, and pivot shift test.

C. Posterior cruciate ligament is usually damaged in violent, usually high–kinetic energy injuries. These usually occur in combination with fractures, specifically to the patella and hip or with other knee ligament injuries. Injury to popliteal artery should be evaluated in this injury with palpation or even arteriography. The test used to diagnose posterior cruciate ligament injury is posterior drawer test.

D. In stance more than 60% of the body's weight is carried on the peripheral aspect of the tibial plateau by meniscal fibrocartilages. In younger persons, the meniscal injuries usually accompany other ligament injuries whereas in elderly, these usually occur in isolation. When a meniscal tear is extensive it can result in block to terminal knee flexion or extension, commonly described by patients as "locking of the knee". A torn meniscus can cause knee swelling and pain as it irritates the joint surface or synovium. Chronic meniscal injuries can result in arthritic joint surface. Joint line tenderness is found in about 50% of these injuries. McMurray test is used to detect tear of the meniscus that can be displaced. It is performed by flexing and extending the knee between 90° and 140° of flexion. One of the examiner's hands rotates the tibia at the ankle while the other hand is placed in front of the joint line. This is followed by the extension of knee in the rotated position. A palpable click indicates an unstable tear of the meniscus. The Apley grind test can help

distinguish between tear in the anterior or posterior portion of the meniscus. MRI or arthroscopy can also be used as diagnostic tools to identify a meniscal lesion.

E. Pes anserine bursa lies between the medial hamstring tendons (sartorius, gracilis, and semitendinosus) and proximal medial tibia. It is inferior to the joint line which helps distinguish from the medial joint line tenderness secondary to meniscal injury.

311. (E)

A. Brachial plexitis is an acute disorder of that almost always begins with unilateral diffuse pain in the shoulder followed by weakness in the proximal muscles. Sensory disturbances are less pronounced than motor deficits. The pain usually subsides after the acute phase. Electrodiagnostic studies can help to establish the diagnosis.

B. Cervical degenerative disc disease can result in diffuse axial pain in the neck or radicular pain along a particular dermatome corresponding to the nerve root involved if associated with a herniated nucleus pulposus.

C. Whiplash injury typically follows a high-impact motor vehicle accident that results in axial neck pain. It has a musculoskeletal component to it and is frequently associated with facet joint involvement.

D. Pancoast tumor is the tumor of the apex of the lung that typically involves the brachial plexus. Pain is a common presenting symptom usually involving the lower cervical nerve roots or trunks. CT scan or MRI can sometimes offer valuable diagnostic information.

E. Thoracic outlet syndrome usually involves impingement of subclavian vessels and lower trunk of brachial plexus resulting in various degrees of vascular or neurologic compromise or both with local supraclavicular pain. The most common etiologies are cervical rib, hypertrophy of scalenus anticus, costoclavicular abnormalities, but nevertheless can result from an acute trauma. The pain and sensory changes are usually aggravated by any activity that extends the brachial plexus, including carrying heavy objects, abducting arms over the head or with repetitive movements of the arm. Motor weakness is seen in intrinsic muscles of the hand. The obliteration of radial pulse with arm extension or abduction or traction can be present and is called Adson or Allen test.

312. **(C)**

   A. H wave responses, in adults can be obtained in lower extremities. H wave response is an electric equivalent of the ankle deep tendon reflex, when the tibial nerve is stimulated.

   B. The tibial nerve behind the knee in the popliteal fossa is stimulated and the impulse travels via afferent fibers to the spinal cord at the S1 level. After synapse in the cord, anterior horn cells produce a motor response that can be recorded in gastrocnemius and soleus muscles.

   C. H waves are true reflexes, F wave is not. Because the H wave has to travel to the level of cord in order to produce a response, the latency is longer compared to F wave.

   D. This is correct as explained in (B).

   E. Since the impulses are conducted through S1 nerve, H reflex is typically prolonged in S1 radiculopathy but may be normal in L5 radiculopathy.

313. **(B)** The spinal cord receives its blood supply from three longitudinal arteries: a single anterior spinal artery and two posterior spinal arteries. The diameter of anterior spinal artery is greatest at the cervical and lower thoracic levels and narrowest at the midthoracic levels from T3-T9. This region of the cord is considered to be the "vulnerable zone" with respect to circulation. The anterior spinal artery is reinforced at a number of segmental levels by feeder arterial branches called anterior medullary feeder arteries. At the thoracic level, there are a total of eight of these feeder arteries, largest of which is called artery of Adamkiewicz or great anterior medullary artery. This artery typically enters the cord on the left side anywhere from T7 to L4, but most commonly at T9-T12.

314. **(C)**

   A. The involvement of deep radial nerve is called posterior interosseous nerve entrapment. The symptoms are similar to radial tunnel syndrome including pain over the proximal dorsal forearm, with maximum tenderness at the site of radial tunnel that is 4 cm distal to the lateral epicondyle over the posterior interosseous nerve. The pain is typically elicited by attempting to resist extension of long finger.

   B. Medial epicondylitis or golfer's elbow results in pain and exquisite tenderness over medial epicondyle that is further aggravated by flexion and pronation of the forearm and the wrist.

   C. Lateral epicondylitis or tennis elbow involves the extensor-supinator muscle mass, including extensor carpi radialis brevis, extensor digitorum communis, extensor carpi radialis longus, extensor carpi ulnaris, and supinator. The extensor carpi radialis is most commonly involved, mostly from repetitive movement of the wrist involving wrist flexion, elbow extension, and forearm pronation. Provocative test involves grasping or extending the wrist against resistance or supinating the forearm when sudden and severe pain is experienced in the area of lateral epicondyle. The patient's being an "avid golfer" is a distractor here.

   D. de Quervain disease or tenosynovitis of the tendon sheath of extensor pollicis brevis and adductor pollicis longus causes swelling and tenderness of anatomic snuff box.

   E. Brachioradialis tendonitis results in pain in the lateral forearm, that is, region of brachioradialis tendon, the provocative tests described above typically do not elicit characteristic symptoms.

315. **(C)** Patients with cervical rheumatoid arthritis develop neck pain exacerbated by movement, with atlantoaxial disease producing pain in upper cervical spine and subaxial involvement producing pain in lower neck and clavicular areas. Neurologic involvement is seen in more advanced cases of spinal cord or nerve root compromise related to deformity and soft

tissue hypertrophy. Plain radiography is useful in showing structural abnormalities and dynamic studies including flexion extension, oblique and open mouth frontal projections in identifying instability. Anterior subluxation of atlantoaxial joint is the most common form of cervical spine derangement followed by sub-axial subluxation (between C3 and C7), lateral subluxation, cranial settling (vertical subluxation), and posterior subluxation. Also, the autoimmune inflammatory changes affect the synovium of zygapophyseal joints resulting in laxity and subsequent instability.

316. **(B)**

A. Trauma to L2 nerve root may cause ipsilateral groin pain, but is not the most likely cause.

B. The most likely cause of the symptoms mentioned in the question is trauma to genitofemoral nerve. In fact, it is the most common complication associated with lumbar sympatholysis, particularly by the lateral approach. The incidence has been reported to be as high as 15%, but may be as low as 4% with a single-needle technique. Most cases are transient and resolve with conservative measures but others may last as long as 6 weeks. Repeat local anesthetic lumbar sympathetic block, TENS (transcutaneous electrical nerve stimulator) unit and intravenous lidocaine have all been described as options for remission of genitofemoral neuralgia.

C. Psoas spasm is also sometimes seen but it typically produces discomfort in ipsilateral low back.

(D) and (E) do not present as groin pain.

317. **(D)** Painful symptoms of Charcot-Marie-Tooth (CMT) disease have been described in the hypertrophic or demyelinating form (CMT-1). Pain may be described shooting, sharp, or burning in their toes, feet, ankles, and knees. Common presentation is in the first or second decade with difficulties walking or running.

318. **(C)** Morton neuroma may be considered in the spectrum of interdigital neuritis (compression neuropathy). It is usually between the third and fourth toes or less often between the fourth

and fifth toes. The pain tends to be experienced more with walking and weight bearing while wearing shoes. The pain is generally alleviated with rest and removal of shoes. The pain may be reproduced by exerting pressure between the two toes implicated. Interdigital injection of local anesthetic relieves the pain.

319. **(B)** MRI, especially with T2-weighted images (though generally more time consuming to obtain) is useful in imaging conditions such as osteomyelitis, discitis, spinal cord compression, and malignancy. T1-weighted images provide reasonably good anatomic detail in imaging of end-plate reactive changes as well as postoperative scarring, but gadolinium-DTPA contrast should be used in postoperative patients to differentiate scarring from intervertebral discs.

320. **(E)** The H reflex is examined utilizing a modified motor nerve conduction study technique. The H reflex is generally present in the soleus muscle and at time forearm flexor muscles. It may be more widespread in hyperreflexic conditions (eg, myelopathy) and pediatrics. Delayed or absence of the tibial H wave may reflect S1 radiculopathy or other neuropathic processes.

321. **(E)** The elderly may seek medical attention for multiple problems with initial complaints of abdominal pain including: dissecting abdominal aortic aneurysm in diabetic ketoacidosis, pneumonia, pyelonephritis, inflammatory bowel disease, mesenteric ischemia, constipation, bowel obstruction, peritonitis, and drug-induced GI mucosal irritation.

322. **(A)** The ulnar nerve may be compressed in the cubital tunnel (cubital tunnel syndrome) which may lead to atrophy of the first dorsal interosseous muscle, clawing of the small finger, weakness of small finger adduction (Wartenberg sign) and eventually in chronic ulnar nerve compromise—with weakness of grip and pinch.

323. **(E)** Tarsal tunnel syndrome is not a common source of foot discomfort and needs to be

distinguished from multiple other causes of pain in the foot including: painful peripheral neuropathies, medial plantar nerve entrapment (which may occur in joggers), posterior tibial nerve entrapment symptoms tend to be located in medial plantar heel area, abductor digiti quinti nerve entrapment (usually with burning pain in heel pad area), and plantar fasciitis. Plantar fasciitis pain may be diffuse or migrate but with time is usually noted at the inferior aspect of the heel (around the medial calcaneal tuberosity) mainly, although typically severe with the first few steps in the morning, tends to diminish through the course of the day (unless intense or prolonged weight-bearing activity is under taken).

324. **(E)** Although, somewhat controversial and different from various proposed research criteria, the diagnosis of CRPS I, includes:

1. The presence of an initiating noxious event or a cause of immobilization.
2. Continuing pain, allodynia, or hyperalgesia with which the pain is disproportionate to any inciting event.
3. Evidence at some time of edema, changes in skin blood flow, or abnormal sudomotor activity in the region of the pain.
4. This diagnosis is excluded by the existence of condition that otherwise would account for the degree of pain and dysfunction.

325. **(E)** Paroxysmal hemicranias may be chronic (CPH) (eg, daily) or episodic (EPH) (eg, discrete headache period or separated by periods of remission) characterized by severe, excruciating, throbbing, boring, or pulsatile pain affecting the orbital, supraorbital, and temporal regions.

The pain tends to be associated with at least one of the following signs or symptoms ipsilateral to the painful side:

1. Conjunctival injection
2. Nasal congestion
3. Lacrimation
4. Ptosis
5. Rhinorrhea
6. Eyelid edema

Attacks may occur at any time—occasionally waking patients from sound sleep and tend to last for 2 to 25 minutes (although may linger a couple of hours). The patient generally has 1 to 40 attacks per day.

326. **(E)**

1. Although thoracic radiculopathy has been described to result from multiple etiologies including tumor, scoliosis, infection, spondylosis, and herniated disc, diabetes mellitus is described as the most common cause.
2. The lower cervical discs are most commonly affected by herniation.
3. The frequency of L4-5 herniation is 45% compared to 42% at the level of L5-S1. With L4-5 herniation, L5 nerve root is most commonly affected.
4. Lower cervical nerve roots of brachial plexus, that is, C8 and T1 nerve roots are most commonly affected in thoracic outlet syndrome.

327. **(C)** Epidural spinal cord compression is compression of spinal cord or cauda equina nerve roots from a lesion outside the dura mater. Epidural spinal cord or cauda equina compression is the second most common neurologic complication of cancer, occurring in up to 10% of patients. The most common tumors causing metastatic epidural compression are breast, lung, prostate, lymphoma, sarcoma, and kidney. Conus medullaris lesions typically cause a rapidly progressive symmetric perineal pain followed by early autonomic dysfunction, saddle sensory loss, and motor weakness. Limited straight leg raise test usually points to an epidural or intradural extramedullary lesion causing root compression, whereas segmental pain and sacral sparing suggest intramedullary disease.

328. **(E)**

1. The incidence of spinal cord pain has been estimated to be in the range of 6.4% to 94% of patients who experience spinal cord injury.
2. Patients may describe a variety of pain types; however, the three most common types are spontaneous steady, spontaneous neuralgic,

and evoked pain including allodynia and hyperpathia. According to a study of 127 patients with spinal cord pain by Boureau and colleagues, 75% of patients reported burning pain.

3. Bowel and bladder dysfunction may be associated with spinal cord injury depending on the level and extent of injury.

4. Onset is typically within 1 to 6 months of the injury. When the onset was delayed beyond 1 year, 56% of the patients were found to suffer from a syrinx.

329. **(A)** Froment sign is positive when ulnar nerve dysfunction is present. Froment sign is tested by placing a piece of paper between patient's thumb and index finger and checking the position of the thumb as the examiner tries to pull the paper away from the patient. Normally the distal joint of the thumb remains in extension but if there is ulnar nerve dysfunction the tip of the thumb flexes significantly to increased pressure in attempt to keep the paper from moving.

330. **(E)** Drug-induced painful neuropathies may include toxoids (especially with doses greater than 200 mg/m^2), cisplatinum, vincristine, amiodarone, metronidazole, and pyridoxine (especially at doses greater than 200-300 mg/d).

331. **(E)** SCS has been utilized by clinicians for a variety of chronic pain issues. Although a large body of work has been published, precise mechanisms of action of SCS remain elusive. Animal studies suggest that SCS triggers release of serotonin, substance P, and γ-aminobutyric acid (GABA) within the spinal cord dorsal horn.

CHAPTER 6

Types of Pain
Questions

DIRECTIONS (Questions 332 through 486): Each of the numbered items or incomplete statements in this section is followed by answers or by completions of the statement. Select the ONE lettered answer or completion that is BEST in each case.

332. A 45-year-old patient with metastatic breast carcinoma is prescribed 30 mg of sustained-release morphine (MS Contin) twice a day and one 15-mg tablet of immediate-release morphine (MSIR) every 6 hours as needed for breakthrough pain. On her routine follow-up visit she reports that she routinely uses MSIR four times a day with satisfactory pain control on most days and no major side effects. What would be your best course of action in this situation?

    (A) Prescriptions should be left unchanged
    (B) MS Contin should be changed to 40 mg of OxyContin twice a day and 5 mg of oxycodone every 6 hours as needed for breakthrough pain
    (C) Fentanyl patch of 25 µg/h should replace MS Contin with 15 mg of MSIR every 6 hours as needed for breakthrough pain
    (D) MS Contin should be increased to 60 mg twice a day with MSIR 15 mg every 6 hours as needed for breakthrough pain
    (E) MS Contin should be increased to 60 mg twice a day, and MSIR should be discontinued

333. Approximately in what percentage of patients with malignancies does pain unrelated to cancer occur?

    (A) Less than 2%
    (B) 3%
    (C) 7.5%
    (D) 11%
    (E) 25%

334. There is a significant incidence of neuropathic pain in a cancer patient with brachial plexopathy. The etiology of the brachial plexopathy in such a patient may be caused by direct tumor infiltration or radiation fibrosis. Electrophysiologic evaluation with nerve conduction velocity (NCV) study and electromyography (EMG) helps to distinguish between the two etiologies. Which of the following findings of NCV/EMG is the most helpful to differentiate between the direct tumor infiltration and the radiation fibrosis etiologies of brachial plexopathy?

    (A) Segmental nerve conduction slowing
    (B) Myokymia
    (C) Fibrillation potentials
    (D) Positive sharp waves
    (E) Decreased amplitude of the compound muscle action potential (CMAP)

335. If bony metastases are present, which primary cancer location has the best 5-year survival prognosis?

    (A) Myeloma
    (B) Breast
    (C) Prostate
    (D) Thyroid
    (E) Kidney

336. The most frequent spinal cord symptom or sign in patients with carcinomatous meningitis is

    (A) nuchal rigidity
    (B) back pain
    (C) reflex asymmetry
    (D) positive straight leg raise test
    (E) weakness

337. Which of the following would most likely be responsible for the central pain syndrome?

    (A) Epidural spinal cord compression
    (B) Metastatic bony destruction of the vertebrae with a nerve root compression
    (C) Metastatic involvement of the cranial nerves
    (D) Carcinomatous meningitis
    (E) Radiation myelopathy

338. The majority of patients with epidural metastasis have the following pattern of pain:

    (A) Local
    (B) Radicular
    (C) Referred
    (D) Funicular
    (E) All of the above

339. All of the following are true about the World Health Organization (WHO) analgesic ladder, EXCEPT

    (A) it is a method for relief of cancer pain based on a small number of relatively inexpensive drugs
    (B) it has three steps
    (C) step one involves the use of opioids
    (D) it suggests to use only one drug from each group at a time
    (E) it is a simple and effective method for controlling cancer pain

340. The following are all true about methadone, EXCEPT

    (A) it has a highly variable oral bioavailability
    (B) it is a low cost medication
    (C) it has no known active metabolites

    (D) it has N-methyl-D-aspartate (NMDA) receptor agonist properties
    (E) it has high lipid solubility

341. 58-years-old patient with metastatic prostate cancer is taking sustained-release morphine (MS Contin) every 8 hours with a total daily dose of 225 mg with optimal pain control. Because of some circumstances, he has to be converted to transdermal therapeutic system fentanyl (TTS-fentanyl). What is the correct dose of fentanyl patch equivalent to the current dose of MS Contin for this patient?

    (A) 25 µg/h every 72 hours
    (B) 50 µg/h every 48 hours
    (C) 75 µg/h every 72 hours
    (D) 100 µg/h every 48 hours
    (E) 125 µg/h every 72 hours

342. Which of the following is true with respect to central pain syndromes?

    (A) The most common cause of central pain state are lesions located in the brainstem
    (B) The Wallenberg syndrome (lateral medullar syndrome) is characterized by contralateral facial sensory loss and Horner syndrome
    (C) The most common lesions that produce thalamic pain syndrome are infarctions
    (D) Spinal cord lesions rarely cause sensory deficits
    (E) Central pain syndromes of spinal origin usually respond to epidural steroids

343. Peripheral neuropathy is a common pain syndrome characterized by which of the following?

    (A) Asymmetric paresthesias and proximal motor impairment
    (B) Proximal more than distal sensory impairment
    (C) Most peripheral neuropathies may be classified as demyelinating, axonal, or mixed

(D) Peripheral mononeuropathy is the most common peripheral nerve disease in patients with long-standing diabetes mellitus

(E) Nerve conduction studies only measure conduction through small unmyelinated fibers, so impairment of the fast conducting fibers may go undetected

344. Events seen in the development of neuropathic pain are

(A) following nerve injury, there is a decreased activity of the sodium channels which allows for abnormal conduction through pain facilitating fibers

(B) wide dynamic range neurons in the dorsal horn respond with increased frequency as the intensity of the repeated afferent stimulus increases

(C) an increase in potassium channels would facilitate an amplified afferent activity

(D) C-polymodal nociceptors are activated by low-threshold mechanical, thermal, and chemical stimuli

(E) γ-aminobutyric acid (GABA) and glycine are released in the dorsal horn and augment the response of second order neurons

345. Examples of neuropathic pain conditions include all, EXCEPT

(A) complex regional pain syndrome (CRPS)

(B) diabetic peripheral neuropathy

(C) postherpetic neuralgia (PHN)

(D) Raynaud phenomenon

(E) phantom limb pain

346. Which of the following conditions is more likely to be associated with neuropathic pain?

(A) Traumatic nerve injury

(B) Stroke

(C) Syringomyelia

(D) Multiple sclerosis

(E) Large myelinated fiber neuropathy

347. A patient with CRPS responds well to sympathetic ganglion block. The results of this block

can lead you to say which of the following about this particular pain condition?

(A) It is vascularly mediated

(B) It is sympathetically mediated

(C) It is sympathetically maintained

(D) It is less severe than previously thought

(E) It will not respond well to spinal cord stimulation

348. Neuropathic pain can result in which of the following condition?

(A) Central sensitization

(B) Allodynia

(C) Hyperalgesia

(D) B and C

(E) A, B, and C

349. Potential neurophysiologic mechanisms underlying the development of neuropathic pain include

(A) microglial activation in the spinal cord

(B) cytokine production in the spinal cord

(C) decreased glutamate release in the spinal cord

(D) A and C

(E) A and B

350. When the stimulus of light touch exerts pain which of the following is exhibited?

(A) Hyperalgesia

(B) Allodynia

(C) Hyperreflexemia

(D) Paresthesia

(E) Hypertouchemia

351. Phantom pain refers to

(A) any sensation of the missing limb, except pain

(B) painful sensations referred to the missing limb

(C) spontaneous movement of the stump ranging from small jerks to visible contractions (jumpy stump)

(D) pain referred to the amputation stump

(E) B and D

352. A 74-year-old male has a left lower extremity amputation after a long bout with uncontrolled diabetes mellitus (DM). What are the chances that this patient will develop phantom pain?

    (A) 33%
    (B) 49%
    (C) 55%
    (D) 90%
    (E) 75%

353. A vascular surgeon consults the pain team on a patient who is scheduled to undergo an amputation secondary to peripheral vascular disease. The patient has read about phantom pain on the Internet and would like to know when it would likely start. You tell the vascular surgeon that

    (A) the onset of phantom pain is usually within the first week after amputation
    (B) most studies have shown that phantom pain will start between 2 and 4 weeks after an amputation for peripheral vascular disease
    (C) the likelihood of her developing phantom pain in the first 6 months after amputation is low, but increases drastically between 6 and 9 months
    (D) the onset will likely be delayed for years
    (E) none of the above

354. The patient mentioned in the previous question develops early and severe phantom pain:

    (A) The patient is more likely to suffer from long-standing pain
    (B) The patient is less likely to suffer from long-standing pain
    (C) The patient is more likely to suffer incapacitating pain for 1 year that will subside rather abruptly
    (D) It is likely that the patient will develop neuropathic pain in the extremity contralateral to the amputation
    (E) The pain will likely be refractory to treatment with anticonvulsants

355. The number of amputees who have severe phantom limb pain is

    (A) 20% to 30%
    (B) 60% to 80%
    (C) 5% to 10%
    (D) 1% to 2%
    (E) 45% to 55%

356. Preamputation pain

    (A) is more likely to lead to phantom pain if the amputation is traumatic
    (B) may sensitize the nervous system, explaining why some individuals may be more susceptible to development of chronic phantom pain
    (C) is more likely to lead to phantom pain if the amputation is secondary
    (D) is similar in character and localization to the subsequent phantom pain in 80% of patients
    (E) is less likely to lead to phantom pain if the amputation is in the upper extremities

357. A 25-year-old left lower extremity amputee returns from Iraq. He experiences phantom pain, but is attempting to move forward in life. To ease his transition back into society which of the following is the next best step?

    (A) He should take as long as possible to grieve before he finds new employment
    (B) He should initially use a cosmetic prosthesis before embarking on the task of learning to use a functional one
    (C) He should absolutely refuse to ever have spinal anesthesia as it may worsen phantom pain
    (D) He should learn coping strategies as phantom pain is a psychological disturbance
    (E) None of the above

358. Stump pain and phantom pain are often confused. There are, however, notable differences. Which of the following is true?

(A) Unlike phantom pain, stump pain occurs in the body part that actually exists, in the stump that remains

(B) Stump pain typically is described as a "sharp," "burning," "electric-like," or "skin-sensitive" pain

(C) Stump pain is usually caused by a neuroma

(D) Surgical revision of the stump or removal of the neuroma is sometimes considered when treating stump pain

(E) All of the above

359. A neuroma is an inflammation of a nerve that is seen universally after a nerve has been cut (ie, during an amputation). They show spontaneous and abnormal evoked activity following mechanical or chemical stimulation from the periphery. This results from

(A) an increased and novel expression of sodium channels

(B) hyperexcitability changes and reorganization of the thalamus

(C) an increase in potassium efflux

(D) increased activity in afferent C fibers

(E) A and D

360. Some amputees show an abnormal sensitivity to pressure and to repetitive stimulation of the stump, which can provoke attacks of phantom pain. Which of the following is the case in humans?

(A) It can be reduced by giving the NMDA antagonist, ketamine

(B) It can only be reduced by terminating the stimulation

(C) It can be attributed to the general excitability of spinal cord neurons, where only C fibers gain access to secondary pain-signaling neurons

(D) Sensitization of the dorsal horn may be mediated by glycine and serotonin

(E) All of the above

361. Of the following, which does not play a role in the mechanism for generating phantom pain?

(A) Peripheral sensitization

(B) Central sensitization

(C) Cortical reorganization

(D) Increased thalamus response to stimulation

(E) Sympathetic inhibition

362. Pharmacologically treating phantom pain is not easy. Which of the following medications has not proven to be effective in well-controlled trials?

(A) Tramadol

(B) Gabapentin

(C) Memantine

(D) Amitriptyline

(E) A and C

363. A 65-year-old Vietnam War veteran with a left below the knee amputation and phantom pain has surgery on an amputation neuroma. He should expect

(A) excellent resolution of his phantom pain

(B) short-term pain relief

(C) a likely infection and subsequent complicated hospital course

(D) decreased pain only if he receives a 40-minute infusion of diphenhydramine within 24 hours of the surgery

(E) none of the above

364. A patient has tingling sensations in a phantom limb that are uncomfortable and annoying but do not interfere with activities or sleep. According to the Sunderland classification of patients with phantom pain, what group is this patient in?

(A) Group I

(B) Group II

(C) Group III

(D) Group IV

(E) None of the above

365. The gate-control theory of pain has been used to explain phantom limb pain. It states that

    (A) following significant destruction of sensory axons by amputation, wide dynamic range neurons are freed by inhibitory control

    (B) self-sustaining neuronal activity may occur in spinal cord neurons

    (C) if spontaneous spinal cord neuronal activity increases by any amount, pain may occur in the phantom limb

    (D) A and B

    (E) A, B, and C

366. All of the following are true about primary dysmenorrhea, EXCEPT

    (A) pain is transmitted via the thoracolumbar spinal segments and pelvic afferents

    (B) the etiology of pain includes myometrial contractions leading to intense intrauterine pressure and uterine hypoxia

    (C) prostaglandins and leukotriene production that sensitizes afferent pelvic nerves is part of its pathogenesis

    (D) endometriosis and adenomyosis are its most common causes

    (E) altered central receptivity of the afferent input from the pelvis is thought to be relevant in its development

367. All of the following are true about chronic endometriosis, EXCEPT

    (A) ovaries, cul-de-sac, uterine tubes, surface of the bowel are among the most common sites of pathologic implantation of the functioning endometrial tissue

    (B) retrograde menstruation, lymphatic spread, and hematogenous spread of the endometrial tissue are all thought to play a role in endometriosis etiology

    (C) pain occurs only with menses

    (D) definitive diagnosis can be made by visualization of the characteristic lesions without a mandatory histologic confirmation

    (E) leuprolide acetate (Lupron) may be an effective treatment of the symptoms of chronic endometriosis

368. All of the following are correct, EXCEPT

    (A) pudendal nerve takes origin from S2, S3, and S4 roots bilaterally

    (B) bilateral denervation of the inferior hypogastric nerves is as effective as a lumbar epidural block with respect to sensory input from the uterus and cervix

    (C) many patients with hymenal neuropathy are so emotional and complain so violently that the pelvic examination is not possible

    (D) patients with sympathetic pelvis syndrome have a deep pain in the pelvis not associated with physically detectable abdominal wall or muscle tenderness

    (E) ilioinguinal and iliohypogastric neuropathy is rarely associated with the surgeries in the lower abdominal wall area

369. All of the common reasons for the inadequate management of acute pain in a hospital setting are true, EXCEPT

    (A) the common idea that pain is merely a symptom and not harmful in itself

    (B) the fact that opioids have no potential for addiction when administered strictly for acute pain

    (C) lack of understanding of the pharmacokinetics of various agents

    (D) lack of appreciation of variability in analgesic response to opioids

    (E) prescription of inappropriately low doses of opioids and thinking that opioids must not be given more often than every 4 hours

370. The following are true about pathologic (nonphysiological) pain, EXCEPT

    (A) it occurs in the context of central sensitization

    (B) it occurs in the context of peripheral sensitization

    (C) it outlasts the stimulus

    (D) it spreads to nondamaged areas

    (E) it is elicited by A-δ and C fibers, but not A-β fibers, which transmit touch sensation

371. Perioperative administration of NSAIDs

    (A) does not reduce the demand for opioids during and after the surgery
    (B) is contraindicated because of increased possibility of bleeding
    (C) has synergistic effect with opioids
    (D) has its analgesic effect only through peripheral mechanisms
    (E) is not associated with the concerns for postoperative bleeding

372. All of the following are true about the NMDA receptors, EXCEPT

    (A) they are involved in development of "windup" facilitation
    (B) NMDA agonists reduce development of tolerance to opioids
    (C) NMDA receptors are involved in development of central sensitization
    (D) NMDA receptors are involved in changes of peripheral receptive fields
    (E) NMDA receptors are involved in induction of oncogenes and long-term potentiation

373. As compared with somatic pain, all of the following are true about visceral pain, EXCEPT

    (A) it may follow the distribution of a somatic nerve
    (B) it is dull and vague
    (C) it is often periodic and builds to peaks
    (D) it is often associated with nausea and vomiting
    (E) it is poorly localized

374. The following statements are true regarding preemptive analgesia, EXCEPT

    (A) preemptive analgesia is helpful in reducing postoperative pain in part by reducing the phenomenon of central sensitization
    (B) early postoperative pain is not a significant predictor of long-term pain
    (C) local anesthetics, opioids, and NSAIDs can be used for preemptive analgesia

    (D) preemptive analgesia may have the potential to prevent the development of chronic pain states
    (E) preemptive analgesia is thought to reduce neuroplastic changes in the spinal cord

375. The following statements are true regarding multimodal analgesia, EXCEPT

    (A) it may include NSAIDs, acetaminophen, local anesthetics, and opioids in the same patient
    (B) it is beneficial because of the synergistic action of the individual medications with different sites of action along the pain pathways
    (C) it is not very valuable owing to an increase in the incidence of side effects
    (D) it facilitates early mobilization of the postsurgical patient
    (E) it expedites return to normal parenteral nutrition

376. All of the following statements about PHN are correct, EXCEPT

    (A) midthoracic dermatomes is one of the most common sites for PHN
    (B) men are affected more often than women in a ratio of 3:2
    (C) ophthalmic division of the trigeminal nerve is one of the most common sites for PHN
    (D) PHN may occur in any dermatome
    (E) PHN has an incidence of 9% to 14.3%

377. PHN is defined as

    (A) any pain associated with the herpes zoster
    (B) pain caused by herpes zoster for more than 1 month
    (C) persistent pain with a significant neuropathic component in a dermatomal distribution
    (D) pain caused by herpes zoster for more than 3 months
    (E) neuropathic pain in midthoracic dermatomes caused by herpes simplex virus

378. Which of the following is true about the management of PHN?

(A) Approximately 40% of patients with PHN have either incomplete or no relief from treatment

(B) Prevention of herpes zoster is not nearly as important as a multimodal treatment of PHN

(C) Current multimodal treatment of PHN is nearly 100% effective, independent of the duration of the symptoms

(D) Current multimodal treatment of PHN is nearly 100% effective as long as it is started within the first month of the symptoms of PHN

(E) Current multimodal treatment of PHN is nearly 100% effective as long as it is started immediately after the first symptoms of herpes zoster

379. The following are true about the use of antidepressants in treatment of PHN, EXCEPT

(A) amitriptyline has been shown to be effective in treatment of PHN, but has significant limitations in the long term because of its side effects

(B) selective serotonin reuptake inhibitors (SSRIs) have been found to be equally or more effective in treatment of PHN than the older generation of tricyclic antidepressants (TCAs) or selective norepinephrine reuptake inhibitors (SNRIs)

(C) SNRIs have been shown to be more effective than placebo in treatment of PHN

(D) antidepressant therapy in PHN is built on sound, scientific basis

(E) one of the significant side effects of TCAs is their anticholinergic properties

380. Which of the following is true about use of opioids in the treatment of PHN?

(A) The use of opioids is not justified for nonmalignant pain

(B) Opioids tend to be less effective for the treatment of neuropathic pain than nonneuropathic pain

(C) Opioids were not found to be useful in the treatment of PHN

(D) The use of opioids should be avoided in combination with antidepressants because of the risk of excessive central nervous system (CNS) suppression

(E) The use of opioids in PHN should be avoided owing to the increased potential of addiction

381. Which of the following is the most common cause of autonomic neuropathy in the developed world?

(A) Leprosy
(B) Diabetes mellitus (DM)
(C) Human immunodeficiency virus (HIV) infection
(D) Heavy metal poisoning
(E) Idiopathic etiology

382. Diabetic amyotrophy

(A) has a poor prognosis
(B) has better prognosis when it involves upper extremities
(C) usually resolves within 1 to 2 years spontaneously
(D) has better prognosis when the symptoms do not involve pain
(E) it is directly related to hyperglycemia

383. The following are true about the distal sensorimotor polyneuropathy, EXCEPT

(A) it is the most common neuropathic manifestation of both type 1 and type 2 diabetes
(B) it starts distally and spreads proximally
(C) initial symptoms may involve numbness and tingling in the toes or feet
(D) it is a length-dependent neuropathy
(E) it is usually asymmetrical

384. The prevalence of diabetic neuropathy in DM patients is

(A) less than 1% at diagnosis of DM, rising to 10% in patients diagnosed for longer than 5 years

(B) about 10% at diagnosis of DM, rising to more than 50% in patients diagnosed for longer than 5 years

(C) about 50% at diagnosis of DM, rising to almost 100% in patients diagnosed for longer than 5 years

(D) about 50% at diagnosis of DM, and does not change significantly with time

(E) no such studies have been done so far

385. Patients with diabetic distal sensorimotor polyneuropathy initially may complain of numbness and tingling in the toes or feet, which then slowly spreads proximally over months to years. Eventually, numbness and tingling appear in the fingertips, as the symptoms of diabetic polyneuropathy progress to

(A) ankle
(B) knee
(C) mid-thigh
(D) buttock and groin
(E) abdomen

386. Which of the following is the most widely accepted cause of trigeminal neuralgia?

(A) Demyelinating conditions, as trigeminal neuralgia is most common in patients with multiple sclerosis

(B) Direct trauma of the trigeminal ganglion at the level of the foramen ovale, before branching into its three branches

(C) Arterial cross-compression of the trigeminal nerve in the posterior fossa

(D) Tumors of the posterior fossae

(E) Poor vascular supply to the affected trigeminal branch

387. Which of the following is true regarding medical management for the treatment of trigeminal neuralgia?

(A) Anticonvulsant medications are usually considered as the second line of treatment

(B) Beneficial effects of carbamazepine are better in elderly patients

(C) Risk of side effects of carbamazepine increase with age

(D) Carbamazepine has proven to be the most effective treatment for trigeminal neuralgia, independently of the side-effect profile

(E) Because of the unlikelihood of serious side effects with surgery, all patients should consider this option first

388. The gasserian ganglion

(A) receives exclusively proprioceptive information from the muscles of mastication

(B) the mandibular branch is located medial to the ophthalmic branch

(C) the two medial branches are sensory while the lateral branch is partially motor

(D) the ganglion lies out of the cranium, in the Meckel cave

(E) the foramen rotundum is used as landmark for the blockage of the trigeminal ganglion

389. Which of the following is true regarding the diagnosis of trigeminal neuralgia?

(A) The diagnosis must be confirmed with magnetic resonance imaging (MRI) to detect vascular trigeminal nerve compression

(B) Sensory evoked potentials is the most sensitive test to perform the diagnosis

(C) The diagnosis is clinical and tests are only necessary to rule out associated conditions

(D) To accurately diagnose the condition, it is necessary to correlate clinical findings with MRI and sensory evoke potential tests

(E) None of the above

390. Giant cell arteritis is characterized by which of the following?

(A) Affects almost exclusively Asian population

(B) As other forms of vasculitis, giant cell arteritis commonly involves skin, kidneys, and lungs

(C) Males are more commonly affected

(D) It is more common in older patients, with a peak incidence between 60 to 75 years of age

(E) Visual loss is the presenting symptom in over 50% of the patients

391. According to the International Headache Society Diagnostic Criteria, analgesic rebound headache is

(A) headache that resolves or reverts within 2 weeks after discontinuation of the suspected medication

(B) headache that worsens after intake of analgesics and reduces in intensity and frequency with reduction in the analgesic dose

(C) the intensity of the headache decreases in intensity proportionally to the decrease in the dose of analgesic

(D) headache greater than 15 days per month that has developed or markedly worsened during medication overuse

(E) headache that increases in intensity with the use of morphine, most likely because of the cerebral vasodilation mediated by histamine release

392. Cluster headaches are characterized by

(A) lancinating unilateral headache that is commonly triggered by stress factors

(B) the pain is strictly unilateral and autonomic symptoms occur ipsilateral to the pain

(C) the onset is slow with progressive worsening of the pain over several hours with an attack usually lasting 3 to 4 days

(D) melatonin is commonly indicated as therapy for the acute attack

(E) cluster headaches are more common in elderly patients

393. Which of the following describes the pathophysiologic changes seen in migraine?

(A) Inflammation of hypothalamic structures leads to low threshold stimulation of vascular and meningeal tissues

(B) Central sensitization mediated by attribution to activation of β-fibers in the trigeminal system, mediates extracranial hypersensitivity

(C) Large cerebral vessels, pial vessels, large sinuses, and the dura, are innervated by fibers originating from the sphenopalatine ganglion

(D) Activation and threshold reduction of the trigeminocervical complex by its most caudal cells

(E) In acute attacks, a marked reduction in vasoactive substances, including substance P, calcitonin gene related peptide (CGRP), and nitric oxide is commonly seen

394. Which of the following is correct regarding headache?

(A) Migraine is the most common form of headache

(B) Tension-type headache (TTH) is commonly aggravated by physical exercise

(C) The presence of nausea, vomiting, photophobia, or phonophobia excludes the diagnosis of TTH

(D) The most common form of migraine is associated with aura

(E) Comorbid conditions associated with chronic migraine include depression, anxiety, and panic disorders

395. Hundred precent oxygen inhalation is a safe and effective method for acute treatment of

(A) chronic daily headache

(B) TTH

(C) migraine with aura

(D) cluster headache

(E) glossopharyngeal neuralgia

396. The Ramsay Hunt syndrome is caused by the infection of the varicella-zoster virus of the

(A) sphenopalatine ganglion

(B) gasserian ganglion

(C) geniculate ganglion

(D) glossopharyngeal ganglion

(E) stellate ganglion

397. Which of the following characterizes the spontaneous intracranial hypotension (SIH)?

(A) Is the same entity as post–dural puncture headache (PDPH)

(B) Headache is consistently unilateral

(C) Orthostatic headache is pathognomonic

(D) Patients complain of bitemporal headache

(E) To confirm the diagnosis, it is required that cerebrospinal fluid (CSF) opening pressures be below 60 mm H_2O

398. A 20-year-old male presents to the clinic with complaints of moderate headaches located bilateral in the forehead, parietal, and occipital areas. The pain is dull and continuous and not associated with nausea, vomiting, photophobia, and phonophobia. The patient recalls that the symptoms started 1 year ago and have been constant since they started. No abnormalities where observed on physical examination, sinus computed tomography (CT), or brain MRI. The patient has occasionally tried over-the-counter analgesics with no relief. Which of the following is the most likely diagnosis?

(A) Status migrainosus

(B) Rebound headache

(C) New daily persistent headache

(D) Cluster headache

(E) Classical migraine

399. Which of the following is a theory that may explain the presence of aura?

(A) Cortical spreading depression

(B) The vascular theory

(C) Hormonal fluctuation

(D) Estrogen withdrawal

(E) Cerebral idiopathic hypertension

400. Chronic low back pain and neck pain persists 1 year or longer in what percentage of patients?

(A) 5% to 10%

(B) 15% to 20%

(C) 20% to 25%

(D) 25% to 60%

(E) 60% to 75%

401. The prevalence of zygapophysial (facet) joint involvement in low back pain is

(A) 5% to 10%

(B) 10% to 15%

(C) 15% to 45%

(D) 50% to 60%

(E) 65% to 70%

402. A 58-year-old with metastatic lung cancer suddenly complains of severe back pain. Symptoms of early spinal cord compression include all of the following, EXCEPT

(A) rapid onset

(B) symmetric and profound weakness

(C) spasticity

(D) increased deep tendon reflexes

(E) urinary retention and constipation

403. Specific indications for discography include all of the following, EXCEPT

(A) further evaluation of abnormal discs to assess the extent of abnormality

(B) patients with persistent, severe symptoms in whom other diagnostic tests have revealed clear confirmation of a suspected disc as the source of pain

(C) assessment of patients who have failed to respond to surgical procedures to determine if there is possible recurrent disc herniation

(D) assessment of discs before fusion to determine if the discs within the proposed fusion segment are symptomatic

(E) assessment of minimally invasive surgical candidates to confirm a contained disc herniation or to investigate contrast distribution pattern before intradiscal procedures

404. The following signs and symptoms are consistently found with cervical radiculopathy, EXCEPT

(A) gait disturbances

(B) normal muscle tone

(C) negative Babinski test

(D) weak tendon reflexes

(E) positive axial compression test (Spurling maneuver)

405. All of the following are reasons associated with smoking as a risk factor for low back pain, EXCEPT

(A) mineral content of the lumbar vertebrae is decreased

(B) fibrinolytic disc activity is altered

(C) blood flow and nutrition to the disc are diminished

(D) disc pH is higher

(E) increased degenerative changes of the lumbar spine

406. All of the following treatments have strong evidence to back their use when treating acute low back pain, EXCEPT

(A) muscle relaxants effectively reduce low back pain

(B) bed rest is effective for treating low back pain

(C) continuing normal activity gives equivalent or faster recovery from acute low back pain

(D) NSAIDs prescribed at regular intervals are an effective treatment for acute low back pain

(E) different types of NSAIDs are equally effective at treating low back pain

407. Age-related changes in the intervertebral discs include all of the following, EXCEPT

(A) the dimensions of the lumbar intervertebral discs decrease with age

(B) collagen lamellae of the annulus fibrosis increases in thickness

(C) distinction between the nucleus pulposus and annulus fibrosis becomes less apparent

(D) the nucleus pulposus is less able to transmit weight directly

(E) 80% of nucleus pulposus cells in the elderly exhibit necrosis

408. Radiculopathy is a neurologic condition associated with all of the following characteristics, EXCEPT

(A) numbness

(B) weakness

(C) pain

(D) compression of axons

(E) ischemia of axons

409. Adverse effects of epidurally administered steroids include all of the following, EXCEPT

(A) Cushing syndrome

(B) osteoporosis

(C) avascular bone necrosis

(D) hypoglycemia

(E) suppression of the hypothalamus-pituitary axis

410. Relative contraindications to epidural steroid injections include

   (A) preexisting neurologic disorder (ie, multiple sclerosis)
   (B) sepsis
   (C) therapeutic anticoagulation
   (D) localized infection at injection site
   (E) patient refusal

411. L4-L5 disk herniation with L5 nerve root involvement includes

   (A) numbness over the medial thigh and knee
   (B) weakness with dorsiflexion of great toe and foot
   (C) difficulty walking on toes
   (D) pain in lateral heel
   (E) quadriceps weakness

412. In patients with chronic low back pain, the prevalence of sacroiliac joint pain is

   (A) 10%
   (B) 15%
   (C) 20%
   (D) 25%
   (E) 30%

Questions 413 to 417

Match the following terms with the correct definitions.

413. Spondylolysis

414. Spondylolisthesis

415. Kissing spines

416. Radiculopathy

417. Radicular pain

   (A) Neurologic condition in which conduction is blocked to the axons of a spinal nerve or its roots. It results in numbness and weakness
   (B) An acquired defect caused by fatigue fracture of the pars interarticularis

   (C) Pain that arises as a result of irritation of a spinal nerve or its roots
   (D) Displacement of a vertebrae or the vertebral column in relationship to the vertebrae below it
   (E) Periostitis of spinous processes or inflammation of the affected ligament

418. Evidence regarding the value of epidural injections for the management of chronic spinal pain demonstrates the following:

   (A) Limited with interlaminar lumbar epidural steroid injections for short-term relief of lumbar radicular pain
   (B) Strong with interlaminar lumbar epidural steroid injections for long-term relief of lumbar radicular pain
   (C) Moderate for lumbar transforaminal epidural steroid injections for short-term relief of lumbar radicular pain
   (D) Strong for lumbar transforaminal epidural steroid injections for long-term relief of lumbar radicular pain
   (E) Strong for caudal epidural steroid injections for short-term relief of lumbar radiculopathy and post–lumbar laminectomy syndrome

419. All of the following statements regarding intervertebral disc innervation are true, EXCEPT

   (A) nerve plexuses that innervate the intervertebral discs are derived from dorsal rami
   (B) in normal lumbar intervertebral discs, nerve fibers are only found in the outer third of the annulus fibrosis
   (C) discs painful on discography and removed with operation have nerve growth deep into the annulus and into the nucleus pulposus
   (D) disc fissuring is a trigger for neo-innervation of a disc
   (E) the anterior and posterior nerve plexuses accompany the anterior and posterior longitudinal ligaments

420. Three days after a lumbar epidural steroid injection was given, a 57-year-old male complains of fever and severe back pain over the site where the injection was given. Two days later, the back pain has progressively worsened, and a severe radiating pain goes down the right leg and knee. Which of the following is the most likely complication of the epidural steroid injection?

(A) Epidural abscess
(B) Epidural hematoma
(C) Arachnoiditis
(D) Anterior spinal artery syndrome
(E) Cauda equina syndrome

421. X-ray imaging is recommended for which of the following cause of low back pain?

(A) Disc bulging
(B) Cauda equina syndrome
(C) Spondylolisthesis
(D) Lateral disc herniation
(E) Spinal cord tumors

422. Which of the following nerve root and muscle motion combinations is correct?

(A) L2—leg extension
(B) L3—heel walking
(C) L4—toe walking
(D) L5—first toe dorsiflexion
(E) S1—hip flexion

423. Which of the following is the most frequent complication of a laminotomy with discectomy?

(A) Recurrent disc herniation
(B) Infection
(C) Dural tear
(D) Neural injury
(E) Failed back surgery syndrome (FBSS)

424. Which of the following includes conservative treatment for FBSS?

(A) Discectomy
(B) Chemonucleolysis
(C) Rehabilitation
(D) Laminectomy
(E) Fusion

425. Favorable prognostic indicators for patients undergoing repeated lumbosacral surgery include all of the following, EXCEPT

(A) female sex
(B) satisfactory outcome from prior surgeries
(C) operative findings of disk herniation
(D) epidural scarring requiring lysis of adhesions
(E) radicular pain

426. Waddell signs were developed to help identify nonorganic causes of low back pain. They include all of the following, EXCEPT

(A) tenderness
(B) stimulation
(C) distraction testing
(D) regional disturbance
(E) underreaction

427. A 25-year-old male presents with progressively worsening neck and back pain and stiffness over 4 months that improves with light exercise and warm showers. Which of the following is the most likely diagnosis?

(A) Rheumatoid arthritis
(B) Ankylosing spondylitis
(C) Psoriatic arthritis
(D) Klippel-Feil syndrome
(E) Reiter syndrome

428. Which of the following is a major criteria for cervicogenic headache?

(A) Bilateral head or face pain without sideshift
(B) Pain is superficial and throbbing
(C) Restricted neck range of motion
(D) Pain relief with digital pressure to cervical vertebrae
(E) Lack of relief from anesthetic blockade

429. Neurogenic claudication can be distinguished from vascular claudication by which of the following?

(A) Leg tightness
(B) Pain alleviated with standing

(C) Pain exacerbated with lumbar flexion

(D) No change in pain with exercise

(E) Pain exacerbated with lying supine

430. Neck pain has been suggested to have a multifactorial origin. Which of the following statements regarding neck pain is true?

(A) Workplace interventions are not effective at reducing neck pain

(B) Normal degenerative changes in the cervical spine are a risk factor for pain

(C) Physical activity does not protect against neck pain

(D) Precision work does not increase the risk of neck pain

(E) Social support in the workplace does not affect neck pain

431. In patients with neck pain, what is more predictive at excluding a structural lesion or neurologic compression than at diagnosing any specific etiologic condition?

(A) MRI

(B) Discography

(C) Blood tests

(D) Physical examination

(E) Electrophysiology

432. All of the following characteristics are associated with a poor prognosis for neck pain, EXCEPT

(A) prior neck pain

(B) pain resulting from an accident

(C) passive coping techniques

(D) middle age

(E) compensation

433. Which of the following is the most common complication of fluoroscopically guided interlaminar cervical epidural injections?

(A) Nonpositional headache

(B) Vasovagal reactions

(C) Increased neck pain

(D) Fever

(E) Dural puncture

434. A 54-year-old female complains suddenly of inability to move her legs after a transforaminal epidural steroid injection. On further examination, she is found to have intact light touch sensation, sphincter disturbance, and loss of pain and temperature sensation. What is the most likely diagnosis?

(A) Cauda equina syndrome

(B) Epidural hematoma

(C) Epidural abscess

(D) Transient paraplegia

(E) Anterior spinal artery syndrome

435. A 57-year-old diabetic male presents with a new onset of neck pain over the past several hours; the pain is beginning to move down each arm equally. Two days ago he had a cervical epidural injection which he receives periodically for a herniated disc. On physical examination, his temperature is 102.4°F, his cervical spine is exquisitely tender to palpation and he complains of radicular pain down both arms. The most likely organism causing this presentation is

(A) *Pseudomonas*

(B) *Escherichia coli*

(C) *Streptococcus pneumoniae*

(D) *Hemophilus influenza*

(E) *Staphylococcus aureus*

436. The following statements are true regarding the pathologic mechanism in HIV-related neuropathy, EXCEPT

(A) HIV is found within endoneurial macrophages

(B) HIV is found within Schwann cells

(C) antisulfatide antibodies are one of the humoral factors responsible for demyelinating diseases in AIDS patients

(D) secretion of cytokines by the HIV-infected glial cells may generate tissue-specific autoimmune attack

(E) the pathologic mechanisms in HIV-related neuropathies are not well understood

437. Pain syndromes of neuropathic nature occur in approximately 40% of AIDS patients with pain. Several types of peripheral neuropathies have been described in patients with HIV and AIDS. The most common painful neuropathy encountered in patients with HIV and AIDS is

(A) mononeuritis multiplex
(B) polyradiculopathy
(C) cauda equina syndrome
(D) painful toxic neuropathy
(E) predominantly sensory neuropathy of AIDS

438. The most important pathophysiologic event in sickle cell anemia, which explains most of its clinical manifestations, is vascular occlusion. The following are the pathophysiologic processes that lead to vascular occlusion in patients with sickle cell disease (SCD), EXCEPT

(A) erythrocyte dehydration
(B) distortion of the shape of erythrocytes
(C) polymerization of the sickle cell hemoglobin on deoxygenation
(D) decreased deformability of erythrocytes
(E) decreased stickiness of erythrocytes

439. A physician has to exercise extra caution when attributing SCD patient's complaints of pain to behavioral deviations, such as drug-seeking behavior, because

(A) patients in real pain, such as sickle cell pain, do not develop addiction to opioids
(B) most patients with SCD have substance abuse and addiction, as they are exposed to opioids early in life
(C) there is a higher incidence of controlled-substance diversion in SCD patients
(D) sickle cell pain could be the prodrome of a serious and potentially fatal complication of SCD
(E) severe pain, such as sickle cell pain, should only be managed by an experienced physician subspecializing in pain management

440. What makes the pain of SCD unique in its acuteness and severity?

(A) SCD patients tend to have a decreased threshold to pain because of prolonged and early exposure to severe pain in life
(B) SCD patients have increased tolerance to opioids and opioid-related hyperalgesia
(C) SCD pain pathophysiology involves a combination of ischemic tissue damage and secondary inflammatory response
(D) Repetitive SCD crises lead to ischemic damage of the CNS and subsequent central sensitization to pain
(E) SCD patients tend to anticipate and respond with a spectacular behavioral manifestation to pain, because of its cyclic feature

441. At initial presentation, objective signs of a painful SCD crisis, such as fever, leukocytosis, joint effusions, and tenderness, occur in

(A) less than 10% of patients
(B) about 25% of patients
(C) about 50% of patients
(D) about 75% of patients
(E) more than 90% of patients

442. What percentage of hospital admissions in adult SCD patients result from acute sickle cell pain?

(A) Less than 10%
(B) About 25%
(C) About 50%
(D) About 75%
(E) More than 90%

443. Which of the following is true regarding treatment of sickle cell pain with NSAIDs?

(A) They should be completely avoided because of potential side effects
(B) They should not be administered continuously for more than 5 days
(C) They should be administered only in combination with opioids
(D) They should not be administered continuously for more than 1 month
(E) Potential morbidity from their side effects in SCD patients is the same as in the general population

444. Pharmacologic management of SCD pain includes three major classes of compounds: nonopioids, opioids, and adjuvants. Nonopioids include acetaminophen, NSAIDs, topical agents, tramadol, and corticosteroids. The following is true about Tramadol, EXCEPT

  (A) it inhibits neuronal reuptake of serotonin and norepinephrine

  (B) it acts as a weak μ-receptor agonist

  (C) it does not have a "ceiling" effect because of its safe side-effect profile

  (D) it is not associated with an addiction potential

  (E) it is a centrally acting analgesic

445. All of the following are true about chronic pain in the spinal cord injury (SCI) patient, EXCEPT

  (A) approximately two-thirds of all SCI patients suffer from chronic pain

  (B) approximately one-third of SCI patients with pain have severe pain

  (C) pain in SCI patients may lead to severe depression and even suicide

  (D) because of the overwhelmingly significant impairment of other important functions, pain is only a minor consideration in an SCI patient

  (E) pain in SCI interferes with rehabilitation and activities of daily living (ADLs)

446. In an SCI patient, chronic pain secondary to overuse is common in

  (A) neck

  (B) lower back

  (C) shoulders and arms

  (D) hips and thighs

  (E) knees and feet

447. Autonomic dysreflexia usually occurs after an SCI at

  (A) any level

  (B) above C4

  (C) above C7

  (D) above T6

  (E) above L1

448. The following is true regarding the visceral pain in an SCI patient, EXCEPT

  (A) it is unlikely that visceral pain may occur in the absence of any abdominal organ dysfunction

  (B) the pattern of visceral pain is not affected in an SCI patient, because it is transmitted through the sympathetic system, which usually bypasses the site of injury

  (C) autonomic dysreflexia cannot be triggered by visceral pain

  (D) visceral pain is always present in an SCI patient as part of the central pain syndrome

  (E) increases in spasticity or autonomic reactions may be the only indications of abdominal organ dysfunction

449. Neuropathic pain in SCI is divided into above-level, at-level, and below-level types. Depending on the type of pain, nerve root injury (peripheral component), and/or SCI (central component) may contribute to the pain. Which of the following is true?

  (A) Below-level pain has only peripheral component

  (B) At-level pain has only peripheral component

  (C) Below-level pain is usually caused by compressive mononeuropathy

  (D) Below-level pain is usually caused by CRPS

  (E) At-level pain may have both peripheral and central components

450. One of the characteristics of stimulus-evoked neuropathic pain in SCI can be temporal summation of pain. Temporal summation of pain is defined as

(A) elicitation of pain by nonnoxious stimulation

(B) pain continuing after stimulation has ceased

(C) an increased pain response to a noxious stimulus

(D) abnormal increase in pain with each repetitive stimulation

(E) pain felt in a place apart from the stimulated area

451. An axonal injury triggers a Wallerian degeneration, which is defined as

(A) degeneration of the portion of the axon separated from the neuronal body by the injury

(B) degeneration of the injured neuron distal and proximal to the level of injury

(C) atrophy of the motor unit supplied by the injured neuron

(D) dying of the body of the neuron, which lost its axon

(E) degeneration of the secondary afferent neuron because of the absence of the input from the injured primary afferent neuron

452. Which of the following is true about the central cord syndrome?

(A) It is the injury of the mid-portion of the spinal cord, usually around T6 level

(B) Upper extremities are affected more than lower

(C) It is very uncommon

(D) Patient usually presents with absent perianal sensation

(E) It is usually associated with complete SCI

453. A common sensory symptom in patients with CRPS is hyperpathia which may be defined as

(A) normally innocuous stimuli are perceived as painful

(B) exaggerated pain perception after a noxious stimulus at the site of injury

(C) exaggerated pain perception after a noxious stimulus in the area surrounding the primary affected skin

(D) exaggerated delayed painful perception after a noxious stimulus

(E) unpleasant abnormal sensation, whether spontaneous or evoked

454. Common findings in patients with CRPS I include

(A) symmetrical distal extremity pain

(B) pain intensity that is usually proportional to the intensity of the initiating event

(C) nearly all patients with CRPS I having sweating abnormalities

(D) sensory abnormalities that are most often proximal

(E) consistency between the inciting lesion and the spatial distribution of the pain

455. Late changes observed in patients with CRPS I include

(A) sensory abnormalities

(B) warm extremities

(C) distal swelling

(D) trophic changes

(E) increased dermal blood flow

456. Which of the following is true in relation to CRPS?

(A) Males are more commonly affected than females

(B) CRPS II is more common than CRPS I

(C) Three bone scan showing unilateral periarticular uptake is mandatory to confirm CRPS diagnosis

(D) The diagnosis of CRPS is mainly clinical

(E) The mean age group is between 15 and 25 years

457. Which of the following is the diagnostic criteria that differentiates CRPS II from CRPS I?

(A) Triple-phase bone scan showing diffuse spotty osteoporosis

(B) Weakness of all muscles of the affected extremity

(C) Sweating abnormalities

(D) Lesion of a peripheral nerve structure is mandatory

(E) Paresis

458. Patients with CRPS exhibit significant psychologic findings, including

(A) the most common psychiatric comorbidities are anxiety and depression

(B) increased incidence of somatization in patients with CRPS than to patients with chronic low back pain

(C) psychiatric problems are the cause of CRPS

(D) CRPS is a psychogenic condition

(E) maladaptive behaviors in CRPS patients indicate the presence of psychopathology

459. The Lewis triple response consists of the following, EXCEPT

(A) activation and sensitization of cutaneous C fibers elicit local edema

(B) reddening of the skin at the site of the stimulus

(C) spreading flare

(D) local peripheral vasoconstriction mediated by the release of substance P

460. The diagnosis of myofascial pain syndrome is confirmed when

(A) the myofascial trigger point is identified by palpation

(B) a patient has a widespread muscle condition

(C) a patient is diagnosed with fibromyalgia first

(D) regional muscle spasms are noted

(E) none of the above

461. Four experienced physicians examine a patient. They all identify the same precise localization of trigger points within a muscle. The minimum criteria that must be satisfied in order to distinguish a myofascial trigger point from any other tender area in muscle are

(A) a taut band and a tender point in that taut band

(B) a local twitch response

(C) referred pain

(D) reproduction of the person's symptomatic pain

(E) A and C

462. A 23-year-old female is found to have a trigger point in the left trapezius muscle. With regard to electrical characteristics of the trigger point, which of the following is false?

(A) A characteristic electrical discharge emanates from the trigger point

(B) Spontaneous EMG activity typical of end-plate noise occurring in myofascial trigger points has been further confirmed in a study of young subjects with chronic shoulder and arm pain

(C) The sympathetic nervous system does not have a modulating effect on the motor activity of the trigger point

(D) End-plate noise without spikes was found at trigger point sites to a significantly greater degree than at end-plate zones outside of trigger points, and not at all in taut band sites outside of an end-plate zone

(E) All the above statements are true

463. Manual therapy is one of the four basic treatment options used for inactivating trigger points. Some practitioners also incorporate the stretch and spray technique. It is therapeutic

- (A) because like with other soothing sprays, the placebo effect is extremely high
- (B) because the vapocoolant spray stimulates thermal and tactile A-β skin receptors, thereby inhibiting C fiber and A-δ fiber afferent nociceptive pathways and muscle spasms, myofascial trigger points, and pain when stretching
- (C) because the vapocoolant is focused specifically on the trigger point
- (D) because therapists don't have to be as liberal when passively stretching patients
- (E) B and D

464. Which of the following is not an effective myofascial release technique?

- (A) Strumming
- (B) Perpendicular and oscillating mobilizations
- (C) Therapeutic ultrasound
- (D) Connective tissue massage
- (E) Pétrissage

465. Trigger points can theoretically be related to underlying articular dysfunction. Joint and muscular dysfunction is closely related and should be considered as a single functional unit. It has been noted that

- (A) restrictions in joint capsules inhibit function for those muscles overlying the particular joint, but muscle dysfunction does not result in joint capsule restrictions
- (B) restrictions in joint capsules do not inhibit adjacent muscles, nor does muscular dysfunction result in joint capsule restrictions
- (C) restrictions in joint capsules inhibit muscle function for those muscles overlying the particular joint. Conversely, muscle dysfunction results in joint capsule restrictions

- (D) restrictions in joint capsules do not severely limit the overlying muscles; however, muscle dysfunction does regulate joint capsule range of motion
- (E) muscle dysfunction does not result in joint capsule range of motion

466. An administrative assistant presents with a number of upper back trigger points. She is scheduled for dry needling. What is the most common indication for this therapeutic modality?

- (A) Relief of an acute myofascial pain syndrome
- (B) To identify a myofascial trigger point as the cause of a particular pain
- (C) To eliminate a trigger point permanently
- (D) Inactivation of myofascial trigger points to facilitate physical therapy
- (E) None of the above

467. Randomized, double-blind, controlled studies have shown that adding which of the following medications to local anesthetics increases the pain relief obtained from myofascial trigger point injections?

- (A) Steroids
- (B) Ketorolac
- (C) Vitamin B_{12}
- (D) Diphenhydramine
- (E) None of the above

468. Which of the following is not a complication of trigger point injections?

- (A) Local hemorrhage into muscle
- (B) Infection
- (C) Transient nerve block
- (D) Syncope
- (E) Torticollis

469. Two days after a trigger point injection, a patient presents to your office irate. He claims that the trigger point injection has not helped him whatsoever. Which one of the following is not a likely reason why you are having this problem?

(A) You missed the trigger point during needling

(B) The patient is not motivated to improve

(C) You injected the secondary or satellite trigger point and not the primary trigger point

(D) Insufficient muscle stretching in the clinic after the injection

(E) Not enough stretching by the patient at home

470. Mechanical precipitating factors can cause unrelenting musculoskeletal pain. The major mechanical factors that practitioners must consider in treating myofascial pain syndrome include anatomic variations, poor posture, and work-related stress. Of the anatomic variations, which of the following are the most common?

(A) Leg length discrepancy and small hemipelvis

(B) Short femur syndrome

(C) Long great toe syndrome

(D) Kyphosis

(E) All of the above

471. What nutritional or hormonal factors have repeatedly been found to be low in persons with persistent myofascial pain?

(A) Iron

(B) Folic acid

(C) Vitamin B_{12}

(D) Thyroid hormone

(E) All of the above

472. Biologic aberrations seen in most patients with fibromyalgia include all of the following, EXCEPT

(A) lowered pain thresholds to pressure induced pain

(B) disordered sleep as evidenced by polysomnography

(C) increased spinal fluid levels of substance P

(D) decreased spinal fluid levels of nerve growth factor (NGF)

(E) no physiological or biochemical evidence for central sensitization

473. Of the following criteria, which are absolutely necessary for the classification of fibromyalgia syndrome?

(A) Widespread pain for at least 3 months

(B) Pain sensitivity to 4 kg of digital pressure at a minimum of 11 of 18 anatomically defined tender points

(C) Diagnosis after the age of 18 years

(D) A and B

(E) A, B, and C

474. Which of the following is not one of the 18 potential locations for tender points in fibromyalgia?

(A) Occiput, at the suboccipital muscle insertion

(B) Low cervical, at the anterior aspects of the intertransverse spaces at C5-C7

(C) Lumbar paraspinal musculature, from the level of L3 to L5

(D) Lateral epicondyle, extensor muscle, 2 cm distal to the epicondyle

(E) Knees, at the medial fat pad proximal to the joint line and condyle

475. A 60-year-old female recently diagnosed with fibromyalgia has been exhibiting signs of anxiety and depression and is now in treatment. This situation

(A) makes perfect sense because fibromyalgia is a psychogenic disorder

(B) relates to the fact that a subgroup of fibromyalgia patients concurrently have depression and anxiety, although an affective disorder is unlikely to cause fibromyalgia

(C) demonstrates a patient who is less likely to exhibit signs of depression than one who has not sought out medical care

(D) exhibits a patient who was probably abused as a child

(E) none of the above

476. Which of the following does not occur often as a clinical manifestation of the fibromyalgia syndrome?

    (A) Irritable bladder syndrome
    (B) Irritable bowel syndrome
    (C) Urinary urgency
    (D) Dizziness and light-headedness
    (E) A and D

477. A 50-year-old female with fibromyalgia complains of trouble sleeping. You are not surprised as it is well-known that these patients

    (A) awaken in the morning feeling stiff, cognitively sluggish, and unrefreshed by their sleep
    (B) commonly awaken feeling distressingly alert after only a few hours of sleep (mid insomnia) and then are unable to sleep soundly again until near morning (terminal insomnia)
    (C) don't have trouble napping during the day
    (D) A and B
    (E) A, B, and C

478. Which one of the following statements is false regarding fatigue in fibromyalgia?

    (A) It should always be attributed to the fibromyalgia itself
    (B) It is rarely induced by medications
    (C) It manifests as a feeling of weakness as opposed to the feeling of tiredness felt in chronic fatigue syndrome
    (D) A and B
    (E) A, B, and C

479. Secondary fibromyalgia refers to

    (A) fibromyalgia that does not interfere with a patient's functioning
    (B) fibromyalgia that occurs in the setting of another painful condition or inflammatory disorder
    (C) a multifocal pain syndrome that occurs only after a patient has been diagnosed with dysthymia

    (D) fibromyalgia that meets all the other characteristics of the disease but only produces between 8 and 10 tender points
    (E) none of the above

480. A very inquisitive 40-year-old female, recently diagnosed with fibromyalgia, states that she has been reading about her condition on the Internet. She wants to know about substance P. You tell her that

    (A) substance P is a pronociceptive neurochemical mediator of pain because it carries or amplifies afferent signals
    (B) substance P levels in the patients with fibromyalgia have been found to be significantly higher in the CSF, serum, and urine
    (C) the elevation of substance P in the CSF is a result of lowered CSF substance P esterase
    (D) the elevation in CSF substance P is indicative of fibromyalgia
    (E) A and B

481. The management objectives for fibromyalgia are

    (A) not specific because there is still no cure
    (B) reestablish emotional balance
    (C) improve sleep
    (D) restore physical function
    (E) all of the above

482. The shared decision concept

    (A) is a method where half of the treatment decisions come from the physician and half come from the ancillary staff (physical therapists, massage therapists, etc)
    (B) improves both patient and physician satisfaction
    (C) must be used on selective patients because cultural background, beliefs, and religion can all inhibit its effectiveness
    (D) A and B
    (E) A, B, and C

483. A 60-year-old female recently diagnosed with fibromyalgia wants to discuss her treatment options. She is adamant about not taking medications. Which one of the following statements is false regarding her alternatives?

(A) Relaxation techniques like progressive muscle relaxation, self-hypnosis, or biofeedback have been recommended

(B) Cognitive behavioral therapies and support groups are efficacious is some patients

(C) Aerobic exercise can yield positive outcomes

(D) Heat and cold applications can provide relief

(E) Deep massage does more harm than good

484. A PhD student comes with questions. She wants to know how dopamine and serotonin play a role in fibromyalgia pathogenesis. You tell her that

(A) dopamine levels directly correlate with pain levels

(B) tryptophan, serotonin, 5-hydroxytryptophan, and 5-hydroxyindole acetic acid have been found to be decreased in fibromyalgia patients

(C) the number of tender points in fibromyalgia patients have not been found to correlate with the concentration of serotonin in the serum

(D) dopamine agonists have been found to decrease pain in fibromyalgia patients

(E) B and D

485. No treatments seem to be working for a 45-year-old female with a 5-year history of fibromyalgia. She has talked to a relative who told her that oxycodone/acetaminophen works for all pain. How do you respond?

(A) Opioids work but only when a short-acting medication is combined with a long-acting medication

(B) In combination with pregabalin and duloxetine, hydromorphone has displayed incredible synergy in extremely depressed fibromyalgia patients

(C) Women with fibromyalgia have reduced μ-opioid receptor availability within regions of the brain that normally process and dampen pain signals

(D) Fibromyalgia is so difficult to treat that you are willing to try anything that she thinks may help

(E) You are not opposed to trying opioids, but the potential hyperalgesia has been found to be significantly worse in patients with fibromyalgia

486. Numerous medications have been used to treat the insomnia associated with fibromyalgia. Which one of the following has not been used?

(A) Amitriptyline
(B) Cyclobenzaprine
(C) Fluoxetine
(D) Clonazepam
(E) Pregabalin

Directions: For Question 487 through 605, ONE or MORE of the numbered options is correct. Choose answer

(A) if only answer 1, 2, and 3 are correct
(B) if only 1 and 3 are correct
(C) if only 2 and 4 are correct
(D) if only 4 is correct
(E) if all are correct

487. Pathophysiologic components of cancer pain can be

(1) somatic (nociceptive) pain
(2) sympathetic pain
(3) neuropathic pain
(4) central pain

488. The skeletal sites most commonly involved in osteolytic metastatic processes are

(1) ribs
(2) humerus
(3) femur
(4) tibia

489. The primary compression of the spinal cord from metastatic deposits occurs in

    (1) the thoracic spine in 70% of patients

    (2) the lumbar spine in 20% of patients

    (3) the cervical spine in 10% of patients

    (4) multiple sites of the spine in 60% of patients

490. In a patient with skeletal metastases, bisphosphonates

    (1) inhibit recruitment and function of osteoclasts

    (2) stimulate osteoblasts

    (3) have greatest effect in breast cancer and multiple myeloma

    (4) have an acute pain-relieving effect

491. The following substance(s) may be useful in treating a patient with a malignant disease:

    (1) Gabapentin

    (2) Amitriptyline

    (3) Samarium 153

    (4) Hydromorphone

492. The following is (are) the possible compilation(s) of a neurolytic celiac plexus block:

    (1) Persistent diarrhea

    (2) Aortic pseudoaneurysm

    (3) Intradiscal injection

    (4) Damage to the artery of Adamkiewicz

493. In a cancer pain patient, the following agent(s) can be used effectively via implantable intrathecal delivery system:

    (1) Opioids

    (2) α_2-Adrenergic agonists

    (3) Local anesthetics

    (4) Ziconotide

494. Which of the following conditions are the possible complications of chemotherapy in a cancer patient?

    (1) Toxic peripheral neuropathy

    (2) PHN

    (3) Avascular necrosis

    (4) Pseudorheumatism

495. As compared to younger subjects which of the following is correct about older people with pain?

    (1) There may be difficulties in determining the etiology of pain in older people

    (2) Older people generally receive significantly lower amounts of opioid analgesia

    (3) There may be increased potency of opioids

    (4) The majority of older people choose quantity of life over quality of life

496. The goals of palliative care can be summarized as follows:

    (1) To help those who need not die to live, and to live with the maximum of freedom from constraints on their quality of life arising from acute and chronic conditions of the body

    (2) To help those who can no longer live to die on time—not too early and not late

    (3) To help the dying, whether in hospital, nursing home, hospice, or at home, to die with dignity and in peace

    (4) To administer euthanasia only to the patients who truly understand the fact that their condition is terminal and who personally request it

497. Peripheral neuropathy(ies) is (are) characterized by

    (1) sensory loss

    (2) fasciculations

    (3) dysesthesias

    (4) chronic pain

498. Area(s) of acute pain processing in cortical and subcortical regions of the brain as determined by functional MRI include

    (1) anterior cingulate cortex

    (2) parietal cortex

    (3) prefrontal cortex

    (4) hypothalamus

499. Small-diameter peripheral neuropathies are commonly painful. Example(s) of these neuropathies include

(1) Ross syndrome (segmental anhidrosis)
(2) Fabry disease
(3) Charcot-Marie-Tooth disease type 1
(4) diabetic neuropathy

500. Chronic renal failure neuropathy is commonly manifested with

(1) restless leg syndrome
(2) painful neuropathy
(3) distal weakness
(4) selective loss of small nerve fibers

501. Animal studies in neuropathic pain conditions have shown

(1) intraplantar injections of interleukin 1(IL-1) reduces mechanical nociceptive threshold
(2) IL-1 hyperalgesia is mediated by bradykinin B-1 receptors
(3) effects of IL-1 on mechanical hyperalgesia seems to be mediated by prostaglandins
(4) IL-1 effects on nociceptions may be mediated by vagal afferents

502. Potential complication(s) of stellate ganglion block include

(1) pneumothorax
(2) lesion of the recurrent laryngeal nerve
(3) neuritis
(4) Horner syndrome

503. Important factor(s) involved in the development of neuropathic pain include

(1) behavioral studies have shown that NMDA is involved in the induction and maintenance of pain-related behaviors
(2) the spinal N-type voltage-dependent calcium channels are the predominant isoform involved in the pre- and postsynaptic processing of sensory nociceptive information

(3) tactile allodynia in the spinal nerve ligation model may be blocked by intrathecal N-type Ca^{2+} blockers like ziconotide
(4) after nerve injury there is upregulation of the NMDA receptors

504. Which of the following is (are) effect(s) of μ-opioid agonists in neuropathic pain conditions?

(1) Decrease dynamic allodynia
(2) Decrease temperature threshold for cold pain
(3) Decrease static allodynia
(4) μ-Opioid agonists do not have any beneficial effects in patients with neuropathic pain conditions

505. Effect(s) of GABA in the modulation of afferent nociceptive input include

(1) $GABA_A$ produces postsynaptic inhibition via metabotropic receptors, which are ligand-gated Cl^- channels
(2) the dominant type of inhibition of glutaminergic excitatory postsynaptic action potential is produce by GABA and/or glycine
(3) $GABA_B$ and adenosine produce postsynaptic hyperpolarization by activation of K^+ channels
(4) GABA and glycine produce slow activation of postsynaptic potentials

506. During the windup process

(1) sustained depolarization may recruit K^+ channels, leading to decrease in the intracellular Ca^{2+} levels
(2) cumulative recruitment of NMDA-receptor current leads to progressive relief of the Mg^{2+} blockade of the NMDA-receptor pore
(3) more intense or sustained noxious peripheral stimulation induces a decrease in the release of neuromodulator peptides, leading to an excitatory state
(4) intracellular calcium levels play a major role in the development of windup

507. In patients with PHN

   (1) histopathologic studies in patients with PHN commonly show ganglion cell loss and fibrosis

   (2) sensory loss function in the affected dermatome with increase heat pain perception is an almost universal finding

   (3) antiviral drugs used in chronic PHN usually are ineffective in alleviating pain

   (4) cold stimuli–evoked pain is more common than heat-evoked pain

508. The Special Olympics has brought together thousands of people with disabilities. Often enough, the race times in these events are significantly better than those of participants in the traditional games. In addition to undergoing the same type of grueling training regimens, however, participants in the Special Olympics often have to deal with difficulties performing activities of daily living as well as comorbidities associated with their primary disease. The likelihood that an amputee in a wheelchair race has phantom limb pain would be decreased if the

   (1) participant is a young child

   (2) participant is a male

   (3) participant is a congenital amputee

   (4) amputation is a below the knee amputation versus an above the knee amputation

509. A triple amputee (bilateral lower extremities, left upper extremity) presents to the pain clinic for work-up and treatment of phantom limb pain. This patient's pain most likely

   (1) occurs intermittently

   (2) is primarily localized to the fingers or palm of the hand in the upper extremity or toes, feet, or ankles in the bilateral lower extremities

   (3) is of stabbing, shooting, or pins and needles character

   (4) presents with attacks that last several minutes to an hour

510. True statement(s) about phantom sensations is (are):

   (1) They are less frequent than phantom pains

   (2) They usually appear 1 month after the amputation

   (3) The phantom sensation usually manifests as enlargement of the missing limb

   (4) A common position of the phantom for upper limb amputees is the fingers clenched in a fist

511. Which of the following is (are) example (s) of how the peripheral nervous system may play a role in phantom pain modulation?

   (1) Dorsal root ganglion (DRG) cells display an altered expression pattern of different sodium channels

   (2) Generation, but not maintenance of phantom pain by the sympathetic nervous system

   (3) Long after limb amputation, injection of noradrenaline around a stump neuroma is reported to be intensely painful

   (4) Phantom pain is directly related to the skin temperature of the stump

512. Phantom pains are often a replica of preamputation pain. It has also been noted that amputees with phantom pain have more often suffered from intense and long-lasting preamputation pain than have patients without phantom pain. These observations led to the premise that preemptive analgesia may help decrease postamputation pain. Of the studies done on this subject matter

   (1) most have been of very poor methodological quality

   (2) the two which included blinding and randomization showed no significant differences versus controls

   (3) the aim has been to thwart spinal sensitization by blocking the cascade of intraneuronal responses that take place after peripheral nerve injury

   (4) the sample size was always greater than 100

513. Which of the following dietary modification(s) should be made to alleviate symptoms of interstitial cystitis?

(1) Restrict spicy foods
(2) Eliminate alcohol intake
(3) Cease smoking
(4) Increase orange juice intake

514. Sodium pentosan polysulfate (Elmiron)

(1) is an antispasmodic medication
(2) is an oral analogue of heparin
(3) alleviates symptoms of interstitial cystitis by relaxing smooth musculature
(4) increases antiadherent surface of the bladder lining

515. Which of the following substance(s) is (are) thought to be involved in descending inhibition?

(1) GABA
(2) Serotonin
(3) Endogenous opioid peptides
(4) Norepinephrine

516. Which of the following is (are) the psychological factor(s) affecting pain response?

(1) Fear and helplessness
(2) Sleep deprivation
(3) Anxiety
(4) Cultural differences

517. Which of the following is (are) psychological method(s) for reducing pain?

(1) Placebo and expectation
(2) Psychological support
(3) Procedural and instructional information
(4) Cognitive coping strategies

518. Gastrointestinal (GI) impairment in a postsurgical patient can be

(1) worsened by increased sympathetic activity because of severe pain
(2) contributed to by administration of opioids

(3) mitigated by early mobilization of the patient
(4) worsened by epidural blockade with local anesthetic

519. Which of the following feature(s) suggest neuropathic pain?

(1) Pain in the area of sensory loss
(2) Good response to opioids
(3) Pain in response to nonpainful stimuli
(4) Absence of Tinel sign

520. The correct corresponding vertebral levels for optimal epidural catheter placement for various surgical procedures are

(1) T10-12 for lower abdominal surgery
(2) T8-10 for upper abdominal surgery
(3) L2-4 for lower extremity surgery
(4) C7-T2 for upper extremity surgery

521. Which of the following medications are useful in an inpatient management of a post–burn injury pain?

(1) Opioids
(2) Ketamine
(3) Benzodiazepines
(4) Nitrous oxide

522. In patients with a traumatic chest injuries thoracic epidural analgesia has been shown to significantly improve inspiratory effort, negative inspiratory force, gas exchange, ability to cough, and ability to clear bronchial secretions. The following finding may be considered relative contraindications for epidural analgesia in a patient with posttraumatic chest injury:

(1) Inadequate coagulation function
(2) Spine fractures
(3) Inadequate intravascular volume resuscitation
(4) Concomitant head injury

523. The most common characteristics of pain in PHN include

   (1) steady burning or aching

   (2) dull and poorly localized

   (3) paroxysmal and lancinating

   (4) usually not aggravated by contact with the affected skin

524. Which of the following group(s) of medications was found to be useful in treatment of PHN?

   (1) Opioids

   (2) Antiepileptic drugs

   (3) Topical agents

   (4) Antidepressants

525. Which of the following is (are) true about interventional therapy for PHN?

   (1) No proven surgical cure for PHN has been found

   (2) Cryotherapy is likely to bring only short-term relief

   (3) Topical lidocaine may provide effective analgesia for PHN

   (4) Transcutaneous nerve stimulation (TENS) has been shown to give an effective symptomatic relief in some patients

526. Antiviral agents in the acute phase of herpes zoster

   (1) competitively inhibit DNA polymerase, terminating DNA synthesis and viral replication

   (2) are generally well tolerated

   (3) hasten healing of the rash

   (4) may reduce the duration of PHN

527. Oral steroids for acute herpes zoster

   (1) are not currently recommended

   (2) may provide pain relief in the acute phase

   (3) have no benefit in prevention of PHN

   (4) have almost no side effects in patients with herpes zoster

528. Which of the following statement(s) is (are) true about diabetic amyotrophy?

   (1) It is commonly associated with pain

   (2) It responds well to a complicated multimodal treatment

   (3) Involves weakness and atrophy of the involved muscles

   (4) Sciatic nerve and its supplied muscles are most commonly affected

529. Charcot joint

   (1) affects primarily weight-bearing joints

   (2) can be caused by multiple causes other than DM

   (3) is related to the destruction of afferent proprioceptive fibers

   (4) is related to the destruction of efferent neural fibers

530. Which of the following statement(s) about treatment of diabetic peripheral neuropathic pain (DPNP) is (are) true?

   (1) Most of the antidepressants are Food and Drug Administration (FDA) approved for the treatment of DPNP

   (2) Most therapies for DPNP result in more than 90% reduction in pain

   (3) Most of the anticonvulsant drugs are FDA approved for the treatment of DPNP

   (4) NSAIDs are the most commonly utilized medications

531. Treatment of painful diabetic neuropathy (PDN) rests on modification of the underlying disease and control of pain symptoms. In turn, the modification of the underlying disease includes strict glycemic control. Which of the following is (are) true?

   (1) Tight glycemic control can halt or slow the progression of distal sensorimotor neuropathy

   (2) Hemoglobin A_{1c} target should be < 6%

(3) Euglycemia is the ideal goal

(4) Weight loss and exercise program is an important part of glycemic control in a diabetic patient

532. The current treatments of the PDN include

(1) antiepileptic drugs

(2) antidepressants

(3) opioids

(4) aldose reductase inhibitors

533. The convulsive tic

(1) is more severe in males

(2) may indicate the presence of a tumor, vascular malformation, or ecstatic dilation of the basilar artery

(3) is because of presence of bilateral facial spasms

(4) is a result of painful periodic unilateral facial contractions

534. Which of the following support(s) the diagnosis of idiopathic trigeminal neuralgia?

(1) Periods of weeks or months without pain

(2) Increase pain by commonly benign stimuli, like talking, eating, or washing

(3) Pain often alleviated by sleep

(4) Bilateral pain in the distribution of the trigeminal nerve, described as shooting or lancinating

535. Which of the following is (are) true regarding trigeminal neuralgia?

(1) Very often, trigeminal neuralgia is the presenting symptom in patients affected with multiple sclerosis

(2) Trigeminal neuralgia is 20 times more common in patients with multiple sclerosis

(3) Trigeminal neuralgia tends to occur in the early stages of multiple sclerosis

(4) Bilateral trigeminal neuralgia is seen more often than expected in patients with multiple sclerosis

536. The retrogasserian glycerol injection

(1) is a selective neurolytic agent with preference for sensory fibers, leaving intact motor neurons

(2) recurrence rates are the highest of all ablative techniques

(3) sensory loss is almost unseen in patients after this procedure

(4) sensory loss is less common than with radiofrequency thermocoagulation

537. Which of the following is (are) true for trigeminal neuralgia?

(1) Trigeminal neuralgia is the most common cranial neuralgia

(2) It is more common in females

(3) The highest incidence is in elderly patients

(4) The disease most frequently linked with trigeminal neuralgia is multiple sclerosis

538. Potential factors involved in the development of trigeminal neuralgia include

(1) ion channel upregulation in the area of the trigeminal injury

(2) focal demyelination

(3) up to 30% of patients with trigeminal neuralgia have arterial cross compression at the level root entry zone

(4) cell body degeneration in the trigeminal complex of the mesencephalon

539. Spontaneous intracranial hypotension (SIH)

(1) the most common site of idiopathic dural tears is the lower lumbar region

(2) congenital subarachnoid or Tarlov cysts are a potential site for dural weakness and rupture

(3) the most obvious difference between PDPH and SIH, is the lack of postural symptoms in the second

(4) are no characteristic findings on MRI

540. A common treatment for patients with PDPH is epidural blood patch (EBP). Which of the following is (are) true regarding this therapy?

(1) Maintenance of supine position for 2 hours after the patch provides higher chances for success

(2) As a result of the predominant caudad spread of the blood after EBP, a level of placement above the suspected dural tear is recommended

(3) The effectiveness of EBP is reduced when the dural tear was caused by a large-size needle

(4) The long-term relief of an initial EBP is close to 98%

541. The incidence of PDPH is between 1% and 75%. Factor(s) that prevent its development at the time of dural puncture include

(1) use of an interlaminar approach

(2) use of intrathecal catheter

(3) bed rest after the puncture

(4) use of small-gauge spinal needle

542. Diagnostic criteria for cervicogenic headache by the International Headache Society and the International Association for the Study of Pain (IASP) include

(1) unilateral headache

(2) relief of acute attacks by blocking the greater occipital nerve with local anesthetic

(3) aggravation of the headache with neck movements

(4) decrease range of neck motion

543. The cervicogenic headache

(1) has a prevalence of 0.4% to 2.5% in the general population and may account for up to 15% to 20% of patients with chronic headache

(2) is more common in females; a female to male ratio of 4 to 1

(3) mean age is the beginning of the fourth decade

(4) is aggravated by neck movement, and alleviated by occipital nerve block

544. The cortical spreading depression

(1) may produce the aura symptoms

(2) produces activation of the trigeminal nerve endings

(3) consist of decreased cerebral blood flow spreading forward from the occipital cortex

(4) is followed by generalized cerebral vascular dilation that explains the headache

545. In terms of migraine which of the following is (are) true?

(1) Migraine with aura is associated with an increase of cerebral blood flow that happens after the headache begins

(2) In migraine with aura there is a decrease of cerebral blood flow that starts after the headache begins

(3) In migraine without aura there is no change in cerebral blood flow

(4) In migraine without aura there is increase of cerebral blood flow before the headache begins

546. Migraine is a risk factor for

(1) major depression

(2) manic episodes

(3) anxiety disorders

(4) panic disorders

547. Migraine happens in 18% of women, 6% of men, and 6% of children. Migraine usually

(1) begins in the first three decades of life

(2) is of higher prevalence in the fifth decade

(3) decrease symptoms in the last trimester of their pregnancy in most females

(4) is improved, common after surgical menopause

548. Tension-type headache

  (1) is the result of sustained contraction of the pericranial muscles with subsequent ischemic pain

  (2) has more common onset during adolescence and young adulthood

  (3) has increased EMG activity in muscles with tenderness

  (4) reduces CNS levels of serotonin that may be responsible for abnormal pain modulation

549. For any structure to be deemed a cause of low back pain, it must have the following characteristic(s):

  (1) A nerve supply

  (2) Be capable of causing low back pain in healthy volunteers

  (3) Be susceptible to disease or injuries known to be painful

  (4) Be shown to be a source of pain in a patient using diagnostic techniques of known reliability and validity

550. Randomized controlled trials (RCTs) have generated evidence-based conclusions for preventive interventions back and neck pain. Which of the following statement(s) is (are) true based on the evidence of RCTs?

  (1) Lumbar supports are not effective in preventing neck and back pain

  (2) Exercise may be effective in preventing neck and back pain

  (3) Back schools are not effective in preventing back and neck pain

  (4) Ergonomic interventions are effective in preventing back and neck pain

551. Anomalies of lumbar nerve roots include which of the following?

  (1) Two pairs of nerve roots arise from a single dural sleeve

  (2) A dural sleeve arises from a lower position in the dural sac

  (3) The vertebral foramen is unoccupied by a nerve or contains a supernumerary set of roots

  (4) Extradural anastomoses between roots in which a bundle of nerve fibers leaves one dural sleeve to enter an adjacent one

552. Low back pain is defined as pain perceived within a region bounded

  (1) superiorly by an imaginary line through the T12 spinous process

  (2) inferiorly by a transverse line through the posterior sacrococcygeal joints

  (3) laterally by the lateral borders of the erector spinae

  (4) within the region overlying the sacrum

553. Complications of cervical transforaminal injections include which of the following?

  (1) Cerebellar infarction

  (2) Cerebral infarction

  (3) Spinal cord infarction

  (4) Anterior spinal artery syndrome

554. Discographic stimulation (formally known as discography) is considered positive if

  (1) adjacent disc stimulation causes pain

  (2) thermal stimulation with a wire electrode causes pain

  (3) pain is reproduced at pressures greater than 80 psi

  (4) pain is reproduced at pressures less than 50 psi and preferably less than 15 psi

555. The use of chemonucleolysis for lumbar disc herniations is indicated for which of the following?

  (1) Contained disc protrusions

  (2) Extruded disc herniations

  (3) Herniations unresponsive to nonsurgical management

  (4) Sequestered disc herniations

556. Causes of FBSS include which of the following?

 (1) Inappropriate selection of patients
 (2) Irreversible neural injury
 (3) Inadequate surgery
 (4) New injury to nerves and spine

557. Selection criteria for elective lumbosacral spine surgery include

 (1) radicular pain with corresponding dermatomal segmental sensory loss
 (2) abnormal imaging study showing nerve root compression
 (3) signs of segmental instability consistent with symptoms
 (4) success of conservative therapy

558. The main types of cervical involvement in rheumatoid arthritis include

 (1) atlantoaxial subluxation
 (2) cranial settling
 (3) subaxial subluxation
 (4) occipital condyle fractures

559. Whiplash and whiplash-associated disorders (WAD) comprise a range of injuries to the neck caused by or related to a sudden distortion of the neck. Characteristics include

 (1) spinal cord injury (SCI)
 (2) referred shoulder pain
 (3) sensory deficits
 (4) headaches

560. Distraction testing allows an examiner to identify neurologic and mechanical abnormalities in the cervical spine. It is characterized by

 (1) relief of neck pain
 (2) lifting head from the chin and occiput
 (3) relief of pressure on zygapophyseal joints
 (4) examiner standing in front of a standing patient

561. A 45-year-old male with complaints of cervical neck pain radiating down his left arm is examined by a physician. With one particular maneuver, his pain is exactly reproduced. The test(s) that can reproduce his symptoms include

 (1) distraction testing
 (2) Valsalva test
 (3) spurling maneuver
 (4) Adson test

562. The following are true about HIV infection–related neuropathies, EXCEPT

 (1) inflammatory demyelinating polyneuropathies occur early in the course of HIV infection
 (2) vasculitis-related neuropathies occur midcourse in HIV infection
 (3) distal sensory neuropathies occur late in HIV infection
 (4) HIV-related neuropathies tend to be nonspecific to the stage of HIV infection

563. Which of the following is (are) true about the predominantly sensory neuropathy of AIDS?

 (1) The predominant symptom is pain in the soles of the feet
 (2) Ankle jerks are often absent or reduced
 (3) As symptoms of the neuropathy progress, they usually remain confined to the feet
 (4) EMG demonstrate sensory, but not motor involvement

564. Which of the following group(s) of medication(s) is (are) useful in treatment of pain in HIV and AIDS patients?

 (1) Opioids
 (2) Anticonvulsants
 (3) Psychostimulants
 (4) Antidepressants

565. Pathophysiologic tissue injury in SCD generates multiple pain mediators. The facilitators of the pain transmission include

 (1) bradykinin
 (2) serotonin
 (3) substance P
 (4) dynorphin

566. Which of the following established four components of SCD is responsible/associated with the patient's pain?

(1) Anemia and its sequelae

(2) Organ failure

(3) Comorbid conditions

(4) Pain syndromes

567. Which of the following statement(s) is (are) true about avascular necrosis (AVN) and SCD?

    (1) Core decompression is an effective treatment of late stages of the AVN

    (2) Treatment of AVN is mostly symptomatic

    (3) AVN affects mostly femoral head

    (4) AVN is the most common complication of SCD in adults

568. Which of the following statement(s) is (are) true about leg ulceration and SCD?

    (1) Leg ulcers occur in 5% to 10% of the adult SCD patients

    (2) Skin grafting is a very effective treatment for chronic leg ulcers in SCD patients

    (3) Many leg ulcers heal within a few months with good localized treatment

    (4) Regranex, used to treat leg ulcers, contains an autologous platelet-derived growth factor

569. Management of painful vasoocclusive crises in SCD patients frequently employs supplemental oxygen. Which of the following is (are) true about the supplemental oxygen administration in SCD patients?

    (1) Supplemental low-flow oxygen is often given to patients with SCD painful crisis in efforts to diminish the number of reversibly sickled cells

    (2) There is little supportive data for the use of supplemental oxygen in SCD patients

    (3) Routine oxygen administration in the absence of hypoxemia may impair reticulocytosis in SCD patients

    (4) Routine oxygen administration in the absence of hypoxemia has no proven benefit in SCD patients

570. Which of the following statement(s) is (are) true about epidemiology of SCD?

    (1) It is the most common hemoglobinopathy in the United States

    (2) The prevalence is significantly higher in the African American population than in the general population

    (3) It occurs in 0.3% to 1.3% of the African American population

    (4) The prevalence of SCD does not depend on the ethnic background of the population

571. Which of the following is (are) the measure(s) used to treat vasoocclusive crises of SCD during pregnancy?

    (1) Aggressive hydration

    (2) Supplemental oxygen in patients with hypoxemia

    (3) Partial exchange transfusions

    (4) Prophylactic transfusions

572. When an opioid-tolerant patient in a sickle cell vasoocclusive crisis is admitted to a hospital, which of the following step(s) should be taken?

    (1) A baseline opioid infusion should be started immediately at an equianalgesic dose to patient's home opioid requirement

    (2) A baseline infusion should be supplemented with a patient-controlled analgesia (PCA) on demand for breakthrough pain

    (3) As patient's new opioid requirement becomes known from the PCA history, conversion to a combination of long- and immediate-release opioid can be undertaken

    (4) Fast opioid dose increases may lead to hypoxemia and/or hypercarbia, which may exacerbate sickling of erythrocytes

573. Autonomic dysreflexia

    (1) is usually triggered by a spontaneous sympathetic discharge above the SCI level
    (2) is rarely associated with headache
    (3) is never life-threatening
    (4) manifests itself with increased blood pressure

574. Which of the following is (are) true about the anterior cord syndrome?

    (1) It is characterized by complete sensory loss
    (2) Prognosis for motor function recovery is very poor
    (3) It is a complete SCI syndrome
    (4) It is characterized by complete motor function loss

575. Which of the following is (are) true about the posterior cord syndrome?

    (1) It is characterized by preservation of temperature sensation
    (2) It is characterized by preservation of normal gait
    (3) It is uncommon
    (4) It is characterized by preservation of proprioception

576. Which of the following is (are) true feature(s) of Brown-Séquard SCI syndrome?

    (1) Ipsilateral motor deficit
    (2) Contralateral pain sensation deficit
    (3) Contralateral temperature sensation deficit
    (4) Uncommonness

577. Anticonvulsants are commonly used for the treatment of neuropathic pain in the SCI patients. Which of the following correctly describe(s) their pharmacologic actions?

    (1) Modulation of calcium channels
    (2) Modulation of sodium channels
    (3) Increase of GABA inhibition
    (4) Blockade of reuptake of norepinephrine

578. Which of the following is (are) the usual symptom(s) of the autonomic dysreflexia?

    (1) Dramatic rise in blood pressure
    (2) Flushing and sweating in areas above the SCI
    (3) Marked reduction in peripheral blood flow
    (4) Decline in heart rate

579. Heterotopic ossification (HO) is commonly seen in patients with traumatic brain injury (TBI), cerebral vascular accident, burns, trauma, total joint arthroplasty, and SCI. Which of the following is (are) true about HO in SCI patients?

    (1) It is always painful
    (2) Hip is the most commonly affected
    (3) It is defined as ossification inside the joint capsule
    (4) Osteoclast inhibitors are use for both treatment and prophylaxis of HO

580. CRPS in the initial stages may be associated with

    (1) neurogenic inflammation
    (2) higher local levels of tumor necrosis factor alpha
    (3) high systemic CGRP levels
    (4) Increase in protein concentration in fluid of affected joints

581. Which of the following is true about motor abnormalities in CRPS?

    (1) Dystonia of the hand or affected foot occurs in about 30% of the patients in the acute stages
    (2) Decrease active range of motion and increase amplitude of physiological tremor is seen in about 50% of the patients
    (3) They are likely related to an abnormal peripheral process
    (4) They may be explained by abnormalities in the cerebral motor processing

582. In terms of CRPS which of the following is (are) true?

    (1) Incidence of CRPS is 20% after brain lesion

    (2) Affected extremities after brain injury are at higher risk of developing CRPS than unaffected

    (3) CRPS following SCI is frequent

    (4) Upper extremities are more commonly affected than lower extremities

583. Which of the following is true regarding bone scintigraphy?

    (1) The three stages of the three-phase bone scan include the perfusion, blood-pool, and mineralization phases

    (2) Homogeneous unilateral hyperperfusion in the perfusion phase is consistent with CRPS

    (3) Homogeneous unilateral hyperperfusion in the blood-pool phase is consistent with CRPS

    (4) Patients with CRPS show increase unilateral periarticular trace uptake in the mineralization phase

584. Which of the following is true regarding C fiber impulses?

    (1) After sensitization, antidromic impulses to peripheral C fiber terminals release vasoactive substance

    (2) Neurally released substances trigger neurogenic inflammation

    (3) Neurogenic inflammation includes axonal reflex, vasodilation, and plasma extravasation

    (4) C fiber activation peripherally releases CGRP and substance P

585. The major peripheral pathologic finding(s) in patients with CRPS is (are)

    (1) patch atrophy of some muscle cells

    (2) capillary microangiopathy

    (3) Wallerian degeneration

    (4) generalized osteopenia

586. Which of the following is (are) true regarding CRPS?

    (1) Medical procedures are the second most common cause of CRPS

    (2) Decrease deep tendon reflexes are a result of muscle atrophy

    (3) Cutaneous dynamic mechanical allodynia is a hallmark of central sensitization

    (4) Hypoesthesia may be rarely seen in patients with CRPS

587. Characteristics of CRPS I in pediatrics include

    (1) CRPS I is more common in girls

    (2) the lower extremity is more often affected

    (3) CRPS may have genetic predisposition

    (4) CRPS is more common in Hispanics

588. Characteristics of CRPS II in pediatrics include

    (1) the incidence is similar in boys and girls

    (2) brachial plexus injury during delivery commonly leads to chronic pain

    (3) Erb palsy do not generally develop CRPS

    (4) patients with Erb palsy need a comprehensive treatment to avoid the development of CRPS II

589. To confirm the diagnosis of CRPS:

    (1) There are no laboratory tests to confirm the diagnosis

    (2) Disturbed vascular scintigraphy is necessary to make the diagnosis of CRPS

    (3) Bone scan is nonspecific for the diagnosis of CRPS

    (4) There is no utility in ordering bone scan in patients with CRPS

590. Which of the following is true regarding movement disorders in CRPS patients?

    (1) Motor dysfunction is the result of voluntary defensive response to protect the limb from painful stimuli

    (2) Deep tendon reflexes in these patients are normal to brisk

    (3) Movement disorders often happen in early stages of the disease

    (4) Akinesia is a prominent finding in CRPS patients

591. In terms of CRPS and dystonia, which is characterized by involuntary contractions of one or more muscles, it can be said that

    (1) dystonia is a prominent feature of CRPS

    (2) dystonia in patients with CRPS typically presents with flexure postures

    (3) tonic dystonia often spares the first two digits

    (4) extensor postures occur early in the development of dystonia

592. Supraspinal regulatory mechanisms that may explain some of the features of CRPS include

    (1) spread of cortical representation of the affected limb

    (2) patients with generalized dystonia have increased intracortical excitability to sensory stimuli

    (3) motor cortical disinhibition

    (4) early increase activity of the thalamus contralateral to the affected limb

593. Which of the following is (are) myofascial trigger point characteristic(s)?

    (1) Weakness with muscle atrophy

    (2) Referral of pain to a distant site upon activation of the trigger point

    (3) Range of motion not restricted

    (4) Autonomic phenomenon, such as piloerection or changes in local circulation (regional blood flow and limb temperature) in response to trigger point activation

594. The definitive goal of treatment of persons with myofascial pain syndrome is (are)

    (1) restoration of function through inactivation of the trigger point

    (2) restoration of normal tissue mobility

    (3) relief of pain

    (4) increased range of motion

595. Inactivation of the myofascial trigger point can be accomplished

    (1) manually

    (2) by direct injection of a local anesthetic into the muscle

    (3) by dry needle intramuscular stimulation of the myofascial trigger point

    (4) by correcting structural mechanical stressors

596. With regard to trigger point injections, botulinum toxin which of the following is true?

    (1) Has been tried unsuccessfully in myofascial trigger point inactivation

    (2) Can cause a flulike myalgia

    (3) Occasionally causes weakness that is confined to the area of injection

    (4) Is a long-lasting trigger point injection capable of about a 3 month inactivation of the trigger point

597. A 40-year-old female with chronic myofascial neck pain wants to go to an acupuncturist. She should know that

    (1) in one study it was found that shallow needling reduced the pain of chronic myofascial neck pain

    (2) in a randomized, double-blind, sham-controlled study, acupuncture was found to be superior to dry needling in improving range of motion

(3) in a randomized, double-blind, sham-controlled study, acupuncture was found to be better than placebo when treating trigger points in chronic neck pain

(4) in a randomized, double-blind, controlled study, acupuncture was found to be better than control only when it was followed by transcutaneous electrical stimulation

598. A 40-year-old woman comes to the pain clinic for initial evaluation. After a thorough history and physical examination, the patient is diagnosed with fibromyalgia. Which symptom(s) would support your diagnosis of fibromyalgia as opposed to myofascial pain syndrome?

(1) Widespread pain
(2) Irritable bowel syndrome
(3) Distal paresthesias
(4) Occipital headaches

599. Which of the following is (are) true of fibromyalgia?

(1) Adult women are twice as likely to be affected as adult men
(2) Prevalence peaks in the fourth decade of life
(3) Many children diagnosed with fibromyalgia will have worsening of their symptoms as they reach adulthood
(4) Affects all ethnic groups

600. Risk factors for the development of fibromyalgia syndrome include

(1) physical trauma
(2) febrile illness
(3) family history of fibromyalgia
(4) history of sexual abuse

601. Sleep disturbances are common in patients with fibromyalgia. Difficulties the patient may encounter include

(1) problems initiating sleep
(2) awakening in the middle of the night
(3) light, unrefreshing sleep
(4) difficulty napping throughout the day

602. Pathophysiologically, fibromyalgia

(1) is a disorder of abnormal processing of sensory information within the CNS
(2) exhibits a narrow array of recognized objective physiological and biologic abnormalities
(3) patients demonstrate abnormally low regional cerebral blood flow in thalamic nuclei and other pain-processing brain structures that is inversely correlated with spinal fluid substance P levels
(4) demonstrates abnormal spinal cord windup

603. That same patient (who happens to be a neurobiology graduate student) starts to ask about the role that cytokines play in fibromyalgia. You tell her that

(1) IL-8 has been found to be significantly higher in the serum of fibromyalgia patients, especially in depressed patients
(2) IL-6 was not found to be increased in the blood of fibromyalgia patients
(3) the production of IL-8 in vitro is stimulated by substance P
(4) cytokines do not play a role in the pathogenesis of fibromyalgia

604. Which of the following medications are FDA approved for the treatment of fibromyalgia?

(1) Cyclobenzaprine
(2) Duloxetine
(3) Tramadol
(4) Pregabalin

605. The pain in fibromyalgia is, at least in part, mediated by central sensitization. Studies have shown that

(1) dextromethorphan and ketamine may improve pain and allodynia in fibromyalgia patients
(2) the majority of patients with fibromyalgia that tried ketamine benefited
(3) ketamine's efficacy was limited because of its side effects
(4) dextromethorphan had a similar side-effect profile

Answers and Explanations

332. (D) If a patient routinely uses breakthrough medications, the daily total amount should be converted to a sustained-release dose and added to the current maintenance dose.

333. (B) Approximately 3% of pain syndromes in cancer patients are unrelated to the underlying malignancy or cancer treatment. Most commonly, pain is caused by degenerative disc disease, arthritis, fibromyalgia, or migraine and has often predated the diagnosis of cancer.

334. (B) Segmental nerve conduction slowing, fibrillation potentials, positive sharp waves, and decreased amplitude CMAPs are all helpful in determining the presence of brachial plexopathy in general. Myokymia is present in 63% of patients with radiation fibrosis induced brachial plexopathy. Brachial plexopathy caused by direct tumor infiltration has a low incidence of myokymia. *Myokymia* is a continuous but brief involuntary muscle twitching that gives the appearance of wormlike rippling of the muscle. It can be determined very distinctly by EMG.

335. (D) A 5-year survival for a cancer patient with documented skeletal metastases varies widely depending on location of the primary tumor: myeloma—10%; breast—20%; prostate—25%; lung—less than 5%; kidney—10%; thyroid—40%; melanoma—less than 5%.

336. (C) Reflex asymmetry occurs in 67% of patients with carcinomatous meningitis and is the most frequent spinal cord–related sign. The frequency of nuchal rigidity, back pain, positive straight leg raise test, and weakness is 11%, 25%, 13%, and 33%, respectively.

337. (E) Central pain syndromes are relatively rare in cancer patients. Although epidural spinal cord compression is almost always painful, central pain is not the predominant symptom. Nociceptive input from progressive bony destruction by metastases is the usual cause of pain, with or without concurrent radicular pain from nerve root compression. Radiation myelopathy is the central pain syndrome.

338. (A) The most common pattern of pain in patients with epidural metastasis is local. *Local pain* over the involved vertebral body, which results from the involvement of the vertebral periosteum, is dull and exacerbated by recumbency.

Radicular pain from compressed or damaged nerve roots is usually unilateral in the cervical and lumbosacral regions and bilateral in the thorax. The pain is experienced in the overlying spine, deep in certain muscles supplied by the compressed root, and in the cutaneous distribution of the injured root.

Referred pain has a deep aching quality and is often associated with tenderness of subcutaneous tissues and muscles at the site of referral. The typical examples of referred pain pattern include buttocks and posterior thigh pain with lumbosacral spine involvement; pain in the flank, groin, and anterior thigh in the upper lumbar spine involvement; midscapular and shoulder pain in the cervicothoracic epidural disease.

Funicular pain usually occurs some distance below the site of compression and it has hot or cold qualities in a poorly localized nondermatomal distribution. It presumably results from compression of the ascending sensory tracts in the spinal cord.

339. **(C)** The WHO analgesic ladder is based on the premise that most patients throughout the world gain adequate pain relief if health care professionals learn how to use a few effective and relatively inexpensive drugs well. Step 1 of the ladder involves the use of nonopioids. If this step is ineffective, go to step 2 and add an opioid for mild to moderate pain. Step 3 substitutes an opioid for moderate to severe pain in step 2. Only one drug from each group should be used at a time. Adjuvant drugs can be used in all steps.

340. **(D)** Methadone has a variable oral bioavailability between 41% and 99% and, therefore, should be started with extra caution (low initial dose and slow subsequent increases). Methadone differs from all other opioids by its noncompetitive antagonist activity at the NMDA receptors. Activation of NMDA receptors has been shown to play a role in development of tolerance to analgesic effects of opioids, as well as in the pathologic sensory states, such as neuropathic pain, inflammatory pain, ischemic pain, allodynia, and spinal states of hypersensitivity.

341. **(C)** As a rough guide for conversion, the 8-hourly dose of MS Contin (225/3 = 75 mg in this case) can be considered equal to the micrograms per hour dose of TTS-fentanyl. In one study, most people had satisfactory pain profiles with frequency of administration of every 3 days. Only in 24% of subjects in the study required different frequency of administration varying from 48 to 60 hours.

342. **(C)**

A. The most common cause of central pain states are spinal cord lesions.

B. The Wallenberg syndrome is usually vascular in origin, and characterized by crossed sensory findings that include ipsilateral facial sensory loss, Horner syndrome, and

contralateral body impairment of pain and temperature loss.

C. The most common lesions that produce thalamic pain syndrome are infarctions, followed by arteriovenous malformations (AVMs), neoplasms, abscesses, plaque of multiple sclerosis, traumatic injury, and others.

D. Spinal cord lesions are the most common cause of central pain syndromes and present with areas of sensory loss resulting from disruption of the spinothalamic tract.

E. The treatment of central pain of spinal origin is complex with poor response to most forms of therapy.

343. **(C)** Sensory symmetric impairment is commonly seen distally with progression to more proximal areas of the limbs as the disease progresses. Peripheral polyneopathy is the most common initial manifestation of diabetes mellitus. The nerve conduction studies measure only the fastest conducting fibers, leaving injury of small-diameter fibers, which transmit pain sensations, undiagnosed.

344. **(B)** Following nerve injury there is an increase in the expression of sodium channels in the neuroma and in the DRG. Consistent with the role of sodium channels in the development of neuropathic pain is blockage of their activity by low plasma concentrations of lidocaine. A reduction in potassium channel activity leads to increased afferent activity. The largest population of afferent axons is C-polymodal nociceptors that are activated by high-threshold mechanical, thermal, and chemical stimuli.

345. **(D)** Raynaud phenomenon is not a neuropathic pain condition, but rather a vascular condition (although, potentially sympathetically mediated and/or sustained).

346. **(C)** Although not completely known some conditions predispose to the development of neuropathic pain. The relative frequency is 5% for patients with traumatic nerve injury, 8% for patients after stroke, 28% for patients with multiple sclerosis, and 75% for patients with syringomyelia. Neuropathies with predominant

involvement of large myelinated fibers are usually not painful.

347. **(C)** We do not know if it is sympathetically mediated (B) from the block since this does not provide evidence of etiology. We do not know the involvement of vascularity since the block is affecting sympathetic outflow and precludes vascular evidence (which could be mediated by a host of other physiologic events). There is no clinical evidence to support a less severe case (D) and, the evidence suggests that it will respond to spinal cord stimulation (E).

348. **(E)** Central sensitization is the reason for many of the symptoms including allodynia and hyperalgesia. Therefore, all are correct.

349. **(E)** Cytokines are inflammatory mediators released by a variety of cells that regulate the inflammatory response. Systemic or local injection of cytokines in animal models causes mechanical and thermal hyperalgesia. Cytokines may cause excitation of nociceptors via the release of other mediators, like prostaglandins. At the level of the CNS, cytokines may be liberated by microglial cells. The best studied excitatory amino acid is glutamate. Glutamate may bind to ionotopic or metabotropic glutamate receptors. Peripheral and central activation of those receptors induces pain behaviors in animals. All basic science evidence suggests (A) and (B), but does not suggest (C).

350. **(B)** Following tissue damage, there is a decrease of the threshold for noxious stimuli (hyperalgesia), which may be associated to perception of pain to normally innocuous stimuli. This phenomenon is termed allodynia. Allodynia is most likely caused by plastic changes at the level of the primary sensory fibers and spinal cord neurons.

351. **(B)** Phantom sensation: any sensation of the missing limb, except pain (A).

Stump contractions: spontaneous movement of the stump ranging from small jerks to visible contractions (jumpy stump) (C).

Stump pain: pain referred to the amputation stump (D).

352. **(E)** While ranges between 2% and 88% are quoted in the literature, most current studies state that between 60% and 80% of patients will develop phantom pain after amputation.

353. **(A)** Prospective studies in patients undergoing amputation mainly because of peripheral vascular disease have shown that the onset of phantom pain is usually within the first week after amputation.

However, in a retrospective study of individuals who were congenital amputees or underwent amputation before the age of 6 years, Melzack and coworkers found that the mean time for onset of phantom limb pain was 9 years in the group of congenital amputees and 2.3 years in the group of individuals with early amputations. [Jensen TS, Krebs B, Nielsen J, et al. Phantom limb, phantom pain, and stump pain in amputees during the first 6 months following limp amputation. *Pain.* 1983 Nov;17(3):243-256.]

[Nikolajsen L, Ilkjaer S, Kroner K, et al. The influence of preamputation pain on postamputation stump and phantom pain. *Pain.* 1997 Sep; 72(3):393-405.]

354. **(A)** Patients who develop early and severe phantom pain are more likely to suffer from chronic pain, whereas individuals who are pain-free at the beginning are less likely to develop significant pain. However, prospective studies with a maximum follow-up period of 2 years suggest that phantom pain may diminish with time.

355. **(C)** While phantom limb pain is seen in 60% to 80% of amputees, only 5% to 10% have severe pain.

356. **(B)** Some retrospective studies, but not all have pointed to preamputation pain as a risk factor for phantom pain. It has been hypothesized that preoperative pain may sensitize the nervous system, explaining why some individuals may be more susceptible to development of chronic pain.

A. It has been noted that patients with traumatic amputations, who had no pain prior to the amputation, develop pain to the same extent as patients with preoperative pain who endure amputations after significant medical pathology.

C. There is no correlation between the development of phantom pain and whether the amputation was primary or secondary. Primary amputation is when the limb is lost at the time of the injury. Secondary amputation is when the limb is surgically removed in a hospital.

D. Phantom pain may mimic preamputation pain in both character and localization. Preamputation pain may persist in some patients, but it is not the case in the majority of patients.

E. Site of amputation has not been found to have a role in determining whether preamputation pain leads to phantom pain.

357. **(E)**

A. Amputees who experienced a long delay between the amputation and return to work, had difficulty in finding suitable jobs, and had fewer opportunities for promotion.

B. The use of a functionally active prosthesis as opposed to a cosmetic prosthesis may reduce phantom pain.

C. Spinal anesthesia in amputees may precipitate transient, difficult to treat phantom pain. Given the low incidence of recurrent phantom limb pain with spinal anesthesia, its transient nature, and the fact that it can be treated if it occurs, it has been concluded that spinal anesthesia is not contraindicated in patients with previous lower limb amputation.

D. While there is no evidence that phantom pain represents a psychological disturbance, it may be triggered and precipitated by psychosocial factors. It has been shown that coping strategies are important for the experience of phantom pain Research has indicated that the way individuals cope with pain may influence pain, and physical and psychological adjustment.

358. **(E)** Stump pain is located at the end of an amputated limb's stump. Unlike phantom pain, it occurs in the body part that actually exists, in the stump that remains. It typically is described as a "sharp," "burning," "electric-like," or "skin-sensitive" pain. Some patients have spontaneous movements of the stump, ranging from slight, hardly visible jerks to severe contractions.

Stump pain results from a damaged nerve in the stump region. Nerves damaged in the amputation surgery try to heal and may form abnormally sensitive regions, called neuromas. A neuroma can cause pain and skin sensitivity. Percussion of neuromas may increase nerve fiber discharge and augmentation of stump and phantom pain.

No one treatment has been shown to be effective for stump pain. Because it is a pain caused by an injured peripheral nerve, drugs used for nerve pain may be helpful.

If the stump pain affects a limb, revision of the prosthesis is sometimes beneficial. Other approaches also are tried in selected cases, including: nerve blocks, transcutaneous electrical nerve stimulation, surgical revision of the stump, or removal of the neuroma (this procedure may fail because the neuroma can grow back; some patients actually get worse after surgery), and cognitive therapies.

Stump pain is common in the early postamputation period. Stump pain can also persist beyond the stage of postsurgical healing. Stump pain and phantom pain are strongly correlated. Phantom pain subsides with resolution of stump pain and that it is more prevalent in patients with phantom pain than in those without it.

Careful sensory examination of amputation stumps may reveal areas of sensory abnormalities such as hypoesthesia, hyperalgesia, or allodynia. However, a correlation between phantom pain and the extent and degree of sensory abnormality has not been established.

359. **(E)** The ectopic and increased spontaneous and evoked activity from the periphery is assumed to be the result of an increased and also novel expression of sodium channels.

Local anesthesia of the stump may reduce or abolish phantom pain temporarily. Decreasing peripheral output by locally anesthetizing stump neuromas with lidocaine reduced tap-evoked stump pain. On the other hand, there was a clear increase in pain when the potassium channel blocker, gallamine was injected in the perineuromal space. Both findings support the premise that abnormal input from peripheral nociceptors plays a role in pain generation.

360. **(A)** The pharmacology of spinal sensitization entails an increased activity in NMDA receptor–operated systems, and many aspects of the central sensitization can be reduced by NMDA receptor antagonists In amputees, the evoked pain from repetitive stimulation can be reduced by the NMDA antagonist ketamine

B. Terminating the stimulation is not the *only* way to reduce the pain.

C. After a nerve is injured, there is an increase in the general excitability of spinal cord neurons, where C fibers and A-δ afferents gain access to secondary pain-signaling neurons.

D. Sensitization of dorsal horn neurons is mediated by release of glutamate and neurokinin. This sensitization may present in several ways including: lowered threshold, increased persistent neuronal discharges with prolonged pain after stimulation, and expansion of peripheral receptive fields.

The central sensitization may also be a result of a different type of anatomical reorganization. Substance P is normally expressed in small afferent fibers, but following nerve injury, it may be expressed in large A-β fibers. This phenotypic switch of large A-β fibers into nociceptive-like nerve fibers may be one of the reasons why nonnoxious stimuli can be perceived as painful

361. **(E)**

E. The sympathetic nervous system may play a role in generating and, in particular, in maintaining, phantom pain.

After limb amputation and deafferentation in adult monkeys, there is reorganization of the primary somatosensory cortex, and while these changes may be unique to the cortex, they may also be, at least in part, the result of changes at the level of the thalamus and perhaps even brain stem or spinal cord. After dorsal rhizotomy, the threshold to evoke activity in the thalamus and cortex decreased, and the mouth and chin invade cortices corresponding to the representation of arm and fingers that have lost their normal afferent input. In humans similar reorganization has been observed. In the thalamus, neurons that normally do not respond to stimulation in amputees begin to respond and show enlarged somatotropic maps. A cascade of events seems to be involved in generating phantom pain and it starts in the periphery, spinal cord, brain stem, thalamus, and finally ends in the cerebral cortex.

362. **(C)**

A. and D. Tramdol and amitriptyline have been found to be efficacious in treating phantom and stump pain in treatment naive patients.

B. Gabapentin has been noted to be better than placebo in reducing phantom pain.

Failure to pharmacologically provide pain relief should not be accepted until opioids have been tried. Intravenous (IV) and oral morphine have been shown to decrease phantom pain. Case reports have indicated that methadone may also be helpful.

Other trials have not reported the same the success with an oral NMDA antagonist, memantine.

Suggestions for the treatment of postamputation pain (no evidence) (*Note*: it is important to differentiate between early postoperative pain and chronic pain [pain persisting more than 4 weeks], and stump and phantom pain):

Early postoperative pain
  Stump pain
    Conventional analgesics
• Acetaminophen
• NSAIDs
• Opioids
    +/– combined with epidural pain treatment
  Stump and phantom pain
  If neuropathic pain clearly exists (paroxysms or abnormal stump sensitivity)—trial with TCAs or anticonvulsants.

Chronic pain

Stump pain

- Local stump surgery: if obvious stump pathology is present, revisions should be considered; surgery should be avoided in cases of sympathetically maintained pain.
- Local medical treatment: topical lidocaine or capsaicin can be tried in those who have stump pain but no obvious stump pathology.

Stump and phantom pain (medical treatment, in order of preference)

- Gabapentin 1200 to 2400 mg/d, slow titration. Max dose of 3600 mg/d.
- TCAs (imipramine, amitriptyline, nortriptyline) 100 to 125 mg/d, slow titration. Check electrocardiogram (ECG) before starting. Monitor plasma levels with dose greater than 100 mg/d. If sedation is wanted, amitriptyline should be used.
- If the pain is mostly paroxysmal, lancinating, or radiating:
  - Oxcarbazepine 600 to 900 mg/d. Start at 300 mg and increase by 300 mg daily.
  - Carbamazepine 450 mg/d. Start dose 150 mg, daily increments of 150 mg. Monitor plasma levels after 10 days on maximum dose.
  - Lamotrigine 100 to 200 mg/d. Start dose 25 mg/d, slow titration with increments of 25 mg/14 days (to avoid rash).
- Opioids (long-acting) or tramadol.
- If none of the above has an effect, refer the patient to the pain clinic.
- In pain center: can perform IV lidocaine trial or ketamine trial. If the lidocaine test is positive—reconsider anticonvulsants. If the ketamine test is positive: consider memantine or amantadine.

Physical therapy encompassing massage, manipulation, and passive range of motion may prevent trophic changes and vascular congestion in the stump. Transcutaneous electrical nerve stimulation, acupuncture, ultrasound, and hypnosis, may have a beneficial effect on stump and phantom pain.

363. **(B)** Surgery on amputation neuromas and more extensive amputation were accepted treatment modalities for stump and phantom pain in the past. Today, stump revision is probably done only in cases of obvious stump pathology, and in properly healed stumps there is almost never an indication for proximal extension of the amputation because of pain. Surgery should be avoided in cases of sympathetically maintained pain. Surgery may produce short-term pain relief but pain often reappears. The results of other invasive procedures such as dorsal root entry zone lesions sympathectomy and cordotomy have generally been nontherapeutic, and most of them have been abandoned.

364. **(B)** Classification of patients with phantom pain:

Group I: Mild intermittent paresthesias that do not interfere with normal activity, work, or sleep.

Group II: Paresthesias that are uncomfortable and annoying but do not interfere with activities or sleep.

Group III: Pain that is of sufficient intensity, frequency, or duration to be distressful; however, some patients in this group have pain that is bearable, that intermittently interferes with their lifestyle, and that may respond to conservative treatment.

Group IV: Nearly constant severe pain that interferes with normal activity and sleep.

365. **(D)**

A. and B. The gate control theory of pain, put forward by Ronald Melzack and Patrick David Wall in 1962, and again in 1965, is the idea that the perception of physical pain is not a direct result of activation of nociceptors, but instead is modulated by interaction between different neurons, both pain-transmitting and non–pain-transmitting. The theory asserts that activation of nerves that do not transmit pain signals can interfere with signals from pain fibers and inhibit an individual's perception of pain. It has been used to explain phantom limb pain. Following marked destruction of sensory axons by amputation, wide dynamic range neurons are freed by inhibitory control.

Self-sustaining neuronal activity may then occur in spinal cord neurons.

C. If the spontaneous spinal cord neuronal activity exceeds a critical level, pain may occur in the phantom limb.

This loss of inhibitory control may lead to spontaneous discharges at any level in the CNS and may explain the lack of analgesia in paraplegics with phantom body pain after complete cordectomy Pain increases after blocking conduction are in line with the theory, as continued loss of peripheral sensory input would lead to further disinhibition. Sodium thiopental perpetuates CNS inhibition and has been reported to end phantom limb pain during spinal anesthesia. Melzack R, Wall PD. Mechanisms: a new theory. A gate control system modulates sensory input from the skin before it evokes pain perception and response. *Science*. 1965;150(3699).

366. **(D)** Primary dysmenorrhea is defined as menstrual pain without pelvic pathology. Endometriosis and adenomyosis are the most common causes of secondary dysmenorrhea.

367. **(C)** The pain of endometriosis can occur with menses or sexual intercourse or can always be present. It can also mimic any known pelvic pathology. Answers A, B, D, and E are all correct.

368. **(E)**

369. **(B)** Opioids have the potential for addiction even when administered for acute pain. However, it is the exaggerated common fear of the potential for addiction to opioids that often interferes with adequate pain management. The rest of the answers are correct.

370. **(E)** It is recognized that long-term changes occur within the peripheral and central nervous system following noxious input. This neuroplasticity alters the body's response to usual peripheral sensory input. In pathologic pain conditions, stimulation of A-β fibers, normally eliciting response to touch, may elicit pain.

371. **(C)** Even though there have been some concerns regarding the risks of perioperative NSAIDs, including intra- and postoperative bleeding, they continue to have a useful role. Combination of NSAIDs and opioids has a synergistic analgesic effect, as they act at the different sites of pain pathways. More new evidence is emerging that NSAIDs exert their analgesic effects also through the central mechanisms.

372. **(B)** It has been demonstrated that the administration of an NMDA *antagonist* reduces the development of tolerance to morphine. The rest of the answers are correct.

373. **(A)** The following are the usual features of the somatic pain: well localized, sharp and definite, often constant (sometimes periodic); it is rarely associated with nausea usually when it is deep somatic pain with bone involvement; it may be following the distribution of a somatic nerve. In contrast, the visceral pain: is poorly localized, diffuse, dull, and vague; it is often periodic and builds to peaks (sometimes constant); it is often associated with nausea and vomiting.

374. **(B)** It has been demonstrated that early postoperative pain is a significant predictor of long-term pain. The rest of the answers are correct.

375. **(C)** Multimodal analgesia makes it possible to significantly reduce the total consumption of opioids intra- and postoperatively. Therefore, opioid side-effects are minimized, including inevitable opioid-induced GI stasis that delays the resumption of normal enteral nutrition after surgery.

376. **(B)** PHN affects women more often than men, in a ratio of approximately 3:2. The rest of the answers are correct.

377. **(B)** PHN is defined as pain caused by herpes zoster for more than 1 month.

378. **(A)** As many as 40% of patients with PHN have either incomplete or no relief from treatment. Because of this, the future may lie with prevention through vaccination and early aggressive treatment of herpes zoster with antivirals and analgesics to reduce the extent of the nerve damage and sensitization that may correlate with PHN.

379. **(B)** Experience with serotonergic antidepressants, such as clomipramine, trazodone, nefazodone, fluoxetine, and zimelidine, in PHN has been disappointing. The evidence supporting the use of noradrenergic agents is more compelling. The rest of the answers are correct.

380. **(B)** There has been evidence that opioids do not relieve neuropathic pain as well as non-neuropathic pain. However, there is also evidence that opioids have been successfully used for the treatment of PHN.

381. **(B)** DM is the most common cause of autonomic neuropathy, and peripheral neuropathy in general, in the United States, as well as in the rest of the developed world. Leprosy is the most common cause of peripheral neuropathy in the world.

382. **(C)** Diabetic amyotrophy starts with pain and involves the lower extremities. It has a good prognosis and usually resolves spontaneously in 12 to 24 months. It is not directly related to hyperglycemia.

383. **(E)** Distal sensorimotor polyneuropathy is a *symmetrical* length-dependent process with dying-back or dropout of the longest nerve fibers—myelinated and unmyelinated. All other answers are correct.

384. **(B)** It is generally agreed that the prevalence of neuropathy is about 10% at diagnosis of DM, rising to 50% or more in patients diagnosed for longer than 5 years.

385. **(B)**

386. **(C)** It is accepted that the most common cause of trigeminal neuralgia is arterial cross-compression of the trigeminal nerve in the posterior fossa, as suggested by Jannetta in 1982. Electron microscopy of trigeminal nerve biopsies taken from patients with trigeminal neuralgia has shown areas of axonal swelling and demyelination adjacent to the area of arterial compression. Although trigeminal neuralgia is more common in patients with multiple sclerosis, only a small portion of patients with trigeminal neuralgia suffer from multiple sclerosis and does not explain the majority of the cases.

387. **(C)** Carbamazepine is likely to be beneficial in up to 70% of the patients. Incidence of side effects is often higher in elderly patients especially if the drug escalation is too fast. Allergic rash is seen in up to 10% of the patients and high concentration of the drug may be associated with fluid retention promoting cardiac problems. Carbamazepine is a potent hepatic enzyme inducer which can potentially lead to undesirable drug-to-drug interactions. Although microsurgical exploration of the posterior fossa is the highly successful, it is a major surgery with 0.5% risk of mortality and major morbidity. The effectiveness of pimozide for trigeminal neuralgia is better than carbamazepine, but the high frequency of side effects limits its clinical use.

388. **(C)** The trigeminal ganglion receives sensation from the oral mucosa, scalp, nasal areas, face, and teeth. Proprioceptive information is transmitted into the ganglion from the mastication and extraocular muscles. The peripheral branches of the ganglion are the ophthalmic, the maxillary, and the mandibular, which are organized somatotropically, with the ophthalmic branch located dorsally, the maxillary branch is intermediate, and the mandibular nerve is located ventrally. The gasserian ganglion lies within the cranium, in the middle cranial fossa. The posterior border of the ganglion includes the dura of the Meckel cave. The landmark to perform the trigeminal ganglion block is the foramen ovale and not the foramen rotundum.

389. **(C)** The diagnosis of trigeminal neuralgia is eminently clinical and further tests are necessary only to rule out associated conditions. When the condition is found, MRI and evoked potential testing are strongly recommended to rule out secondary causes. Clinically the onset of trigeminal neuralgia is around the age of 50 years, more common in females, almost exclusively unilateral with a paroxysmal nature.

390. **(D)** The giant cell arteritis affects almost exclusively the white population although it can occur in worldwide. Unlike other forms of vasculitis it rarely affects skin, kidneys, or lungs. Females are affected 3 times more often than males. Visual loss is now considered to affect between 6% to 10% of patients in most series.

391. **(D)** Analgesic rebound headache resolves or reverts to its previous pattern within 2 months of discontinuing of the overused medication.

392. **(B)** The first statement better describes trigeminal neuralgia. Cluster headache affects more males than females with a 5:1 ratio and can begin at any age. Attacks are severe, stabbing, screwing, unilateral pain, occasionally preceded by premonitory symptoms, with sudden onset, and rapid crescendo. Therapeutic interventions for the acute attack include oxygen, triptans, dihydroergotamine, ketorolac, chlorpromazine, or intranasal lidocaine, cocaine, or capsaicin. Melatonin has been found to be moderately effective as a preventive treatment in episodic and chronic cluster headache.

393. **(D)** Sterile neurogenic inflammation is often seen after stimulation of the trigeminal ganglion, which innervates large cerebral vessels, pial vessels, large sinuses, and the dura via unmyelinated C fibers. In acute attacks of migraine, substance P, CGRP, and nitric oxide mediate the neurogenic inflammation.

394. **(E)** TTH is the most common type of headache. Aura is present in only 20% of patients suffering from migraine. Although chronic daily headache diagnostic criteria for probable TTH requires no nausea or vomiting as one of the criteria or absence of photophobia, or phonophobia, nausea may be seen in 4.2% of patients with TTH, while phonophobia is reported in 10.6% of them.

395. **(D)** Inhalation of 100% oxygen at 7 to 12 L/min is effective in treating the majority of cluster headache sufferers when used continuously for 15 to 20 minutes. Generally oxygen inhalation is not considered to be effective in any other form of primary neurovascular headache.

396. **(C)**

397. **(C)** PDPH and SIH are two distinct clinical entities with similar presentation. The headache is always bilateral, located in the occipital and/or frontal area. Although low CSF pressure is often noted, it is not necessary to confirm the diagnosis.

398. **(C)** New daily persistent headache is a chronic, unremitting headache of sudden onset, daily pattern. The duration of the headache should be at least 3 months. Some important features include its moderate severity, bilateral location, and lack of nausea, vomiting (N/V), photophobia, and phonophobia (P/P). On the other hand, status migrainosus is a severe debilitating migraine, associated with N/V, P/P, and with duration longer than 72 hours but that typically do not exceed 2 weeks. The other diagnoses are not consistent with the symptoms.

399. **(A)** The previously known classic migraine (migraine with aura) is preceded by visual aura that starts 20 to 40 minutes before the migraine and is characterized by spreading scintillations reflecting a slow propagation of neuronal and glial excitation emanating from one occipital lobe. Cortical spreading depression (CSD) presents with dramatic shifts in cortical steady potential (DC), temporary increases in extracellular ions and excitatory neurotransmitters (glutamate), and transient raise, followed by sustained decrease in cortical blood flow. The vascular theory proposed that migraine with aura is caused by intracranial cerebral vasoconstriction and the headache by reactive vasodilation. Despite that, the theory can not explain the prodromal symptoms or why some antimigraine medications are not effective. Hormonal fluctuations and estrogen withdrawal may explain the higher incidence of migraine in female patients during their reproductive years, but are not related to the presence of aura. Cerebral idiopathic hypertension is a form of headache of unknown etiology.

400. **(D)** The published literature commonly states that 80% to 90% of low back pain resolves in about 6 weeks, irrespective of the administration or type of treatment, with only 5% to 10% of patients developing persistent back pain.

Contrary to this assumption, actual analysis of research evidence shows that chronic low back and neck pain persist 1 year or longer in 25% to 60% of adult and/or elderly patients.

401. **(C)** Based on evaluations utilizing controlled diagnostic blocks, the prevalence of zygapophysial or facet joint involvement has been estimated to be between 15% and 45% in heterogeneous groups of patients with chronic low back pain.

402. **(E)** The clinical picture of metastatic epidural spinal cord compression is uniformly reported as pain, weakness, sensory loss, and autonomic dysfunction. Metastatic epidural spinal cord compression initially presents with severe back pain in 95% of cases. After weeks of progressive pain, the patient may develop weakness, sensory loss, autonomic dysfunction, and reflex abnormalities. Bladder and bowel dysfunction are rarely presenting symptoms, but may appear after sensory symptoms have occurred. The exception to this generalization develops with compression of the conus medullaris, which presents as acute urinary retention and constipation without preceding motor or sensory symptoms.

403. **(B)** Patients with severe, persistent symptoms (discogenic in origin) that have been confirmed by other diagnostic evaluations do not need to undergo further evaluation by discography. Specific uses for discography include, but are not limited to: further evaluation of demonstrably abnormal discs to help assess the extent of abnormality or correlation of the abnormality with clinical symptoms (in case of recurrent pain from a previously operated disc and a lateral disc herniation); patients with persistent, severe symptoms in whom other diagnostic tests have failed to reveal clear confirmation of a suspected disc as the source of pain; assessment of patients who have failed to respond to surgical procedures to determine if there is painful pseudoarthrosis or a symptomatic disc in a posteriorly fused segment, or to evaluate possible recurrent disc herniation; assessment of discs before fusion to determine if the discs within the proposed fusion segment are symptomatic and to determine if discs adjacent to this segment are

normal; and assessment of minimally invasive surgical candidates to confirm a contained disc herniation or to investigate contrast distribution pattern before intradiscal procedures.

404. **(A)** Gait disturbances are a feature of cervical myelopathy, not radiculopathy. Other signs and symptoms of cervical radiculopathy include upper extremity sensory disturbances and muscle weakness.

405. **(D)** Experimental studies have given support to the hypothesis that blood flow and nutrition to the disc are diminished in smokers, the pH of the disc is lowered, disc mineral content is lower, fibrinolytic activity is changed, and there are increased degenerative changes seen in the lumbar spine.

406. **(B)** There is strong evidence from randomized controlled trials that bed rest is not effective for treating acute low back pain.

407. **(A)** Narrowing of the intervertebral discs has long been considered one of the signs of pathologic aging of the lumbar spine, but recent data has shown that notion to be untrue. Large-scale postmortem analysis have shown lumbar disc height and diameter to actually increase with age. The anterior-posterior diameter increases by about 10% in females and 2% in males. Disc height has been shown to increase by about 10% in most lumbar discs.

408. **(C)** Radiculopathy is a condition in which conduction within the axons of a spinal nerve or its roots are blocked. It can result in numbness and weakness secondary to conduction block in sensory and motor neurons respectively. Conduction blockade can be caused by compression or ischemia. It is important to make the distinction that radiculopathy does not cause pain. It may, however, be associated with pain.

409. **(D)** The major theoretical complications of corticosteroid administration include suppression of pituitary-adrenal axis, hypercorticism, Cushing syndrome, osteoporosis, avascular necrosis of bone, steroid myopathy, epidural

lipomatosis, weight gain, fluid retention, and hyperglycemia.

410. **(A)** Absolute contraindications to epidural steroid injections include sepsis, infection at injection site, therapeutic anticoagulation, and patient refusal. Relative contraindications include preexisting neurologic conditions, prophylactic low-dose heparin, thrombocytopenia, and uncooperative patients.

411. **(B)** L4-L5 disc herniation with L5 nerve root involvement involves: pain over the sacroiliac joint, hip, lateral thigh, and leg; numbness over the lateral leg and first three toes; weakness with dorsiflexion of great toe and foot; difficulty walking on heels; possible foot drop; and internal hamstring reflex diminished or absent. Numbness over the medial thigh and knee, and quadriceps weakness are indicative of L3-L4 disc herniation with L4 nerve root involvement. Difficulty walking on toes and lateral heel pain are common with L5-S1 disk herniation involving the S1 nerve root.

412. **(B)** Fifteen percent of patients with chronic low back pain have sacroiliac joint pain.

413 to 417. 413 (B); 414 (D); 415 (E); 416 (A); 417 (C) Spondylolysis is an acquired defect that results from a fatigue fracture of the pars interarticularis (the part of the lamina that intervenes between the superior and inferior articular processes on each side). Spondylolisthesis is the displacement of a vertebrae or the vertebral column in relationship to the vertebrae below. Kissing spines (also known as Baastrup disease) affects the lumbar spinous processes. Excessive lumbar lordosis or extension injuries to the lumbar spine cause adjacent spinous processes to clash and compress the intervening interspinous ligament. This results in a periostitis of the spinous process or inflammation of the affected ligament. Radiculopathy is a neurologic condition in which conduction blocks the axons of a spinal nerve or its roots that results in numbness and weakness. Radicular pain is pain that arises as a result of irritation of a spinal nerve or its roots.

418. **(E)** In managing lumbar radicular pain with interlaminar lumbar epidural steroid injections, the evidence is strong for short-term relief and limited for long-term relief. In managing cervical radiculopathy with cervical interlaminar epidural steroid injections, the evidence is moderate. The evidence for lumbar transforaminal epidural steroid injections in managing lumbar radicular pain is strong for short-term and moderate for long-term relief. The evidence for cervical transforaminal epidural steroid injections in managing cervical nerve root pain is moderate. The evidence is moderate in managing lumbar radicular pain in post–lumbar laminectomy syndrome. The evidence for caudal epidural steroid injections is strong for short-term relief and moderate for long-term relief, in managing chronic pain of lumbar radiculopathy and post–lumbar laminectomy syndrome.

419. **(A)** The sources of the nerve endings in the lumbar discs are two extensive microscopic plexuses of nerves that accompany the anterior and posterior longitudinal ligaments. The nerve plexuses that innervate intervertebral discs are derived from the lumbar sympathetic trunks. The dorsal rami supply innervation to the muscles of the back and zygapophysial joints. In normal lumbar intervertebral discs, nerve fibers are only found in the outer third of the annulus fibrosis. Discs painful on discography and removed with operation have nerve growth deep into the annulus and into the nucleus pulposus. Disc fissuring is a trigger for neoinnervation and neovascularization of a disc.

420. **(A)** Development of an epidural abscess is a very rare complication of epidural steroid injections. It needs to be recognized and treated quickly to avoid irreversible injury. Symptoms of an epidural abscess include severe back pain that is followed by radicular pain 3 days later. The initial back pain may not become evident for several days after the injection.

421. **(C)** Plain x-rays are recommended for possible fractures, arthropathy, spondylolisthesis, tumors, infections, stenosis, and congential deformities. CT images are recommended for bone/joint pathologies, lateral disc herniations, stenosis

(ie, spinal canal, neuroforaminal, lateral recess), and for those in which an MRI is contraindicated. MRI is recommended for disc herniations, spinal stenosis, osteomyelitis, tumors (ie, spinal cord, nerve roots, nerve sheath, paraspinal soft tissue), and cauda equine syndrome.

422. (D) The L2 nerve root is involved with hip flexion, L3 with leg extension, L4 with heel walking, L5 with first toe dorsiflexion (and heel walking), and S1 with toe walking.

423. (C) Laminotomy with discectomy has a low infection rate, statistically. The most frequent complication is a dural tear. Neural injury may occur as a result of a dural tear and may cause long-term pain and neurologic deficit. Recurrence of the herniation occurs in approximately 5% of cases. Infection and neural injury occurs in less than 0.5% of cases.

424. (C) Conservative treatment is usually the first treatment of choice for patients presenting with FBSS. It consists of medical management of contributing factors (ie, depression, obesity, smoking), rehabilitation, and behavior modification (ie, alcohol or drug dependency).

425. (D) Many prognostic indicators have been implicated in patients undergoing repeat lumbosacral spine surgery. They may or may not be significant for each patient and should be taken into context for the particular patient. Women have been found to have better outcomes than men. Patients with a history of favorable outcomes from prior surgeries tend to have better outcomes as well. A history of few previous surgeries, operative/myelographic findings of disc herniation, and a history of working immediately prior to surgery are all favorable prognostic indicators. Less favorable prognostic indicators include epidural scarring that requires lysis of adhesions and pseudoarthrosis of a prior fusion.

426. (E) Waddell signs are used to help diagnose nonorganic low back pain complaints. Each of the five findings is considered positive if present. Three positive findings are considered highly suggestive of a nonorganic source of pain:

1. Tenderness: does not follow dermatomal or referral patterns and is hard to localize.
2. Stimulation testing: stimulating distant sites should not cause discomfort.
3. Distraction testing: findings when testing the same site are inconsistent when the patient's attention is distracted.
4. Regional disturbance: motor and sensory testing yield nonanatomic findings.
5. Overreaction: inappropriate verbal remarks or facial expressions, withdrawal from touch, or posturing inconsistent with touch.

427. (B) Ankylosing spondylitis is characterized by pain and stiffness in young males (typically ages 17-35 years) more often than females. It is worse in the morning and improves with mild exercise. The pain will typically last for at least 3 months and be diffuse in nature affecting the low back and spine. Rheumatoid arthritis is an inflammatory polyarthritis that affects middle-aged women more often than men. It typically presents with morning stiffness that improves as the day progresses, and the spine is not affected until late in the disease. Psoriatic arthritis is characterized by inflammation of the skin and joints that typically presents in the fourth and fifth decades of life. Klippel-Feil syndrome is a congenital disorder that is characterized by abnormal fusion of two or more bones in the cervical spine. Reiter syndrome is a reactive arthritis that is characterized by a triad of symptoms: nongonococcal urethritis, conjunctivitis, and arthritis.

428. (C) The three major criteria for cervicogenic headache include (1) signs and symptoms of neck involvement (precipitation of head pain by: neck movement and/or sustained awkward head positioning, by external pressure over the upper cervical or occipital region on the symptomatic side; restriction of the range of motion in the neck; ipsilateral neck, shoulder, or arm pain of a rather vague nonradicular nature or, occasionally, arm pain of a radicular nature); (2) confirmatory evidence by diagnostic anesthetic blockades; and (3) unilaterality of the head pain without sideshift. Head pain characteristics include moderate-severe, nonthrobbing, and nonlancinating pain, usually starting in the neck, episodes of varying duration, or fluctuating, continuous pain. Other characteristics of some importance: only marginal effect or lack of effect of indomethacin, only marginal effect or lack of effect of ergotamine and sumatriptan, female sex, not infrequent occurrence of head, or indirect neck trauma by history, usually of more than only medium severity.

429. **(D)** Neurogenic claudication pain is secondary to nerve root compression rather than lack of blood supply that is seen with vascular claudication. The pain is exacerbated by standing erect and downhill walking. Improvement comes with lying supine more than lying in the prone position, sitting, squatting, and lumbar flexion. Neurogenic claudication is not made worse with biking, uphill walking, and lumbar flexion, unlike vascular claudication. It is not alleviated with standing.

430. **(A)** Neck pain has been suggested to have multifactorial etiologies. Risk factors for neck pain that cannot be modified include age, sex, and genetics. There is no evidence that normal cervical spine degenerative changes are a risk factor for neck pain. Modifiable risk factors for neck pain include smoking and exposure to environmental tobacco. Participation in physical activity seems to offer a protective effect. High quantitative job demands, low social support at the workplace, inactive work position, repetitive work, and meticulous work increases the risk of neck pain. There is a lack of evidence that workplace interventions are successful in decreasing neck pain in employees.

431. **(D)** In patients with neck pain, the physical examination is more predictive at excluding a structural lesion or neurologic compression than at diagnosing any specific etiologic condition in patients with neck pain. Other assessment tools (ie, electrophysiology, imaging, injections, discography, functional tests, and blood tests) lack validity and utility.

432. **(B)** Most people with neck pain do not experience a complete resolution of symptoms. Between 50% and 85% of those who experience

neck pain at some initial point will report neck pain again 1 to 5 years later. These numbers appear to be similar in the general population, in workers, and after motor vehicle crashes. The prognosis for neck pain also appears to be multifactorial. Younger age was associated with a better prognosis, whereas poor health and prior neck pain episodes were associated with a poorer prognosis. Poorer prognosis was also associated with poor psychologic health, worrying, and becoming angry or frustrated in response to neck pain. Greater optimism, a coping style that involved self-assurance, and having less need to socialize, were all associated with better prognosis. Specific workplace or physical job demands were not linked with recovery from neck pain. Workers who engaged in general exercise and sporting activities were more likely to experience improvement in neck pain. Postinjury psychologic distress and passive types of coping were prognostic of poorer recovery in WAD. There is evidence that compensation and legal factors are also prognostic for poorer recovery from WAD.

433. **(C)** The reported complications of fluoroscopically guided interlaminar cervical epidural injections are increased neck pain (6.7%), nonpositional headaches (4.6%), insomnia the night of the injection (1.7%), vasovagal reaction reactions (1.7%), facial flushing (1.5%), fever on the night of the procedure (0.3%), and dural puncture (0.3%). The incidence of all complications per injection is 16.8%.

434. **(E)** Anterior spinal artery syndrome classically presents in older patients with abrupt motor loss, sphincter disturbance, and nonconcordant sensory examination with preservation of sensation to light touch but loss of pain and temperature. It may also occur during aortic procedures. When anterior spinal artery syndromes occur during or after transforaminal epidural steroid injection, the patient may have abrupt back or abdominal pain after injection. An MRI will demonstrate a T2 signal change consistent with cord ischemia/infarct. Anterior spinal artery ischemia may be caused by arteriosclerosis, tumors, thrombosis, hypotension, air or fat embolism, toxins, or other causes.

Particulate (steroid) substances, arterial injury, or vascular spasm are other potential causes and have been implicated as significant possibilities for the occurrence of ischemic events after transforaminal epidural steroid injections.

435. **(E)** A spinal epidural abscess must be recognized promptly and treated quickly, otherwise extreme morbidity can result. It may be separate or associated with vertebral osteomyelitis. Diabetic, alcoholic, IV drug using patients, and immunocompromised patients are all at increased risk. *Staphylococcus aureus* is the most common organism involved. An affected patient usually presents with neck pain that rapidly progresses to radicular symptoms. Quadriplegia can result if left untreated. Treatment involves surgical removal and antibiotic management.

436. **(B)** The pathophysiology of HIV-related neuropathies is still not well understood. The current understanding is that it is not related to the direct effect of the virus itself. HIV is *not* found within ganglionic neurons of Schwann cells, but only in endoneurial macrophages, which may generate a tissue-specific autoimmune response by secretion of cytokines, which, in turn, promotes trafficking of activated T cells and macrophages within the endoneurial parenchyma.

437. **(E)** The predominantly sensory neuropathy of AIDS affects up to 30% of people with HIV infection and AIDS and is the most commonly encountered.

438. **(E)** The primary process that leads to vascular occlusion is the polymerization of sickle cell hemoglobin on deoxygenation, which in turn results in distortion of the shape of red blood cells (RBCs), cellular dehydration, decreased deformability, and increased stickiness of RBCs, which promotes their adhesion to and activation of the vascular endothelium.

439. **(D)** SCD is unlike other pain syndromes where the provider can make decisions on treatment based solely on the pain and its associated behavior. A primary care physician, for example, taking care of a middle-aged patient with job-related low back pain may decide to expel the patient from his or her care if the patient in question demonstrates suspicious drug-seeking behavior. Doing the same with patients who have SCD could be counterproductive. There are anecdotes of patients with SCD who were dismissed from certain programs only to be found dead at home within 24 hours after dismissal or to be admitted to other hospitals with serious complications. Sickle cell pain could be the prodrome of a serious and potentially fatal complication of SCD in some patients.

440. **(C)** Tissue ischemia caused by vascular occlusion resulting from in situ sickling causes infarctive tissue damage, which in turn initiates a secondary inflammatory response. The secondary response may enhance sympathetic activity by means of interactions with neuroendocrine pathways and trigger release of norepinephrine. In the setting of tissue injury, this release causes more tissue ischemia, creating a vicious cycle. It is the combination of ischemic tissue damage and secondary inflammatory response that makes the pain of SCD unique in its acuteness and severity.

441. **(C)** Objective signs of a painful crisis, such as fever, leukocytosis, joint effusions, and tenderness, occur in about 50% of patients at initial presentation.

442. **(E)** Pain is the hallmark of SCD, and the acute sickle cell painful episode (painful crisis) is the most common cause of more than 90% of hospital admissions among adult patients who have SCD.

443. **(B)** NSAIDs have potentially serious, systemic adverse effects. They include gastropathy, nephropathy, and hemostatic defects. It is advisable not to administer them continuously for more than 5 days to patients with SCD.

444. **(D)** Tramadol is a synthetic, centrally acting analgesic that is not chemically related to opioids. It acts as a weak agonist with preferential affinity to the μ-receptors. Moreover, it inhibits neuronal reuptake of both serotonin and norepinephrine and stimulates the release of serotonin. Thus, it has functional properties of an

opioid and an antidepressant. This drug received an initial enthusiastic reception based on the perception that it was not associated with clinically significant respiratory depression or addiction potential. However, this enthusiasm waned after reports indicated that seizures may be an adverse effect and that abuse potential is increasing.

445. (D) Chronic pain is a major complication of SCI. Epidemiologic studies indicate that approximately two-thirds of all SCI patients suffer from chronic pain out of which one-third have severe pain. Pain interferes with rehabilitation, daily activities, quality of life, and may have significant influence on mood leading to depression and even suicide.

446. (C) Musculoskeletal pain is common in both the acute and chronic phase of SCI. Chronic pain secondary to overuse is common in shoulders and arm, and vertebral column pain may occur because of the secondary changes following fractures and fixation, mechanical instability, and osteoporosis.

447. (D) Autonomic dysreflexia may complicate SCI patients with a lesion above the splanchnic outflow (sixth thoracic level).

448. (E) Visceral pain usually presents as dull or cramping abdominal uncomfortable and painful sensations, which may be associated with nausea and autonomic reactions. It is likely that visceral pain may occur in the absence of any abdominal organ dysfunction, and may in some cases represent a neuropathic type of pain. SCI patients may not have the typical signs of abdominal illness, and they should be carefully examined whenever any new pain or changes in existing pain occur. Increases in spasticity, pain at any location, or autonomic reactions may be the only indications of abdominal organ dysfunction.

449. (E) Above-level neuropathic pain includes pain caused by compressive mononeuropathies (particularly carpal tunnel syndrome) and CRPS. While below-level pain is considered to be a central pain caused by the spinal cord

trauma, at-level pain may have both peripheral (nerve root) and central (spinal cord) components that are difficult to separate.

450. (D) Answers (A), (B), (C), and (D) define allodynia, aftersensation, hyperalgesia, and referred pain, respectively.

451. (A)

452. (B) Central cord syndrome is one of the incomplete SCI syndromes. It is the most common pattern of injury, representing central gray matter destruction with preservation of only the peripheral spinal cord structures, the sacral spinothalamic and corticospinal tracts. The patient usually presents as a quadriplegic with perianal sensation and has an early return of bowel and bladder control. Any return of motor function usually begins with the sacral elements (toe flexors, then the extensors), followed by the lumbar elements of the ankle, knee, and hip. Upper extremity functional return is generally minimal and is limited by the degree of central gray matter destruction.

453. (D) Sensory symptoms and signs in CRPS include spontaneous pain, hyperpathia, allodynia, and hyperalgesia. Answer (A) is the definition of allodynia, answer (B) defines primary hyperalgesia, and answer (C) is secondary hyperalgesia. Answer (E) is the definition of dysesthesia. Dysesthesia maybe spontaneous.

454. (C) CRPS I is a painful condition following an injury, which may not even be a neuropathic pain, as not obvious lesion is present. Patients with this condition develop asymmetrical distal extremity pain, which is disproportionate to the intensity of the initiating event. Sensory abnormalities appear early in the course of the disease and are more pronounced distally. No clear relationship between the injury and the area of pain distribution exist. Sweating abnormalities, whether hypohidrosis or hyperhidrosis are present in nearly all patients with CRPS I.

455. (D) Trophic changes, particularly abnormal hair growth, fibrosis, decreased dermal blood flow, thin glossy skin, and osteoporosis are more common in long standing cases, while the others described present in acute phases of the disease.

456. **(D)** The diagnosis of CRPS I and II follows the IASP clinical criteria. Bone scintigraphy may be a valuable tool to rule out other conditions. CRPS I is more common than CRPS II and the female to male ratio is from 2:1 to 4:1.

457. **(D)** The symptoms of CRPS II are similar to those of CRPS I, except that in CRPS II, there must be a lesion of a peripheral nerve structure and subsequent focal deficit are mandatory for the diagnosis.

458. **(A)** The majority of patients with CRPS present with significant psychologic distress, being the most frequent anxiety and depression. Current evidence is against the theory that CRPS is a psychogenic condition. The pain in CRPS is the cause of psychiatric problems and not vice versa. When compared to patients with low back pain, CRPS patients showed a higher frequency of somatization, but other psychologic parameters were similar.

459. **(A)** Activation and sensitization of cutaneous C fibers elicit a response consisting of a wheal (local edema), a reddening of the skin at the site of stimulus, and a spreading flare, were the responses described by Lewis (1927). [Lewis T. *The blood vessels of the human skin and their responses.* London: Shaw. 1927.]

460. **(A)** Muscle pain tends to be dull, poorly localized, and deep in contrast to the precise location of cutaneous pain. The diagnosis of myofascial pain syndrome is confirmed when the myofascial trigger point is identified by palpation. An active myofascial trigger point is defined as a focus of hyperirritability in a muscle or its fascia that causes the patient pain.

B. Myofascial pain syndrome is usually thought of as a regional pain syndrome in contrast to fibromyalgia as a widespread syndrome; however, as many as 45% of patients with chronic myofascial pain syndrome have generalized pain in three or four quadrants. Hence, regional pain syndromes

should raise a suspicion of myofascial pain syndrome, but patients with widespread musculoskeletal pain can also have myofascial pain syndrome.

C. The American Pain Society showed general agreement with the concept that myofascial pain syndrome exists as an entity distinct from fibromyalgia.

D. Systemic palpation differentiates between myofascial taut bands and general muscle spasms.

461. **(A)** The minimum criteria that must be satisfied in order to distinguish a myofascial trigger point from any other tender area in muscle are a taut band and a tender point in that taut band. The existence of a local twitch response, referred pain, or reproduction of the person's symptomatic pain increases the certainty and specificity of the diagnosis.

462. **(C)**

D. This statement is true. End-plate noise is characteristic of, but not restricted to, the region of the myofascial trigger point. Hence, an objective EMG signature of the trigger point is now available for diagnostic and research purposes.

463. **(B)**

A. There is no reason to believe that the placebo effect is unusually high with this or other soothing sprays.

B. The stretch and spray technique combines the use of a vapocoolant spray with passive stretching of the muscle. Application of vapocoolant spray stimulates temperature and touch A-β skin receptors, thereby inhibiting C fiber and A-δ fiber afferent nociceptive pathways and muscle spasms, myofascial trigger points, and pain when stretching

C. The patient is positioned comfortably and the muscle involved is sprayed with a vapocoolant spray, and then the muscle is stretched passively. With the muscle in the stretched position, the spray is applied again over the skin overlying the entire muscle, starting at the trigger zone and proceeding in the direction of, and including, the referred pain zone. After, the area is heated with a moist warm pack for 5 to 10 minutes. The patient is encouraged to perform full range of motion exercises with the body part. This technique can be used in physical therapy as a separate modality or following myofascial trigger point injections.

D. It is expected that therapists can be more liberal once the spray has been applied owing to less patient discomfort.

464. **(C)** Myofascial release techniques and sustained pressure may soften and relax contracted and hardened muscles. The principle of the least possible force is applied, instead of applying high stress to the muscle. Effective myofascial release techniques include strumming. Strumming is when a finger runs across a taut band at the level of the trigger point over the nodules from one side of the muscle to the other. The operator's fingers pull perpendicularly across the muscle rather than along the length of the fibers. When the nodule of the trigger point is encountered, light pressure is maintained until the operator senses tissue release. Other techniques include perpendicular and oscillating mobilizations, tissue rolling, connective tissue massage, and deep muscle massage consisting of effleurage (stroking massage technique) and pétrissage (kneading massage technique).

After superficially passing over the muscles and adjacent muscles, massage therapy can be applied directly to the taut band and trigger points. Exercise and massage helped to reduce the number and intensity of trigger points, but the addition of therapeutic ultrasound did not improve the outcome.

465. **(C)** When treating myofascial pain, the physician must evaluate and, if indicated, treat both soft tissue and joint dysfunction. Restrictions in joint capsules hinder the function of the muscles that overlie the joint, while muscle irregularities result in joint capsule restrictions. Zygapophyseal joints may have pain referral patterns that are analogous to myofascial trigger points. The limited range of motion and weakness that results from

this somatic dysfunction that affects muscles and joints can be reversed easily by manual therapy.

466. **(D)** Answers A., B., and D. are the therapeutic, diagnostic, and adjunctive indications for myofascial trigger point needling, respectively, with D. being the most common appropriate use of this technique. Rarely is dry needling done to eliminate a trigger point permanently, although, this can happen when the myofascial pain syndrome is acute.

Inactivation of the myofascial trigger point appears to be the result of the mechanical action of the needle in the trigger point itself, because it also occurs when no medication is used. However, using local anesthetics is more comfortable for the patients and results in longer lasting pain reduction.

After pinpointing and manually stabilizing the trigger point in the taut band with the fingers, the needle is quickly passed through the skin and into the trigger zone. A local twitch response or a report of referred pain indicates that the trigger zone has been entered. One-tenth to 0.2 mL of local anesthetic can be injected. The needle is pulled back to just below the skin, the angle is changed, and it is once again inserted through the muscle to another trigger zone. In this way a funnel-shaped volume of muscle can be evaluated without withdrawing the needle through the skin. The trigger zone is explored this way until no further local twitch responses are obtained. By this time, the taut band is usually gone and the spontaneous pain of the trigger point has subsided. Experienced patients know when trigger points have been inactivated.

467. **(E)**

A., B., and C. While direct needling of myofascial trigger points appears to be an effective treatment, there is insufficient evidence that needling therapies have efficacy beyond placebo. These researchers also found no evidence to suggest that the injection of one material was more effective than another. They found no advantage to adding steroids, ketorolac, or vitamin B_{12} to local anesthetic. Steroids actually have the disadvantage that they are locally myotoxic and that repeated administration can produce all the unwanted side effects associated with steroids. For those who are allergic to local anesthetics, saline or dry needling can be used.

D. No studies have been done to confirm or refute that diphenhydramine increases the efficacy of myofascial trigger points.

468. (E) Complications of trigger point injections:

- Local bleeding into muscle
- Local swelling
- Painful contraction of a taut band from inadequate myofascial trigger point inactivation (missing the trigger point)
- Infection
- Perforation of a viscous body, most commonly the lung
- Nerve injury from direct trauma by the needle
- Transient nerve block
- Syncope
- Allergic reaction from the anesthetic

Torticollis is a contraction, often spasmodic, of the muscles of the neck, chiefly those supplied by the spinal accessory nerve; the head is drawn to one side and usually rotated so that the chin points to the other side. While missing the trigger point during needling can cause a painful contraction of a taut band, torticollis has not been noted.

469. (B) Answers (A), (C), (D), and (E) are all causes of trigger point failure.

C. Myofascial adhesions can possibly develop with secondary or "satellite" trigger points in nearby muscles. Trigger points appearing in muscles that are part of a functional unit must be treated together. Muscles that work together as agonists or in opposition as antagonists, constitute a functional muscle unit. For example the trapezius and levator scapula muscles work together as agonists in elevation of the shoulder, but are antagonists in rotation of the scapula, the trapezius rotating the glenoid fossa upward and the levator scapula rotating it downward.

470. (A) The most common anatomic variations that constitute mechanical factors precipitating myofascial pain are: leg length discrepancy and small hemipelvis, short upper arm syndrome, and the long second metatarsal syndrome.

The leg length disparity syndrome produces a pelvic tilt that results in a cascade of chronic contraction and activation of a chain of muscles in an attempt to straighten the head and level the eyes. The quadratus lumborum and paraspinal muscles contract to correct the deviation of the spine caused by the pelvic tilt. Unwarranted loading perpetuates myofascial trigger points and may result in low back, head, neck, and shoulder pain. Trigger points in these persistently shortened and constantly contracted muscles are not easily inactivated until the muscles are unloaded. The quadratus lumborum is less likely to develop trigger points during the teenage years, and typically, unilateral low back pain is located on the side of the shorter leg because of early shrinking of the ipsilateral annulus fibrosis. In adults, it occurs on the side of the longer leg, caused by later spondylitic changes and quadratus lumborum shortening. A true leg length incongruity can be corrected by placing a heel lift on the shorter leg. The asymmetry caused by a small hemipelvis is corrected by placing an ischial or "butt" lift under the ischial tuberosity.

Short upper arms cause forward shoulder roll, pectoral muscle shortening, and abnormal loading of the neck and trunk muscles as the individual attempts to find a comfortable position when seated.

A long second metatarsal bone obscures the stable tripod support of the foot produced by the first and second metatarsal bones anteriorly and the heel posteriorly. In contrast, in this condition, weight is carried on a knife-edge from the second metatarsal head to the heel, overstressing the peroneus longus that attaches to the first metatarsal bone. Diagnostic callus formation takes place in the abnormally stressed areas: under the second metatarsal head, and on the medial aspect of the foot at the great toe and first metatarsal head. Correction is accomplished with support under the head of the first metatarsal.

471. (E)

A. In women with chronic coldness and myofascial pain, ferritin has been found to be below 65%, largely because of an iron intake that is insufficient to replace menstrual loss. GI blood loss caused by anti-inflammatories and parasitic diseases can also cause ferritin to be low. Ferritin represents the tissue bound nonessential iron stores in the body that supply the essential iron for oxygen transport and iron-dependent enzymes. Fifteen to 20 ng/mL is low and anemia is common at levels of 10 ng/mL or less. The association between depleted iron and chronic myofascial pain hints that iron-requiring enzymatic reactions may be limited in these people, which may produce an energy crisis in muscle when it is overloaded and thereby produce metabolic stress. Myofascial trigger points will not easily resolve in such instances, and iron supplementation in patients with chronic myofascial pain syndrome and serum ferritin levels below 30 mg/mL prevents or corrects these symptoms.

B. and C. Folic acid and vitamin B_{12} function not only in erythropoiesis but also in central and peripheral nerve formation. Preliminary studies have shown that 16% of patients with chronic myofascial pain syndrome either were deficient in vitamin B_{12} or had insufficient levels of vitamin B_{12}, and that 10% had low serum folate levels.

D. Hypothyroidism can be suspected in chronic myofascial pain syndrome when coldness, dry skin/hair, constipation, and fatigue are also present. One study, found that under these circumstances (chronic) it occurred in 10% of patients. The myofascial trigger points tend to be more extensive in hypothyrotic patients. Hormone replacement may resolve many myofascial complaints and perpetuate a more permanent healthy state by allowing the implementation of physical therapy and trigger point inactivation.

Also common in chronic musculoskeletal pain: low vitamin D, recurrent candida yeast infections, elevated uric acid levels, parasitic infections (especially amebiasis), Lyme disease, osteoarthritis, rheumatoid arthritis, Sjögren syndrome, carpal tunnel syndrome, and peripheral neuropathy secondary to DM.

The postlaminectomy syndrome is frequently caused by myofascial trigger points.

472. (D) Biologic abnormalities that are detected in most fibromyalgia patients include

- Dysfunctional sleep by polysomnography
- Physiological or biochemical evidence for central sensitization
- Temporal summation or second pain
- Lowered thresholds to pressure-induced pain detected by brain imaging
- Low levels of the biogenic amines to drive descending inhibition of nociception
- Elevated spinal fluid levels of substance P
- In primary fibromyalgia *only*, elevated spinal fluid levels of NGF

473. (D) The American College of Rheumatology sanctioned a study that led to the criteria for diagnosing fibromyalgia: a history of widespread pain for at least 3 months and pain sensitivity to 4 kg of digital pressure at 11 or more of 18 anatomically defined tender points. The criteria displayed sensitivity and specificity of 88.4% and 81.1%, respectively, for patients with fibromyalgia against normal control and disease control subjects with other painful conditions.

474. (C) In addition to the four areas mentioned in the question stem, five other locations exist:

1. Trapezius, at the middle of the upper muscle border
2. Supraspinatus, near the origins, above the spine of the scapula
3. Second rib, upper surface just lateral to the second costochondral junction
4. Gluteal, in upper outer quadrants of buttocks in anterior fold of muscle
5. Greater trochanter, posterior to the trochanteric prominence

475. (B)

   A. and B. Fibromyalgia is no longer considered a psychogenic disorder, however, there is a subgroup of fibromyalgia patients with associated depression or anxiety.

   C. It is believed that fibromyalgia patients who have had medical treatment are more apt to exhibit symptoms of depression than those in the community who have not.

   D. Sexual abuse in childhood is no longer considered a legitimate hypothesis for the origination of fibromyalgia.

476. (E) The female urethral syndrome or irritable bladder syndrome constitutes urinary frequency, dysuria, suprapubic discomfort, and urethral pain despite sterile urine.

477. (E)

   A., B., and C. Most patients (90%) with fibromyalgia have trouble sleeping. Some have difficulty getting to sleep (initial insomnia), while the majority awaken feeling alarmingly alert after only a few hours of sleep (mid insomnia) and are then unable to sleep soundly again until near morning (terminal insomnia). They usually awaken in the morning feeling incredibly stiff (lasts 45 minutes to 4 hours), mentally listless, and unrefreshed by their sleep. Hence, it is surprising that they have difficulty napping during the day.

   Moldofsky (2002) observed that 60% of fibromyalgia patients exhibit an electroencephalogram (EEG) pattern of sleep architecture called alpha wave intrusions of deep, delta wave, non–rapid eye movement sleep, which relates to subjective fatigue and psychologic distress but is not specific for fibromyalgia. Its prevalence in the healthy general population or in those with insomnia or dysthymia is only 25%. [Moldofsky H. Management of sleep disorders in fibromyalgia. *Rheum Dis Clin North Am.* 2002 May;28(2):353-65.]

478. (E) Approximately 80% of patients with fibromyalgia have fatigue, while a small percentage of these actually meet the criteria for chronic fatigue syndrome (CFS). CFS is thought to affect approximately 4 per 1000 adults. For unknown reasons, CFS occurs more often in women and in adults in their 40s and 50s. The illness is estimated to be less prevalent in children and adolescents, but study results vary as to the degree. CFS often manifests with widespread myalgia and arthralgia, cognitive difficulties, chronic mental and physical exhaustion, often severe, and other characteristic symptoms in a previously healthy and active person. There remains no assay or pathologic finding which is widely accepted to be diagnostic of CFS. It remains a diagnosis of exclusion based largely on patient history and symptomatic criteria, although a number of tests can aid diagnosis. The fatigue of CFS is a feeling of weakness, while the fatigue of fibromyalgia is a feeling of tiredness. Fatigue may result from sedating medications (ie, TCAs being used for the treatment of insomnia in fibromyalgia). The rest of the differential diagnosis is quite extensive and must take into account:

- Sleep disorders
- Chronic infections
- Autoimmune disorders
- Psychiatric comorbidities
- Neoplasia

479. (B) The rest of the answers are blatantly wrong. Secondary fibromyalgia may not be clinically distinguishable from that of primary fibromyalgia.

   Examples of secondary fibromyalgia:

- Rheumatoid arthritis patients have fibromyalgia 30% of the time
- Systemic lupus erythematosus (SLE) 40%
- Sjögren syndrome 50%
- Lyme disease 20%; the symptoms of fibromyalgia may develop 1 to 4 months after infection, often in association with Lyme arthritis. The signs of Lyme disease will normally resolve with antibiotics, but the fibromyalgia symptoms can persist
- Chronic hepatitis
- Inflammatory bowel disease
- Tuberculosis
- Chronic syphilis
- Bacterial endocarditis

- AIDS
- Hypothyroidism
- Hypopituitarism
- Hemochromatosis

Patients with rheumatic disease and concomitant fibromyalgia experience joint pain out of proportion to their synovitis. The practitioner should treat each of the conditions separately, because increasing the dosage of antirheumatic medications in the absence of active inflammation might have minimal effect on the pain augmented by the fibromyalgia.

480. (A)

A. There are several neurochemical mediators of pain that appear to be factors in the pathogenesis of fibromyalgia:

- Substance P
- NGF (elevated in primary fibromyalgia, but not secondary)
- Dynorphin A (normal or elevated in fibromyalgia)
- Glutamate
- Nitric oxide
- Serotonin (decreased in fibromyalgia)
- Noradrenaline (its inactive metabolite is significantly lowered in fibromyalgia)

Substance P, NGF, dynorphin A, glutamate, and nitric oxide are considered pronociceptive because they transmit or intensify afferent signals, leading to the brain perceiving increased pain. On the other hand, serotonin, noradrenaline, the amino terminal peptide fragment of substance P, and endogenous opioids are considered to be antinociceptive because they hinder the transmission of nociceptive signals.

B. All studies on substance P in fibromyalgia patients have found significantly higher average concentrations (two- to threefold) of substance P than in the CSF of healthy control subjects. However, the levels in other bodily fluids like saliva, serum, and urine, have been normal in fibromyalgia.

C. The increased substance P is not because of decreased CSF substance P esterase activity,

because the rate of cleavage of labeled substance P was found to be normal. In primary fibromyalgia, it is believed that NGF may be responsible for the elevated CSF substance P through its effects on central sensitization and neuroplasticity.

D. Increased CSF substance P is not specific to fibromyalgia as it is also seen in painful rheumatic diseases irrespective of whether they have fibromyalgia. In patients that were status post–total hip replacement, elevated substance P prior to the procedure normalized after the surgery when the pain was gone. Certain chronic conditions such as low back pain and diabetic neuropathy present with lower than normal CSF substance P levels.

481. (E) There is no current cure for fibromyalgia, so its management is

- Nonspecific
- Multimodal
- Expectant
- Symptomatic

The goals are to

- Decrease pain
- Enhance sleep
- Reinstate physical function
- Maintain social interaction
- Restore emotional balance
- Decrease the excessive use of health care resources

The best way to achieve these goals is through a multidisciplinary approach of

- Education
- Exercise
- Physical therapy
- Medications
- Social support

482. (B) The shared decision concept emphasizes the importance of simultaneous exchange of information until an agreement between the doctor and patient can be achieved concerning available diagnostic and treatment approaches. It improves both patient and physician satisfaction, is preferred by patients, and sets the stage for better outcomes.

A. The shared decision concept involves the physician and the patient.

C. The physician may outline the treatment options with associated risks and benefits, while the patient may disclose information about their culture, fears, expectations, beliefs, and attitudes.

483. (E)

A. All these techniques have been recommended for some patients with fibromyalgia. Progressive muscle relaxation was developed by Jacobson, who argued that since muscular tension accompanies anxiety, one can reduce anxiety by learning how to relax the muscular tension. Jacobson trained his patients to voluntarily relax certain muscles in their body in order to reduce anxiety symptoms. He also found that the relaxation procedure is effective against ulcers, insomnia, and hypertension. Self-hypnosis is a naturally occurring state of mind which can be defined as a heightened state of focused concentration (trance), with the willingness to follow instructions (suggestibility). Biofeedback is a form of alternative medicine that involves measuring a subject's quantifiable bodily functions such as blood pressure, heart rate, skin temperature, sweat gland activity, and muscle tension, conveying the information to the patient in real time. This raises the patient's awareness and conscious control of their unconscious physiological activities. By providing the user access to physiologic information about which he or she is generally unaware, biofeedback allows users to gain control of physical processes previously considered an automatic response of the autonomous nervous system.

B. Cognitive-behavioral therapies have improved pain scores, pain coping, pain behavior, depression, and physical functioning over several months in fibromyalgia patients. It is suspected that follow-ups with booster sessions may prolong the effects. While some think that support groups perpetuate griping, a resource-oriented self-support group can help a fibromyalgia patient come to terms with an illness and provide invaluable patient education.

C. Aerobic exercise is one of the first nonpharmacologic strategies promoted for patients with fibromyalgia. Low-impact aerobics of sufficient intensity to produce cardiovascular stimulation can decrease pain, enhance sleep, improve mood, increase energy, advance cognition, and better a patient's overall outlook. Fibromyalgia patients who exercise deal better with the disease. However, a fibromyalgia patient can also experience increased pain if the exercise regimen is too strenuous or carried out during an inopportune time in the treatment. These patients should begin with low-impact exercises (ie, aqua therapy). Continuing the patient on the exercise regimen becomes easier as the patient's pain decreases.

D. Heat helps fibromyalgia patients with tenderness, stiffness, and cephalgia. It can also calm muscles, ease exercising, and accentuate a sense of well-being. Cold application also works.

E. Some patients do obtain relief by light massages that progress to more deep sedative ones.

484. (E)

A. and D. Dopamine is a neurotransmitter best known for its role in the pathology of schizophrenia, Parkinson disease, and addiction. There is also strong evidence for a role of dopamine in restless leg syndrome, which is a common comorbid condition in patients with fibromyalgia. In addition, dopamine plays a critical role in pain perception and natural analgesia. Accordingly, musculoskeletal pain complaints are common among patients with Parkinson disease, which is characterized by drastic reductions in dopamine owing to neurodegeneration of dopamine-producing neurons, while patients with schizophrenia, which is thought to arise, at least partly, from hyperactivity of dopamine-producing neurons, have been shown to be relatively insensitive to pain. Interestingly, patients with restless legs syndrome have also been demonstrated to have hyperalgesia to static mechanical stimulation. Fibromyalgia has been commonly referred to as a "stress-related disorder" owing to its frequent onset and worsening of symptoms in the context of stressful events. It was therefore proposed that fibromyalgia may represent a condition characterized by low levels of central dopamine that likely results from a combination of genetic factors and exposure to environmental stressors, including psychosocial distress, physical trauma, systemic viral infections, or inflammatory disorders (eg, rheumatoid arthritis, systemic lupus erythematosus). This conclusion was based on three key observations: (1) fibromyalgia is associated with stress; (2) chronic exposure to stress results in a disruption of dopamine-related neurotransmission; and (3) dopamine plays a critical role in modulating pain perception and central analgesia in such areas as the basal ganglia including the nucleus accumbens, insular cortex, anterior cingulate cortex, thalamus, periaqueductal gray, and spinal cord. In support of the "dopamine hypothesis of fibromyalgia," a reduction in dopamine synthesis has been reported after using positron emission tomography (PET) and demonstrated a reduction in dopamine synthesis among fibromyalgia patients in several brain regions in which dopamine plays a role in inhibiting pain perception, including the mesencephalon, thalamus, insular cortex, and anterior cingulate cortex. A subsequent PET study demonstrated that, whereas healthy individuals release dopamine into the caudate nucleus and putamen during a tonic experimental pain stimulus (ie, hypertonic saline infusion into a muscle bed), fibromyalgia patients fail to release dopamine in response to pain and, in some cases, actually have a reduction in dopamine levels during painful stimulation. Moreover, a substantial subset of fibromyalgia patients respond well in controlled trials to pramipexole, a dopamine agonist that selectively stimulates dopamine D2/D3 receptors and is used to treat both Parkinson disease and restless legs syndrome.

B. Tryptophan is decreased in the serum and CSF of fibromyalgia patients. Serotonin is low in fibromyalgia serum. 5-Hydroxytrytophan, the intermediary between tryptophan and serotonin, and 5-hydroxyindole acetic acid, the by-product of serotonin metabolism, are both low in the CSF of patients with fibromyalgia. The excretion in urine of 5-hydroxyindole acetic acid was lower than normal in patients with fibromyalgia, lower in females versus males, and lower in females with fibromyalgia versus females who don't have fibromyalgia.

C. The numbers of active tender points in fibromyalgia patients directly correlated with the concentration of serotonin in fibromyalgia sera.

485. (C) Fibromyalgia, a common chronic pain condition characterized by widespread pain, is thought to originate largely from altered central neurotransmission. In this study, a sample of 17 fibromyalgia patients and 17 age- and sex-matched healthy controls, were compared using μ-opioid receptor PET. PET scans measure blood flow in the brain. It was demonstrated that fibromyalgia patients display reduced μ-opioid receptor binding potential within several regions known to play a role in pain modulation, including the nucleus accumbens, the amygdala, and the dorsal cingulate.

The reduced availability of the receptors could result from a reduced number of opioid receptors, enhanced release of opioids that are produced naturally by the body, or both. These findings indicate altered endogenous opioid analgesic activity in fibromyalgia and suggest a possible reason for why exogenous opiates appear to have reduced efficacy in this population. The reduced availability of the receptor was associated with greater pain among people with fibromyalgia.

Answers (A), (B), (D), and (E) have no merit.

486. **(C)**

A. and B. The sedating tricyclic biogenic amine reuptake drugs, such as amitriptyline and cyclobenzaprine, are the most commonly prescribed medications for fibromyalgia insomnia. These medications are mostly used in low doses to improve sleep and to enhance the effects of analgesics (amitriptyline 10-25 mg at night and cyclobenzaprine 5-10 mg at night). Patients can develop tachyphylaxis to them, but a 1-month holiday from the drugs may help restore effectiveness.

C. SSRIs are so stimulating that they can interfere with sleep, and should never be taken at bedtime.

D. Benzodiazepine decrease anxiety and allow less troubled sleep (alprazolam, clonazepam). Clonazepam in particular can help control nocturnal myoclonus when it is associated with fibromyalgia.

E. Pregabalin is a sedative in addition to an antinociceptive medication.

487. **(E)**

488. **(B)** In osteolytic bone metastases, the most commonly involved sites are vertebrae, pelvis, ribs, femur, and skull. Upper and lower extremity bones, except femur, are not commonly involved.

489. **(A)** Multiple sites of metastatic epidural spinal cord compression occur in 17% to 30% of all patients. This is particularly common in prostatic and breast carcinoma and uncommon in lung cancer.

490. **(E)** Bisphosphonates decrease resorption of bone directly, by inhibiting the recruitment and function of osteoclasts, and indirectly, by stimulating osteoblasts. In patients with bony metastases, they are the standard therapy for hypercalcemia after rehydration, and have the greatest effect in patients with breast cancer and multiple myeloma. Bisphosphonates also have an acute pain-relieving effect, which is thought to be derived from the reduction of various pain-producing substances.

491. **(E)** Both gabapentin, an antiepileptic drug, and amitriptyline, TCA, are widely used in treating neuropathic pain, which is often a significant component of a cancer pain syndrome.

Samarium 153 belongs to the group of bone-seeking radiopharmaceuticals emitting medium- to high-energy beta particle radiation. The most commonly used agent in this group is Strontium 89 with a documented pain-relieving effect in patients with bony metastases. Samarium 153, rhenium 186, and phosphorus 32 are also available for clinical use.

492. **E)**

493. **(E)** Both gabapentin (an antiepileptic drug) and amitriptyline (a TCA) are widely used in treating neuropathic pain, which is often a significant component of a cancer pain syndrome.

Samarium 153 belongs to the group of bone-seeking radiopharmaceuticals emitting medium- to high-energy beta particle radiation. The most commonly used agent in this group is Strontium 89 with a documented pain-relieving effect in patients with bony metastases. Samarium 153, rhenium 186, and phosphorus 32 are also available for clinical use.

494. **(E)**

495. **(E)**

496. **(A)**

497. **(B)** In clinical practice, most peripheral neuropathies do not produce chronic pain as impairment of nerve fibers carrying nociception should result in decrease pain perception. In most neuropathies, all components of the peripheral nervous system are affected, presenting with variable sensorimotor deficit and autonomic dysfunction.

498. **(B)** The most commonly activated areas during acute processing of pain in humans are S-I, S-II, anterior cingulated cortex, insular cortex, prefrontal cortex, thalamus, and cerebellum.

499. **(B)** Many studies suggest that axonal injury along the nociceptive fiber in the peripheral

nervous system is the main cause of neuro-pathic pain. Several conditions where the small fibers are spared support this concept. The Charcot-Marie-Tooth disease also known as hereditary motor and sensory neuropathy where the demyelination is limited to large myelinated fibers, do not manifest with pain. Segmental anhidrosis or Ross syndrome where only autonomic fibers are affected, is also not painful. On the other hand, conditions affecting the small nerve fibers, like diabetic neuropathy or Fabry disease, a rare lipid-storage disorder, commonly present with pain.

500. **(A)** Chronic renal failure is associated with selective loss of large nerve fibers which is rarely painful. Common symptoms include restless leg syndrome, distal numbness, and paresthesias, with distal weakness usually in the lower extremities.

501. **(E)** Cytokines, a heterogeneous group of pep-tides activate the immune system and mediate inflammation. They form a complex bidirec-tional system that communicates between the immune system and the CNS. IL-1 is the most extensively studied cytokine. Intraplantar as well as intraperitoneal injections of IL-1 reduce mechanical and probably thermal nociceptive threshold, which may be blocked by local cyclooxygenase inhibitors, supporting the role of prostaglandins in the process. The commu-nicating pathway between the peripheral cytokines and the brain may involve vagal afferents terminating in the nucleus tractus soli-tarius and circumventricular sites that lack a blood-brain barrier.

502. **(A)** Blockade of the sympathetic innervation of the head can be documented by the pres-ence of Horner syndrome, which is character-ized by myosis, ptosis, and enophthalmus. Associate findings include conjunctival injec-tion, nasal congestion, and facial anhidrosis. Horner syndrome is an expected finding after blockade of the sympathetic afferents to the face and can not be considered a complication.

503. **(E)** Behavioral studies have shown that activa-tion of NMDA receptors are required for the development and maintenance of pain-related behaviors. Calcium channels are the key ion involved in the release of transmitters. Different subtypes of calcium channels (L-, N-, and P/Q-types) may have a differential role depending on the nature of the pain state. The N-type voltage-dependent calcium channels appear to be the predominant isoform involved in the pre- and postsynaptic processing of sensory nociceptive inputs. Animal and clinical studies have shown partial pain relief with the use of a specific N-type calcium channel blocker synthetically derived from a conotoxin, SNX-111. The generic name of this substance derived from the snail's natural conotoxin is Ziconotide.

504. **(A)** The effectiveness of opioid agonists in the management of neuropathic pain has created significant controversy over the last two decades. Recent studies have increased our understanding about this topic. In patients with SCI and stroke, IV morphine showed poor effects in reducing spontaneous pain, but sig-nificantly reduced stroking allodynia. Other studies used alfentanil in the treatment of neu-ropathic pain independently of the etiology and observed decrease in dynamic, stroking allodynia, and spontaneous pain, while increase the temperature at which heat pain was detected and decrease the temperature at which cold pain was detected.

505. **(A)** Action potentials in the dorsal horn neu-rons are mediated by glutaminergic excitatory postsynaptic potentials, this activity may be inhibited predominantly by the inhibition pro-duced by GABA and/or glycine which causes fast inhibition of postsynaptic potentials. GABAA and glycine receptors are ligand-gated Cl^- channels, while GABAB, adenosine, and opioids exert their typically produced postsy-naptic hyperpolarization by activation of K^+ channels.

506. **(C)** More intense or sustained noxious periph-eral stimulation induce primary afferent noci-ceptors to discharge at higher frequencies and to release from central nociceptor terminals neuromodulator peptides like CGRP, substance P, and glutamate. As more and more dorsal

horn neurons get depolarized, NMDA receptors open by removing the Mg2+ blockade, allowing for intracellular calcium levels to increase. The end result of these intracellular signaling cascades is windup.

507. **(B)** Histopathological studies in patients with PHN have found ganglion cell loss and fibrosis and atrophy of the dorsal horn, DRG, dorsal root, and peripheral nerves. Up to 30% of patients with PHN have no loss of sensation in the affected dermatome demonstrating minimal or no loss of neuronal function and interestingly thermal sensory thresholds are not affected or even decreased. Antiviral drugs have shown disappointing results in patients with chronic PHN. Heat hyperalgesia is more common than cold hyperalgesia, which only occurs in less than 10% of the patients.

508. **(B)** Phantom pain is equally frequent in men and women and is not influenced by age in adults, side or level of amputation, and cause (civilian versus traumatic) of amputation. Phantom pain is less frequent in young children and congenital amputees.

509. **(A)** Phantom pain is usually intermittent. Only a few patients are in constant pain. Episodes of pain are most often reported to occur daily, or at daily or weekly intervals.

Phantom pain is usually localized to the distal parts of the missing limb. Pain is normally felt in the fingers and palm of the hand in upper limb amputees and toes, foot, or ankle in lower limb amputees. This may be because of the larger cortical representation of the hand and foot as opposed to the lesser representation of the more proximal parts of the limb.

The character of phantom pain is usually described as shooting, pricking, burning, stabbing, pins and needles, tingling, throbbing, cramping, and crushing.

510. **(D)** Phantom sensations are more common than phantom pain, and are experienced by nearly all amputees. The incidence of phantom sensations ranges from 71% to 90%, 8 days to 2 years after amputation. Duration and frequency, but not incidence, decrease as time passes. Phantom sensations are less common in congenital amputees and in patients who underwent amputation before the age of 6 years

Nonpainful sensations normally appear within the first days after amputation. The amputee often wakes up from anesthesia with a feeling that the amputated limb is still there. Just after the amputation, the phantom limb often resembles the preamputation limb in shape, length, and volume. As time passes, the phantom fades, leaving back the distal parts of the limb. For example, upper limb amputees may feel hand and fingers, and lower limb amputees may feel foot and toes.

Commonly, upper limb amputees feel the fingers clenched in a fist, while the phantom limb of lower limb amputees is often described as toes flexed In some cases, phantom sensations include feeling of movement and posture; however, in others only suggestions of the phantom are felt.

Telescoping (shrinkage of the phantom) is reported to occur in about one-third of patients. The phantom progressively approaches the stump and eventually becomes attached to it. It has even been experienced within the residual limb. Phantom pain does not retard shrinkage of the phantom.

511. **(B)** Changes occur in the DRG cells, after a complete nerve cut. Cells in the DRG show similar abnormal spontaneous activity and increased sensitivity to mechanical and neurochemical stimulation. Local anesthesia of neuromas abolished tap-induced afferent discharges and tap-induced accentuation of phantom pain, but spontaneous pain and recorded spontaneous activity were unchanged which is consistent with the activity in DRG cells. DRG cells exhibit major changes in the expression of sodium channels, with an altered expression pattern of different channels.

The sympathetic nervous system may play a role in generating and especially in maintaining phantom pain. It was noted that application of noradrenaline or activation of the postganglionic sympathetic fibers excites and sensitizes damaged, but not normal nerve fibers. Injecting noradrenaline into the skin can reestablish neuropathic pain that has just been relieved with a sympathetic block and injecting into a neuroma is reported to be intensely painful.

The catecholamine sensitivity may also manifest itself in the skin with a colder limb on the amputated side, and it has been implied that phantom pain intensity is inversely related to the skin temperature of the stump.

512. **(A)**

1. Numerous studies on preemptive analgesia using epidural, epidural/perineural, and just perineural administration have been conducted. Only two were noted to utilize proper patient randomization and blinding.

2. Persistent pain has been reported in up to 80% of patients after limb amputation. The mechanisms are not fully understood, but nerve injury during amputation is important, with evidence for the crucial involvement of the spinal NMDA receptor in central changes. The study objective was to assess the effect of preemptively modulating sensory input with epidural ketamine (an NMDA antagonist) on postamputation pain and sensory processing.

3. The aim of preemptive analgesia is to avoid spinal sensitization by blocking, in advance, the cascade of intra-neuronal responses that take place after peripheral nerve injury. True preemptive treatment is not likely possible in patients scheduled for amputation as most have been suffering from ischemic pain and are almost certainly presenting with preexisting neuronal hyperexcitability. To conclude: epidural blockade has been shown to be effective in the treatment of preoperative ischemic pain and postoperative stump pain.

513. **(A)** Acidic foods, such as orange juice, carbonated drinks, tomatoes, and vinegar may aggravate the symptoms of interstitial cystitis. Spicy food, alcohol, coffee, chocolate, tea, cola, and smoking should also be either restricted or completely eliminated.

514. **(C)** Sodium pentosan polysulfate (Elmiron) is an oral analogue of heparin. Inside the bladder, it acts as a synthetic glycosaminoglycan layer and fortifies bladder wall defenses from bacteria by increasing the antiadherent surface of the bladder mucosa.

515. **(E)** Endogenous opioid peptides as other neurotransmitters, such as serotonin, norepinephrine, and GABA, are thought to be involved in descending inhibition.

516. **(E)** Anxiety, fear, helplessness, and sleep deprivation are part of the vicious cycle of pain. Cultural background has been shown to play a significant role in the individual's pain response.

517. **(E)**

518. **(A)** There is evidence that pain-related impairment of intestinal motility may be relieved by epidural local anesthetics.

519. **(B)** Pain in the area of sensory loss, also called deafferentation pain, or anesthesia dolorosa, is a prominent sign of a neuropathic pain. Neuropathic pain generally responds less well to opioid treatment than somatic pain. One of the significant signs of neuropathic pain is also allodynia-a painful response to nonpainful stimuli. Tapping of neuromas produces radiating electric shock sensation in the distribution of the damaged nerve is called Tinel sign—another feature of a neuropathic pain.

520. **(E)**

521. **(E)** Post–burn injury pain has two components: a constant background pain and an intermittent procedure-related pain. Continuous infusion of opioids is useful for control of the background component of pain. Pain related to wound care, dressing changes, and others (procedure-related pain) may require brief but profound analgesia. This may be achieved by administration of supplemental IV opioids, or addition of the adjuvant drugs, such as IV ketamine, IV benzodiazepines, inhaled nitrous oxide-oxygen mixture, or even general anesthesia.

522. **(E)** All answers are correct. A concomitant head injury may be associated with increased intracranial pressure, which could be considered a contraindication for an epidural catheter placement.

523. **(B)** Two types of pain may be found in PHN: a steady burning or aching, the other, a paroxysmal, lancinating pain. Both may occur spontaneously and are usually aggravated by any contact with the involved skin.

524. **(E)** All of the listed groups of medication were found to be effective to some extent in the treatment of PHN. A multimodal approach seems to be more effective because of the synergistic effect different modes of action.

525. **(E)**

526. **(E)**

527. **(A)** Oral steroids may provide pain relief in acute phase of herpes zoster, as well as shorten the time to full crusting of lesions. However, controlled trials showed no benefit in the prevention of PHN. With the development of antiviral agents, the use of oral steroids is currently not recommended because of more frequent side effects.

528. **(B)** Diabetic amyotrophy is a condition occurring in diabetic patients, more commonly with type-2 diabetes, which begins with pain in the thighs, hips, and buttocks. Weakness and atrophy of the proximal pelvic muscles groups, iliopsoas, obturator, and adductor muscles follows the painful manifestations. It usually does not involve sciatic nerve, or distal muscles of the lower extremity. The therapy for diabetic amyotrophy is primarily supportive.

529. **(A)** Neuropathic arthropathy (Charcot joint) develops most often in weight-bearing joints. The predominant cause is DM, but also associated with neuropathic arthropathy are leprosy, yaws, congenital insensitivity to pain, spina bifida, myelomeningocele, syringomyelia, acrodystrophic neuropathy, amyloid neuropathy, peripheral neuropathy secondary to alcoholism and avitaminosis, SCI, peripheral nerve injury, postrenal transplant arthropathy, intraarticular steroid injections, and syphilis. The etiology of Charcot joint is believed to be related to the destruction of afferent proprioceptive fibers and subsequent unrecognized trauma to the joint.

530. **(D)** A cross-sectional, community-based survey of 255 patients with DPNP recruited through the offices of endocrinologists, neurologists, anesthesiologists, and primary care physicians found that NSAIDs were the most commonly used medications, with 46.7% reporting their use. This is despite the fact, that there is little evidence to support the efficacy of NSAIDs in DPNP, and that NSAIDs have a high potential for renal impairment in patients with diabetic neuropathy.

531. **(E)**

532. **(A)** Given the frequency of imperfect glycemic control, attempts have been made to identify oral medications which can target downstream metabolic consequences of hyperglycemia, thereby preventing production of reactive oxygen species, which are felt to contribute to diabetic neuropathy. Unfortunately, trials of aldose reductase inhibitors, which decrease aberrant metabolic flux, have been disappointing (eg, sorbinil, zopolrestat).

533. **(B)** The combination of trigeminal neuralgia and hemifacial spasm is known as convulsive tic. It is reported to be more severe in women than in men. Occasionally, strong spasms involve all of the facial muscles unilaterally almost continuously. Seldom, facial weakness may be present. Convulsive tic may indicate the presence of a tumor, vascular malformation, or ecstatic dilation of the basilar artery, compressing the trigeminal or facial nerves.

534. **(A)** The diagnostic criteria for trigeminal neuralgia are: shooting, electric-like, sharp, severe pain which last for seconds but sometimes experienced together with pain-free intervals. The pain is periodic with weeks or months without pain. The pain is typically unilateral and triggered by light touch, eating, talking, or washing.

535. (D) Rarely, trigeminal neuralgia is the presenting symptom of multiple sclerosis. More often, trigeminal neuralgia presents in patients with advanced stages of multiple sclerosis.

536. (C) Glycerol is a nonselective neurolytic agent. Although less common than with radiofrequency thermocoagulation, the frequency of patients affected by sensory loss is high. Recurrence rate is the highest among all ablative techniques.

537. (E) The trigeminal neuralgia is the most common cranial neuralgia and its most frequent form is idiopathic. The incidence of trigeminal neuralgia is 5.7 per 1000 females and 2.5 per 1000 in males. Patients with multiple sclerosis have a higher risk for trigeminal neuralgia. Other potential relation was found in patients with family history.

538. (A) The trigeminal neuralgia is a primary axonal degenerative disease. The ignition hypothesis combines the current knowledge of the role of ion channels in the development of neuropathic pain. Focal demyelination adjacent to the area of arterial compression has been shown by electron microscopy in patients undergoing posterior fossa surgery. In up to 30% of patients with arterial cross compression, there is a groove or an area of discoloration lateral where the root entry zone would be expected.

539. (C) SIH and PDPH have similar presentation, pathophysiology, and treatment. The most important distinction is the initiating event, which is obvious in PDPH. MRI of the brain with gadolinium enhancement in patients with SIH shows meningeal enhancement, and thickening, and a possible caudad shift of the brain toward the foramen magnum. The most common location of spontaneous dural tear is the thoracic region followed by the cervicothoracic and thoracolumbar junction regions.

540. (B) It has been shown that keeping a supine position for 2 hours after the EBP provides higher chances of success when compared with 30 minutes. Although initial relief is very high (close to 100%), the overall long-term relief of

PDPH after EBP is between 61% and 75%. The effectiveness of EBP is reduced when the dural tear was caused by a large-size needle.

541. (C) Two important factors in the prevention of PDPH are the use of small and blunt bevel spinal needles. Other factors that may prevent the development of PDPH include the use of paramedian approach (with angles of 35° or greater) and the use of intrathecal catheters. Bed rest as a preventive measure is not effective.

542. (E) Cervicogenic headache is defined as headache that arises from painful disorders of structures in the upper neck, which generates irritation of the upper cervical roots or their nerve branches. The current classification by the IHS and the IASP accepts these headaches to be unilateral or bilateral. All the other options in the questions are true.

543. (E) According to the International Headache Society and the IASP, cervicogenic headache (CGH) is a pain originated in the neck, mostly unilateral although it may be bilateral, exacerbated by neck movement, and alleviated by local anesthetic block of the occipital nerve. The prevalence of CGH is 0.4% to 2.5% in the general population and may account for up to 15% to 20% of patients with chronic headache, more common in females with a 4:1 ratio and mean age of patients with 42.9 years.

544. (A) During the aura in classic migraine a decrease in cerebral blood flow decreases spreads from the occipital cortex. The variation in the cerebral blood flow causes the aura and activates trigeminal nerve endings. It is possible that cortical spreading depression may stimulate peripheral nerve terminals of the nucleus caudalis trigeminalis.

545. (B) During the aura in classic migraine there is a decrease in cerebral blood flow.

In patients with classic migraine (migraine with aura), there is increase of cerebral blood flow that happens after the headache begins and this change persist until the headache resolves. In migraine without aura, there is no change in cerebral blood flow.

546. **(E)** Migraine is a risk factor for affective disorders. When comparing with nonmigraineurs, patients with migraine have a 4.5-fold increased risk of major depression, a sixfold risk of manic episodes, a threefold increase in anxiety disorder, and a sixfold prevalence in panic disorder.

547. **(A)** Although migraine begins in the first three decades of life, the higher prevalence is in the fifth one. Family history is a common finding, and pregnant females often experience worsening symptoms in the first trimester and improvement during the third. Many women experience improvement of their symptoms after natural, but not surgical menopause.

548. **(C)** Muscle tenderness is common in patients suffering from TTH, but is not secondary to pericranial muscle contraction or ischemic pain in response to emotion or stress. Increased EMG activity is independent of tenderness and pain. Reduced pain threshold observed in chronic TTH may be the result of low CNS levels of serotonin. Although TTH can begin at any age, the most common onset is during adolescence and young adulthood. The prevalence of TTH decreases with increasing age.

549. **(E)** For any structure to be considered as a source for low back pain it must have the following characteristics: a nerve supply, the capability of causing low back pain similar to what is seen clinically (ideally in healthy volunteers), a susceptibility to disease or injuries known to be painful, and should be able to be shown as a source of pain using diagnostic techniques of known reliability and validity.

550. **(A)** There have been RCTs showing that lumbar supports and back schools are not effective in preventing back pain. Exercise has been proven by RCTs to prevent back pain. To date, there are no RCTs on the effectiveness of ergonomics in preventing back pain.

551. **(E)** The most significant anomalies of the lumbar nerve roots are aberrant courses and anastomoses between nerve roots. Type 1 anomalies are aberrant courses of which there are two kinds. Type 1A describes two pairs of nerve roots arising from a single dural sleeve, whereas type 1B defines a dural sleeve arising from a low position on the dural sac. Type 2 anomalies include those in which the number of roots in the intervertebral foramen varies. An empty foramen is classified as type 2A, and a foramen with extra nerve roots is known as a type 2B. Type 3 anomalies are those involving extradural anastomoses between roots in which a bundle of nerves leaves on dural sleeve to enter one nearby. Type 3 anomalies may coexist with type 2 anomalies.

552. **(E)** The IASP published standardized terms to define low back pain as pain perceived to arise for lumbar spinal pain and/or sacral spinal pain. Lumbar spinal pain is defined as pain perceived to arise from the region bordered superiorly by an imaginary line through the T12 spinous process, inferiorly by a line through the S1 spinous process, and laterally by the lateral borders of the erector spinae. Sacral spinal pain is that defined as pain perceived to arise from the region bordered laterally by imaginary vertical lines through the posterior superior and posterior inferior iliac spines, superiorly by a transverse line through the S1 spinous process, and inferiorly by a transverse line through the posterior sacrococcygeal joints.

553. **(E)** Transforaminal injections have been the cause of some of the most worrisome recent complications. These included cerebellar and cerebral infarct, SCI, and infarction, massive cerebral edema, paraplegia, visual defects with occlusion following particulate depo-corticosteroids, anterior spinal artery syndrome, persistent neurologic deficits, transient quadriplegia, cauda equina syndrome, subdural hematoma, and paraplegia following intracordal injection during attempted epidural anesthesia under general anesthesia.

554. **(C)** Despite its controversial history, disc stimulation (formerly known as discography) remains the only means by which to determine whether or not a disc is painful. The test is positive if upon stimulating a disc the patient's pain is reproduced provided that stimulation of

adjacent discs does not reproduce their pain. Discs are also considered to be symptomatic only if pain is reproduced at injection pressures less than 50 psi and preferably less than 15 psi. At injection pressures greater than 80 psi, some discs are painful in normal individuals. The stimulation of discs has been complemented by another approach, heating a wire electrode that has been inserted into a disc annulus. Heating a disc evokes pain that is perceived in the back. This pain may also radiate to the lower extremities and be responsible for referred pain in the thigh and leg.

555. **(B)** Chemonucleolysis is indicated for contained disc protrusions causing sciatic pain that have been unresponsive to conservative management. The injection is contraindicated for extruded and sequestered disc herniations, and in patients with cauda equine syndrome. Relative contraindications include previous chymopapain injections, previous surgery for lumbar disc herniation, spinal stenosis, severe degenerative disc or facet osteoarthritis, and spondylolisthesis.

556. **(E)** Inappropriate or premature selection of patients for surgery is the most common cause of FBSS. The second most common cause is persistence of pain secondary to irreversible neural injury. A less common cause is inadequate surgery. Lastly, a variant of FBSS results from new pathologic processes initiated by the initial surgery.

557. **(A)** The American Association of Neurological Surgeons and the American Academy of Orthopedic Surgeons have published criteria for patient selection for elective lumbosacral spine surgery. They are applicable to new patients, as well as FBSS patients. They include the following:

1. Failure of conservative therapy.
2. An abnormal diagnostic imaging study showing nerve root or cauda equina compression and/or signs of segmental instability consistent with the patient's signs/symptoms.

Radicular pain with one or more of the following: (a) corresponding dermatomal segmental sensory loss, (b) corresponding dermatomal motor loss, (c) abnormal deep tendon reflexes consistent with appropriate dermatomes.

558. **(A)** There are three main types of cervical spine involvement in rheumatoid arthritis: atlantoaxial subluxation, cranial settling, and subaxial subluxation. The inflammatory changes affecting synovial joints and bursae target structures lined with a synovial membrane in the cervical spine. Patients with cervical spine involvement are thought to have a more severe form of rheumatoid arthritis, and their prognosis is usually worse. Occipital condylar fractures result from a full-energy blunt trauma complemented with axial compression, lateral bending, or rotational injury to the alar ligament.

559. **(E)** The *Québec Task Force* (QTF) was a task force sponsored by the Société de l'assurance automobile du Québec, the public auto insurer in Quebec, Canada. In 1995, the QTF submitted a report on WADs which made specific recommendations on prevention, diagnosis, and treatment of WAD. These recommendations have become the base for *Guideline on the Management of Claims Involving Whiplash-Associated*, a guide to classifying WAD and guidelines on managing the disorder. The full report titled *Redefining "Whiplash"* was published in the April 15, 1995 issue of *Spine*. An update was published in January 2001.

Four grades of WAD were defined by the QTF:

Grade 1: Complaints of neck pain, stiffness or tenderness only but no physical signs are noted by the examining physician.

Grade 2: Neck complaints and the examining physician finds decreased range of motion and point tenderness in the neck.

Grade 3: Decreased range of motion plus neurologic signs, such as decreased deep tendon reflexes, weakness, insomnia, and sensory deficits.

Grade 4: Neck complaints and fracture or dislocation, or injury to the spinal cord.

560. **(A)** The distraction test is performed with an examiner standing behind a seated patient, lifting their head from the chin and occiput, and removing the weight of the head from the neck. If relief of neck pain occurs, the test might point to foraminal intrusion on a nerve root as the source of pain.

561. **(A)** Spurling maneuver is used to identify nerve root compression or irritation. The head is tilted toward the affected side and manual pressure is applied to the top of the head. Radicular pain should be reproduced with this maneuver. Valsalva test allows a patient to experience painful or sensory changes when bearing down. The test increases intrathecal pressure and exacerbates compression within the cervical canal caused by tumors, infections, disc herniations, or osteophyte changes. The distraction test is performed with an examiner standing behind a seated patient, lifting their head from the chin and occiput, and removing the weight of the head from the neck. If relief of neck pain occurs, the test might point to foraminal intrusion on a nerve root as the source of pain. Adson test is used to assess vascular compromise because of subclavian artery impingement from thoracic outlet syndrome.

562. **(D)** Peripheral neuropathic pain syndromes in patients with HIV infection tend to be specific to the stage of HIV infection as outlined in answers (1) through (3).

563. **(A)** In patients with predominantly sensory neuropathy of AIDS, the complaints are mostly sensory. However, the NCV and EMG studies demonstrate both sensory and motor involvement.

564. **(E)** Psychostimulants, such as dextroamphetamine, methylphenidate, may be useful agents in patients with HIV infection or AIDS who are cognitively impaired. Psychostimulants enhance the analgesic effects of the opioid drugs. They are also useful in diminishing sedation secondary to opioids. In addition, psychostimulants improve appetite, promote sense

of well-being, and improve feelings of weakness and fatigue in patients with malignancies.

565. **(B)** Tissue injury generates several major pain mediators, including, but not limited to IL-1, bradykinin, K^+, H^+, histamine, substance P, and CGRP. The pathway for painful stimuli is subject not only to activators, sensitizers, and facilitators but also to inhibitors. Serotonin, enkephalin, β-endorphin, and dynorphin are endogenous central pain inhibitors.

566. **(E)** SCD is a quadrumvirate of: (1) pain syndromes, (2) anemia and its sequelae, (3) organ failure, including infection, and (4) comorbid conditions. Pain, however, is the insignia of SCD and dominates its clinical picture throughout the life of the patients. Pain may precipitate or be itself precipitated by the other three components of the quadrumvirate.

567. **(C)** Avascular necrosis is the most commonly observed complication of SCD in adults. Although it tends to be most severe and disabling in the hip area, it is a generalized bone disorder in that the femoral and humeral heads and the vertebral bodies may be equally affected. Treatment of avascular necrosis is symptomatic and includes providing nonopioid or opioid analgesics in the early stages of the illness; advanced forms of the disease require total joint replacement. Core decompression appears to be effective in the management of avascular necrosis if performed during its early stages.

568. **(B)** Leg ulceration is a painful and sometimes disabling complication of sickle cell anemia that occurs in 5% to 10% of adult patients with SCD. With good localized treatment, many ulcers heal within a few months. Leg ulcers that persist beyond 6 months may require skin grafting, although results of this treatment have been disappointing. Recent advances in management include the use of platelet-derived growth factor, prepared either autologously (Procuren) or by recombinant technology (Regranex).

569. **(E)**

570. **(A)** Sickle cell anemia affects millions throughout the world. It is particularly common among people whose ancestors come from sub-Saharan Africa; Spanish-speaking regions (South America, Cuba, Central America); Saudi Arabia; India; and Mediterranean countries such as Turkey, Greece, and Italy.

571. **(E)** General management of vasoocclusive crisis during pregnancy begins with aggressive hydration to increase intravascular volume and decrease blood viscosity. Supplemental oxygen is essential in those patients with hypoxemia. Partial exchange transfusions are used to reduce polymerized hemoglobin S. Prophylactic transfusions may reduce the incidence of severe sickling complications during pregnancy.

572. **(E)** Some patients with SCD are opioid-tolerant secondary to their home opioid management. Therefore, the home opioid requirement should be taken into account for faster and more efficient pain control of sickle crisis pain. Opioid titration, however, may require some additional care because hypoxemia and hypercarbia further exacerbate sickling of erythrocytes.

573. **(D)** Autonomic dysreflexia is a potential life-threatening condition, which is triggered by sensory input below the lesion and manifests itself with increased blood pressure, headache, and a risk of cerebral hemorrhage and seizure.

574. **(C)** Anterior cord syndrome is a common incomplete cord syndrome. A patient with anterior cord syndrome may exhibit complete motor and incomplete sensory loss, with the exception of retained trunk and lower extremity deep pressure sensation and proprioception. This syndrome carries the worst prognosis for return of function, and only a 10% chance of functional motor recovery has been reported.

575. **(B)** Posterior cord syndrome is a rare incomplete cord syndrome consisting of loss of the sensations of deep pressure and deep pain and proprioception, with otherwise normal cord function. The patient ambulates with a foot-slapping gait similar to that of someone afflicted with tabes dorsalis.

576. **(E)** Brown-Séquard syndrome is an uncommon incomplete spinal cord syndrome. It is anatomically a unilateral cord injury, such as a missile injury. It is clinically characterized by a motor deficit ipsilateral to the SCI in combination with contralateral pain and temperature hypesthesia. Almost all these patients show partial recovery, and most regain bowel and bladder function and the ability to ambulate.

577. **(A)** Anticonvulsants have several pharmacologic actions, such as modulation of sodium and calcium channels, increasing GABA inhibition, and suppressing abnormal neuronal hyperexcitability, which suggest an effect in neuropathic pain.

578. **(E)** Patient with autonomic dysreflexia usually exhibit decline in heart rate, dramatic changes in blood pressure, flushing and sweating above the level of the injury, and a marked reduction on peripheral blood flow through the reflex pathways in the preserved vagus nerves.

579. **(C)** HO is the formation of mature, lamellar bone in nonskeletal tissue, usually occurring in soft tissue surrounding joints. The bone formation in HO differs from other disorders of calcium deposition in that HO results in encapsulated bone between muscle planes, not intra-articular or connected to periosteum.

In neurogenic HO secondary to TBI or SCI, the hip is the most common joint affected.

Even though the most common symptom of HO is pain, it may be painless in patients with complete SCI.

Etidronate disodium, a bisphosphonate, is an osteoclast inhibitor. It is structurally similar to inorganic pyrophosphate and is shown to delay the aggregation of apatite crystals into large, calcified clusters in patients with TBI and SCI. The recommended prophylactic treatment for HO in SCI is 20 mg/kg/d for 2 weeks, then 10 mg/kg/d for 10 weeks. The current treatment recommendation for established HO is 300 mg IV daily for 3 days followed by 20 mg/kg/d for 6 months in spinal cord patients.

580. **(E)** Localized neurogenic inflammation may explain the acute edema, vasodilation, and sweating observed in early stages of CRPS. Increased protein concentration and synovial hypervascularization is observed in the intra-articular fluid of affected joints. Findings that support the role of neurogenic inflammation in the generation of CRPS include elevated systemic levels of CGRP and local increase of IL-6 and tumor necrosis factor alpha in artificially produced blisters.

581. **(C)** Up to 50% of CRPS patients show decrease range of motion, increase amplitude of physiologic tremor, and reduce active motor force, with dystonia of the affected limb observed in only 10% of the chronic cases. Those motor changes are unlikely associated with a peripheral process and more likely the result of changes of activity in the motor neurons which point to abnormalities of cerebral motor processing.

582. **(C)** It is estimated that the risk of CRPS after fractures is 1% to 2% and 12% after brain lesions. Retrospective studies in large cohorts shows a distribution in the upper and lower extremity from 1:1 to 2:1. CRPS following SCI are rare. Affected extremities after brain injury are more likely affected than unaffected ones.

583. **(E)** The three stages of the three-phase bone scan include the perfusion phase 30 seconds postinjection, the blood-pool is 2 minutes postinjection, and mineralization phases is evaluated 3 hours postinjection. Homogeneous unilateral hyperperfusion in the perfusion and blood-pool phase is consistent with CRPS and excludes the differential diagnosis of osteoporosis because of inactivity. The mineralization phase in patients with CRPS shows elevated unilateral periarticular uptake.

584. **(E)**

585. **(A)** The major peripheral pathologic findings in CRPS patients include (a) patchy atrophy of some muscle cells, secondary to disuse and nerve damage; (b) capillary microangiopathy, with accelerated turnover of endothelial cells

and pericytes; (c) Wallerian degeneration of several types of axons; and (d) focal osteopenia in the territory innervated by a damaged nerve, and synovial cell disorganization and edema.

586. **(B)** Medical procedures are the second most common cause of CRPS. The finding of exaggerated deep tendon reflexes in CRPS patients has been attributed to cortical disinhibition. Focal deficit of touch (hypoesthesia) were present in 50% of patients. Brushing skin activates low threshold mechanoreceptors which under normal circumstances has no connections with central pain neurons. Brush evoked pain (cutaneous dynamic mechanical allodynia)is a hallmark of central sensitization.

587. **(A)** In contrast to CRPS II which has similar frequencies in boys and girls, CRPS I is more common in girls with a ratio of 4:1. The lower extremity is more affected (5:1 ratio). CRPS I is more common in Caucasians. There is also evidence that CRPS may have a genetic predisposition, with increase incidence in patients with HLA A3, B7, and DR2.

588. **(B)** The gender distribution of CRPS II in the pediatric population is roughly similar in boys and girls. Even though patients with brachial plexus injury during delivery (Erb palsy) is common and can lead to prolonged motor weakness, they rarely develop pain. Interestingly most of these patients do better without treatment.

589. **(B)** The diagnosis of CRPS remains a clinical decision based on findings in the history and physical examination. There are no laboratory tests that can absolutely confirm or exclude the diagnosis. Although controversial, most of the authors find that bone scans are quite nonspecific for the diagnosis of CRPS. Patients with a clinical diagnosis of CRPS may have bone scans showing hypofixation or hyperfixation or may be normal. The primary utility of the bone scan could be in ruling out some underlying orthopedic abnormality that might be triggering neurovascular changes that may confused the findings with those of CRPS.

590.   (C) Movement disorders are an essential feature of patients with CRPS. Motor dysfunction is not simply a voluntary defensive response to protect the limb from painful stimuli, but may represent the interaction of peripheral and central mechanisms. Deep tendon reflexes are often brisk. The prevalence of movement disorders increases with the duration of the disease. One characteristic form of these movement disorders is the presence of inability to start a movement (akinesia).

591.   (A) Dystonia in CRPS patients causes twisting movements or abnormal postures of the affected body parts. The most prominent motor feature is flexor postures (tonic dystonia) of the fingers, feet, and wrist. Extensor postures occur but are rare.

592.   (E) Supraspinal mechanisms play a major role in the abnormal sensory perception of patients with CRPS. Segmental dystonia is characterized by spread of the cortical representation of the affected extremity and its corresponding synaptic connections to adjacent cortical areas. On the other hand, generalized dystonia have increased intracortical excitability to sensory stimuli, and motor cortex disinhibition has been confirmed in CRPS I. PET scan and SPET have shown increased activity of the contralateral thalamus in patients in early stages of CRPS and hypoperfusion in advanced stages.

593.   (C) Myofascial trigger point characteristics:

- Focal severe tenderness in a taut band of muscle
- Referral of pain to a distant site upon activation of the trigger point
- Contraction of the taut band (local twitch response) upon mechanical activation of the trigger point
- Reproduction of the pain by mechanical activation of trigger point
- Restriction of range of motion
- Weakness without muscle atrophy
- Autonomic phenomenon such as piloerection or changes in local circulation (regional blood flow and limb temperature) in response to trigger point activation

Individual features of the trigger point are differentially represented in different muscles. An examiner should not expect to find each feature of the trigger point in every muscle by physical examination.

594.   (A) Inactivation of the trigger point is a means to achieve pain relief, to improve biomechanical function, and then to improve the ability of the patient to better perform whatever tasks have been selected as goals. Relief (not elimination) of pain or increased range of motion, both of which can be the result of trigger point inactivation, are not in themselves the goals of treatment.

595.   (E) While chronic myofascial pain syndrome is best treated with a multidisciplinary team approach including the patient, physicians, psychologists, clinical social workers, occupational therapists, physical therapists, ergonomists, massage therapists, and others actively involved in patient care; patients with acute myofascial pain syndrome may only require treatment by physicians and physical therapists. Too frequently, patients with chronic myofascial pain are started too soon on isotonic training and conditioning, causing further aggravation of active trigger points and an increase in pain and dysfunction.

The acute treatment plan may be divided into a pain-control phase and a training or conditioning phase. During the pain-control phase, the most essential component is inactivation of the trigger point. Patients must change their behaviors and avoid overstressing their muscles without becoming excessively inactive. The pain-control phase must have a definitive endpoint. If patients do not move beyond the pain-control phase to the conditioning phase, patients can be restricted in their functional abilities and be at greater risk of reinjury. The training or conditioning phase follows and it involves therapeutic exercises, movement reeducation, and overall conditioning.

596.   (C) Botulinum toxin has been tried successfully in myofascial trigger point inactivation; however, it can cause a flu-like myalgia that lasts days to a week and sporadically causes weakness beyond the area of injection. It functions as a long-lasting trigger point injection that can provide up to 3 months of relief in contrast to the days to 1-week effect of traditional trigger point injection with local or no anesthetic.

597. (A)

1. Japanese acupuncture or shallow needling reduced the pain of chronic myofascial neck pain in one study.
2. and 3. These have been found to be true.
4. While this study does not exist, a technique of dry needling called intramuscular stimulation does exist. It involves the insertion of the needle into the taut band without necessarily considering the actual trigger point. It may be combined with electrical stimulation delivered through the needle (percutaneous electroneutral stimulation).

598. (E)

599. (D) Fibromyalgia has been found among all cultures throughout the world with an incidence of 2% to 12% of the population. In adulthood, women are affected four to seven times as often as men. The frequency of fibromyalgia increases with age and peaks in the seventh decade of life. In childhood, boys and girls are affected equally. In contrast to adults, children's symptoms may resolve with age.

600. (A) Although research is ongoing, the development of fibromyalgia appears to be increased if the patient has had a febrile illness, a history of physical trauma, or a family history of fibromyalgia syndrome. Approximately one-third of patients with fibromyalgia report that another member of their family has previously been diagnosed with fibromyalgia.

601. (E) Greater than 90% of patients with fibromyalgia suffer from chronic insomnia. Some patients may have problems falling asleep. Other may awaken a few hours after going to sleep and feel alert, thus disrupting their sleep throughout the remainder of the night. After a night of sleep, patients with fibromyalgia may feel stiff, tired, and "cognitively sluggish." These patients also encounter difficulty napping throughout the day. Patients with fibromyalgia have disrupted sleep architecture with alpha wave intrusions in deep, delta wave sleep.

602. (E)

3. In fibromyalgia patients, CT has revealed unusually low cerebral blood flow in the thalamic nuclei, the left and right heads of the caudate nucleus, and the cortex that correlates with spinal fluid substance P levels.
4. Windup is a frequency-dependent increase in the excitability of spinal cord neurons, evoked by electrical stimulation of afferent C fibers. Glutamate (NMDA) and tachykinin NK1 receptors are required to generate windup and therefore a positive modulation between these two receptor types has been suggested. Whatever the mechanisms involved in its generation, windup has been interpreted as a system for the amplification in the spinal cord of the nociceptive message that arrives from peripheral nociceptors connected to C fibers. This probably reflects the physiological system activated in the spinal cord after an intense or persistent barrage of afferent nociceptive impulses. On the other hand, windup, central sensitization and hyperalgesia are not the same phenomena, although they may share common properties. Spinal cord windup is abnormal in fibromyalgia syndrome.

Physical trauma or a fever/infection may be provisionally related to the onset of fibromyalgia in over 60% of cases.

603. (B) The levels of serum IL-8 were higher in fibromyalgia patients, and IL-6 was statistically higher in cultures of fibromyalgia peripheral blood mononuclear cells compared with in controls. The IL-8 increase was most dramatic in depressed patients, but there was also a correlation with the duration of fibromyalgia and the pain intensity. The production of IL-8 in vitro is stimulated by substance P.

604. (D) Pregabalin has the potential to raise the threshold for pain fiber depolarization. It is a ligand for the α2δ subunit of voltage-dependent calcium channel receptors, which has analgesic, anxiolytic-like, and anticonvulsant activity. It decreases the release of numerous neuropeptides, including noradrenaline, glutamate, and substance P. It has already been approved for treating partial seizures, pain following the rash of shingles and pain associated with diabetes nerve damage (diabetic neuropathy). Two double-blind, controlled clinical trials, involving about 1800 patients, support approval for use in treating fibromyalgia with doses of 300 or 450 mg/d. It is effective in reducing the severity of body pain, improving quality of sleep, and reducing fatigue in fibromyalgia patients. Pregabalin was approved by the FDA for use in fibromyalgia patients on June 21, 2007.

The most common side effects of pregabalin include mild to moderate dizziness and sleepiness. Blurred vision, weight gain, dry mouth, and swelling of the hands and feet also were reported in clinical trials. The side effects appeared to be dose-related. Pregabalin can impair motor function and cause problems with concentration and attention. The FDA advises that patients talk to their doctor or other health care professional about whether use of pregabalin may impair their ability to drive.

1. Cyclobenzaprine, have been used in the past with success in fibromyalgia patients, they have not been approved by the FDA.
2. Duloxetine is an FDA-approved treatment for major depression, neuropathic pain from diabetic peripheral neuropathy, and generalized anxiety disorder. The drug is a serotonin and norepinephrine reuptake inhibitor that exhibits nearly equal serotonin and noradrenaline reuptake inhibition. A trial of duloxetine for patients with chronic pain and/or major depression indicated that for the fibromyalgia patients, 80% of the observed effect on pain is a direct analgesic effect rather than an indirect antidepressant effect. Common adverse events were: nausea, headache, dry mouth, insomnia, constipation, dizziness, fatigue, somnolence, diarrhea, and hyperhidrosis. Two placebo-controlled randomized studies

on the treatment of fibromyalgia-associated pain with duloxetine have been published. Both studies demonstrated that duloxetine treatment improved fibromyalgia-associated pain in women. However, the medication has not yet been approved for the treatment of fibromyalgia. Another type of serotonin and noradrenaline reuptake inhibitor is represented by milnacipran, where noradrenaline reuptake inhibition is favored over that of serotonin. Some reports state that milnacipran may also be effective in treating fibromyalgia body pain.

3. Tramadol has only recently been shown to improve the pain of patients with fibromyalgia. It combines weak μ-agonist with NMDA antagonist and noradrenaline and serotonin reuptake inhibition. In the combination preparation that comes with acetaminophen, a considerable synergy has been noticed. Nausea and dizziness can be limiting at first in about 20% of patients, but starting with just one tablet at bedtime for 1 to 2 weeks can decrease the prevalence and allow later increases but about one tablet every 4 days to full therapeutic levels. A typical tramadol regimen for fibromyalgia is 300 to 400 mg/d in three or four divided dosages, concomitant with acetaminophen at 2 to 3 g/d in divided doses.

Administering 5-hydroxytryptophan can augment the synthesis of serotonin. One-hundred milligrams, orally, three times daily has been shown to be an effective dose in treating fibromyalgia.

605. **(B)** Central sensitization can be inhibited by NMDA receptor blockade. Two NMDA receptor antagonists, ketamine and dextromethorphan (an oral preparation) have been found to exhibit favorable effects on pain and allodynia in fibromyalgia patients. With ketamine, 50% of patients benefited. Fibromyalgia subgroups of responders and nonresponders were perpetuated by these findings because all the fibromyalgia patients in the study were otherwise comparable. Ketamine's effectiveness was limited because of its frequently occurring psychotropic side effects, such as feelings of unreality, altered body image perception, aggression, anxiety, nausea, dizziness, and modulation of hearing and vision.

Dextromethorphan has a better side-effect profile than ketamine. It was administered with tramadol to increase the antinociceptive effect, to hold adverse effects low, and to decrease the development of opioid tolerance. A good response was obtained in 58% of the fibromyalgia patients who tried this regimen. It may be a consideration for the patients who respond positively to IV ketamine.

CHAPTER 7

Pain Assessment
Questions

DIRECTIONS (Questions 606 through 614): Each of the numbered items or incomplete statements in this section is followed by answers or by completions of the statement. Select the ONE lettered answer or completion that is BEST in each case.

606. Regarding Minnesota Multiphasic Personality Inventory (MMPI) which of the following statement is true?

    (A) It has 547 questions

    (B) Conversion V is often present in patients with chronic pain

    (C) It can be interpreted by anyone treating the patient

    (D) Is not commonly used in evaluation of patients for spinal cord stimulation (SCS) trial

    (E) Can point out reliably the psychogenic part of the pain behavior

607. Visual analogue scale (VAS)

    (A) correlate highly with pain measured on verbal and numerical rating scales

    (B) is minimally intrusive

    (C) assumes that pain is a unidemnsional experience

    (D) measures the intensity of pain

    (E) all of the above

608. Which of the following tests is used as a more objective determination of disability?

    (A) The most thoroughly studied is the Sickness Illness Profile

    (B) Physical examination is an objective and consistent method of assessing impairment

    (C) McGill Pain Questionnaire

    (D) Patient's subjective report of pain

    (E) MMPI

609. What is the Symptom Checklist 90 (SL-90) and its revised version (SLR-90-R)?

    (A) Is a screen for psychologic symptoms and overall levels of distress

    (B) Self-report measure of patient's perception of his or her general health status

    (C) It is a 136-item scale

    (D) It is a measure of one's mood state

    (E) It is the most widely used personality test

610. Which of the following tests assess limitations in activities of daily living (ADL)?

    (A) Spielberger State-Trait Anxiety Inventory

    (B) Oswestry Low Back Pain Disability Questionnaire

    (C) Beck Depression Inventory

    (D) SL-90

    (E) MMPI

611. Beck Depression Inventory

    (A) is used to look at basic coping styles

    (B) is a 21-item self-report measure of depression for the last 30 years

    (C) is not commonly used in pain literature

    (D) is a measure of malingering

    (E) all of the above

612. In pain assessment

    (A) patient's self-report of pain is the most valid measure of the pain experience
    (B) behavioral measure of pain is the most valid measurement
    (C) the health care provider's observation is the most valid measurement
    (D) none of the above
    (E) all of the above

613. A conscious exaggeration of physical or psychologic symptoms for some easily recognized goal or secondary gain is

    (A) symptom magnification
    (B) malingering
    (C) hysteria
    (D) hypochondriasis
    (E) depression

614. McGill Pain Questionnaire

    (A) consists of three major measures
    (B) was developed by McGill
    (C) is not widely used
    (D) is a single-dimensional pain scale
    (E) does not ask about the location of pain

DIRECTIONS: For Question 615 through 625, ONE or MORE of the numbered options is correct. Choose answer

    (A) if only answer 1, 2, and 3 are correct
    (B) if only 1 and 3 are correct
    (C) if only 2 and 4 are correct
    (D) if only 4 is correct
    (E) if all are correct

615. McGill Pain Questionnaire assesses

    (1) location of the pain
    (2) pattern of the pain over time
    (3) sensory, effective component of pain
    (4) intensity of the pain

616. Advantages of MMPI-2 include:

    (1) It provides 10 clinical scales, 3 validity scales
    (2) Is considered the gold standard
    (3) Is well-normed and extensively researched
    (4) Its test results are easy to interpret

617. In evaluating patients for SCS using MMPI Richard North's group noted that

    (1) patients with high scores on scale 1 (hypochondriasis)t ended to proceed from SCS trial to implant
    (2) patients with higher scores on scale 3 (hysteria) were not offered SCS trial
    (3) patients with higher scores on scale 3 (hysteria) had positive short-term but not long-term outcome
    (4) patients with high score on scale 1 (hypochondriasis) tended not to proceed from SCS trial to implant

618. In regard to MMPI as a predictor of treatment outcome

    (1) it is standardized on chronic pain patients
    (2) it is based on common diagnoses of 1930s
    (3) can be used alone in assessment of pain patients
    (4) items overlapping a great degree across the 10 clinical scales

619. Multidimensional pain assessment inventories include

    (1) pain disability index
    (2) illness behavior questionnaire
    (3) Sickness Impact Profile, West Haven-Yale Multidimensional Pain Inventory
    (4) Dallas Pain Questionnaire

620. Regarding pain scores on the numeric rating scale

   (1) decreased pain scores suggest positive outcome from the treatment of pain

   (2) it should be used only occasionally

   (3) it correlates highly with pain measured on in verbal scale and VAS

   (4) correlates highly with anxiety and depression

621. Regarding SF-36

   (1) yields scores on 10 health scales relating to physical, social, and emotional factors

   (2) is easily administered

   (3) does not have gender or age norms

   (4) has been used to compare patient and surgeon assessment regarding the outcome of lumbar disc surgery

622. Physiologic correlations of pain (eg, heart rate and blood pressure)

   (1) are nonspecific to pain

   (2) many habituate with time despite presence of pain

   (3) occur under conditions of general arousal and stress

   (4) is a great way of measuring the intensity of pain

623. According to Melzack and Casey (1968) the three major psychologic dimensions of pain are

   (1) sensory discriminative

   (2) cognitive evaluative

   (3) motivational affective

   (4) past experiences

624. The most frequently used self-rating instruments for measurement of pain in a clinical setting are

   (1) VAS

   (2) behavioral observational scales

   (3) McGill Pain Questionnaire

   (4) physiologic responses

625. Cognitively impaired elderly patients

   (1) do not respond to pain assessment questionnaire

   (2) do respond appropriately if given VAS or numerical rating scale (NRS)

   (3) malingering by an elderly patient may be an attempt to divert attention away from possible need for institutionalization

   (4) there are guidelines available for elderly patients with dementia

Answers and Explanations

606. (B) The MMPI is a long test and has 566 questions. It does not reliably distinguish between the psychologic and physical pain. It needs expertise to review the test results, and the conversion V (hypochondriasis, depression, and hysteria) is seen in patients with chronic pain and does respond to treatment. The MMPI is commonly used in evaluating patients for SCS trial.

607. (E) The VAS-like verbal and numerical rating scales assumes that pain is a unidimentional experience and measures the intensity of the pain. Although pain intensity is a salient dimension of pain, it is clear that there are many dimensions to pain.

608. (A) The most commonly studied instrument is the Sickness Illness Profile. This has been used in many studies to demonstrate the effect of a variety of treatment methods in patients with pain.

Studies have shown poor reproducibility between physicians in evaluating patients with back pain especially regarding nonneurologic findings like muscle spasm and guarding. At present time there is no reliable test to measure patient's subjective feeling of pain.

609. (A) The SL-90 or Sl-90-R screens for psychologic symptoms and levels of distress. It is one of the personality test and has 90 items describing a physical or psychologic symptom. This is one not categorized as mood test. The most widely used personality test is MMPI.

610. (B) Spielberger State-Trait Anxiety Inventory is a 40-item self-report questionnaire that measures anxiety levels.

Oswestry Low Back Pain Disability Questionnaire assesses limitations in ADL. Ten multiple choice items cover nine aspects of daily functioning including personal care, lifting, walking, sitting, standing, sexual activity, and traveling. The patient chooses from among six statements relating to impact of pain on a particular activity. A percentage score is derived allowing for classification of patients ranging from mildly to profoundly impaired.

Beck Depression Inventory is a self-report measure of depression.

The SL-90 or Sl-90-R screens for psychologic symptoms and levels of distress.

MMPI is commonly used personality test to gain an overall picture of the patient's general psychologic status.

611. (B) Beck Depression Inventory is one of the most commonly used instruments in pain literature. It is a 21-item self-report measure of depression and has been in use for 30 years. Responses require the endorsement of one of a series of four statements, rank ordered according to the severity of content. The scores on each item are tabulated to yield a total depression score. It is not a measure of coping styles or malingering.

612. (A) The studies point to obtaining multiple measures of soft pain and because pain is a subjective phenomenon the patient's self-report is the most valid measure of the experience.

613. (B) Malingering is a conscious exaggeration of physical or psychologic symptoms for some easily recognized goal or secondary gain. It should be differentiated from symptom exaggeration or magnification that could be secondary to personality characteristics such as hysteria or conditioning factors.

614.   **(A)** McGill Pain Questionnaire was developed in 1975 by Ronald Melzack at McGill University in Canada. It consists of three major measures: pain rating index, total number of words chosen, and the present pain intensity. This is a multidimensional scale for measurement of pain. The questionnaire tries to assess the there components of pain postulated by the gate theory: the sensory, the affective, and the evaluative dimensions.

615.   **(E)** There are two types of tools for assessment of pain. Unidimentional single-item scales or multidimensional measure scales. The former includes the VAS or the VNS, the Verbal Descriptor Scale (VDS), and the Pain Thermometer. Each of these single-item scales measures only the intensity of the pain experienced. The multidimensional prototype is McGill Pain Questionnaire. It assesses the location of pain; the pattern of pain over time; the sensory, effective, evaluative, and miscellaneous components of pain; and the intensity of pain.

616.   **(A)** MMPI-2 measures psychologic traits and overall psychologic status. It is considered the gold standard and is scored by a computer. MMPI-2 has 10 clinical scales, 3 validity scales, and numerous other subscales. It is well-normed and highly researched and provides data about patient's test-taking approach; however, it is not normed on pain patients, scales 1 to 3 often evaluated in pain patients (this may unfairly label patients as neurotic). MMPI-2 requires highly skilled evaluator to interpret the test results.

617.   **(B)** MMPI has been widely used in patients undergoing SCS. North's group noted that patients with higher scores on hypochondriasis tended to proceed from trial to implantation; however, scale 3 (hysteria) tended to correlate with a positive short-term but not long-term outcome.

618.   **(C)** Keller and Butcher reinforced the lack of support found in the literature for using the MMPI as a predictor of treatment outcome. Common disadvantages of MMPI are that it is not standardized to chronic pain or medical

patients; it is based on common diagnoses of 1930s; the items bear no face validity in regard to underlying psychotherapy; items overlap to a great degree across the 10 clinical scales; and it is excessively long.

619.   **(E)**

620.   **(B)** The numerical rating scale correlates with scores on VAS or verbal rating scales. It should be used at each evaluation. It is sensitive to pharmacologic procedures that affect the pain intensity.

621.   **(C)** The Medical Outcome Survey (MOS), the 36-item Short Form Health Survey (SF-36) is a 36-item generic questionnaire that yields scores on eight health scales relating to physical, social, and emotional factors. It is easily administered and has gender and age norms based on large US populations, having been applied to more than 260 medical and surgical studies. It has been used to compare patient and surgeon assessment regarding the outcome of lumbar disc surgery.

622.   **(A)** Physiologic correlates of pain that can be measured include blood pressure, heart rate, electrodermal activity, electromyographic activity, and cortical-evoked potentials. Despite initial correlation between onset of pain and changes in these parameters, many patients habituate over time despite the persistence of pain. These responses are also nonspecific to pain and occur under general arousal or stress. Studies have shown that although there are many physiologic responses that occur with the experience of pain, many appear to be general responses to stress and are not unique to pain.

623.   **(A)** Research on pain in the 20th century has been dominated by the notion that pain is purely a sensory experience. Yet pain has an unpleasant affective component to it. It motivates the person to do something to get rid of it. Higher cortical processes such as evaluation of past experience exert control over the other two dimensions.

624.   **(B)** The VAS and the McGill Pain Questionnaire are the two most frequently used self-rating instruments for measurement of pain in clinical

and research testing. McGill Pain Questionnaire is designed to assess the multidimensional nature of pain experience and has been demonstrated to be valid, reliable, and consistent measurement tool. Because of complex nature of pain, measurements from the behavioral observational scales and physiologic responses may not show high concordance.

625. **(A)** Assessing pain in cognitively elder patients is very challenging and there are no guidelines available. The cognitively impaired do not respond quickly to pain assessment questionnaires but can respond to easy to read and follow scales like the VAS or NSR. In assessing pain in patients with dementia one needs to be able to differentiate between pain as a result of pathophysiologic processes and pain symptoms manifesting in an attempt to mask impaired mental processes because of the fear of being institutionalized and losing independence.

Pain Management Techniques
Questions

626. Which of the following is the most common microbe that grows in cultures of infected intrathecal pump wounds?

    (A) *Pseudomonas* species
    (B) *Escherichia coli*
    (C) *Staphylococcus aureus*
    (D) *Staphylococcus epidermidis*
    (E) None of the above

627. You think a patient has developed an intrathecal catheter-tip inflammatory mass. What signs and symptoms would support this finding?

    (A) Diminishing analgesic effects
    (B) Pain that mimics nerve root compression
    (C) Pain that mimics cholecystitis
    (D) A and B
    (E) A, B, and C

628. Advantages of intrathecal drug-delivery are

    (A) the first-pass effect can be avoided
    (B) intrathecal morphine is 300 times as effective as oral morphine for equipotent pain treatment
    (C) the number of central nervous system (CNS) derived side effects can be reduced
    (D) B and C
    (E) A, B, and C

629. Which one of the following is not an item to contemplate prior to placing an intrathecal pump?

    (A) Does the patient have an acceptable physiologic explanation for the pain syndrome
    (B) Does the patient have a life expectancy of 3 months or longer
    (C) Psychologic clearance is not needed in the patient with cancer pain
    (D) How old is the patient
    (E) Has the patient been reasonably compliant with past treatment recommendations

630. Prior to implanting an intrathecal pump many practitioners perform an intrathecal medication trial. Significant parameters to consider include

    (A) delivery site
    (B) type of medication
    (C) whether the patient should be admitted
    (D) A and B
    (E) A, B, and C

631. When dealing with an infection, which of the following would favor explanting the intrathecal device?

    (A) Associated bleeding
    (B) The presence of a seroma
    (C) The presence of a hygroma
    (D) The presence of necrotic tissue around the wound
    (E) All of the above

632. You have separately tried maximum doses of morphine and hydromorphone, in a patient's intrathecal pump without any efficacy. According to the 2007 Polyanalgesic Consensus Guidelines, which one of the following would not be an accepted "next" step?

(A) Switch to morphine plus bupivacaine

(B) Switch to ziconotide

(C) Switch to clonidine

(D) Switch to fentanyl

(E) Switch to hydromorphone plus ziconotide

633. Ziconotide was approved for infusion into the cerebrospinal fluid (CSF) using an intrathecal drug-delivery system by the Food and Drug Administration (FDA) in 2004. Its proposed mechanism of action is

(A) it blocks sodium channels

(B) it blocks $\alpha2\delta$ voltage-gated calcium channels

(C) it blocks N-type calcium channels

(D) it blocks γ-aminobutyric acid ($GABA_B$) receptors in the spinal cord

(E) none of the above

634. Neurology consults you on a 65-year-old female with breast cancer that has diffusely metastasized to her bones. She has had an intrathecal pump for 4 months, and has just been diagnosed with meningitis. Which of the following is true?

(A) The pump must be removed

(B) Enteral antibiotics must be initiated immediately

(C) If the infection is sensitive to vancomycin, and the patient refuses pump removal, intrathecal vancomycin may be administered

(D) Intravenous (IV) vancomycin plus epidural vancomycin has not been found to be effective in resolving infection

(E) All of the above

635. A 72-year-old male with end-stage metastatic prostate cancer has a life expectancy of 6 months. Which of the following is true with regards to managing his intrathecal drug-delivery system?

(A) Treatment decisions should be made based on the 2007 Polyanalgesic Consensus Guidelines for management of chronic, severe pain

(B) Fentanyl is considered a first-line medication

(C) Droperidol may be used, intrathecally, as a first-line medication for nausea

(D) A different algorithm is applied when a patient's life expectancy is less than 18 months

(E) None of the above

636. Granulomas have been found to occur with all medications used intrathecally, EXCEPT

(A) clonidine

(B) sufentanil

(C) baclofen

(D) fentanyl

(E) B and D

Questions 637 to 643

Match the associated side effects with the intrathecal medication that causes it. Each choice can be used once, more than once, or not at all, and each question can have more than one answer.

637. Urinary retention

638. Extrapyramidal side effects

639. Hypotension

640. Auditory disturbances

641. Sedation

642. Nausea

643. Worsening of depression

(A) Opioids

(B) Bupivacaine

(C) Baclofen

(D) Clonidine

(E) Droperidol

(F) Ketamine

(G) Midazolam

644. A 43-year-old female has 8-month history of axial low back pain and pain radiating to the left leg. The magnetic resonance imaging (MRI) of lumbosacral spine shows severe degenerative disc disease at L3-4 through L5-S1 with mild disc protrusions at these levels. She is a possible candidate for

(A) transforaminal epidural steroid injection

(B) facet joint medial branch diagnostic block

(C) spinal cord stimulator (SCS) trial

(D) all of the above

(E) none of the above

645. The causes of axial low back pain are

(A) sacroiliac (SI) arthropathy

(B) internal disc disruption

(C) quadratus lumborum and psoas syndrome

(D) all of the above

(E) none of the above

646. The false-positive rate of diagnostic lumbar facet medial branch blocks are

(A) 8% to 14%

(B) 15% to 22%

(C) 3% to 5%

(D) 25% to 41%

(E) 41% to 50%

647. Percentage of cases where the pain relief is caused by placebo response following interventional procedures are

(A) 12%

(B) 35%

(C) 20%

(D) 15%

(E) 28%

648. The complication of sphenopalatine ganglion radiofrequency thermocoagulation is

(A) infection

(B) epistaxis

(C) bradycardia

(D) all of the above

(E) none of the above

649. The complication of third occipital nerve (TON) radiofrequency thermocoagulation is

(A) change in taste

(B) ataxia

(C) dysphagia

(D) all of the above

(E) none of the above

650. Positive lumbar provocative discogram for mechanical disc sensitization includes reproduction of patient's pain with injection of the contrast in nucleus pulposus at what pressure above the "opening pressure"?

(A) < 30 psi

(B) < 100 psi

(C) < 10 to 15 psi

(D) < 50 psi

(E) < 70 psi

651. The technique of cervical discography includes needle entry through the skin from the

(A) anterior right side of the neck

(B) posterior right side of the neck

(C) anterior left side of the neck

(D) posterior left side of the neck

(E) median posterior side of the neck

652. When performing intralaminar cervical epidural steroid injections without fluoroscopic guidance, the chances of having false positive loss of resistance are close to

(A) 15%

(B) 25%

(C) 35%

(D) 50%

(E) 40%

653. When performing intralaminar cervical epidural steroid injections, the unilateral contrast (and medication) spread is expected in what percentage of cases?

   (A) 50%
   (B) 30%
   (C) 25%
   (D) 10%
   (E) 40%

654. Which of the following is a complication of lumbar sympathetic block?

   (A) Genitofemoral neuralgia
   (B) Retrograde ejaculation
   (C) Intravascular injection
   (D) All of the above
   (E) None of the above

655. What is the best method for evaluating the adequacy of lumbar sympathetic block?

   (A) Increase in temperature by 2°F
   (B) Increase in temperature by 5°F
   (C) Increase in temperature by 10°F
   (D) Temperature change
   (E) Decrease in temperature by 2°F

656. Stellate ganglion is located between the

   (A) C6-C7
   (B) C7-T1
   (C) C5-C7
   (D) C5-C6
   (E) T1-T2

657. In relation to the stellate ganglion the subclavian artery is located

   (A) anteriorly
   (B) posteriorly
   (C) laterally
   (D) medially
   (E) none of the above

658. Despite satisfactory stellate ganglion block for sympathetic-mediated pain, the pain relief in upper extremity is inadequate. The technical explanation for this may lie in inadequate spread of local anesthetics to

   (A) C5 nerve root
   (B) inferior cervical ganglion
   (C) first thoracic ganglion
   (D) T2 and T3 gray communicating rami
   (E) C7 nerve root

659. When performing lumbar discography, the "opening pressure" is the recorded pressure signifying

   (A) first appearance of the contrast in nucleus pulposus
   (B) opening of the annular tear to the contrast
   (C) reproduction of concordant pain
   (D) resting pressure transduced from the nucleus
   (E) a dural leak

660. Intradiscal electrothermal coagulation (IDET) outcomes are adversely affected by

   (A) appearance of the disc on T2-weighted MRI images
   (B) obesity
   (C) age
   (D) coexisting radicular pain
   (E) gender

661. When performing lumbar discography, in relation to the laterality of pain, which of the following should be the needle entry site?

   (A) Ipsilateral
   (B) Contralateral
   (C) Laterality does not make a difference
   (D) Guided by MRI images
   (E) None of the above

662. A patient with painful sacroiliac joint syndrome had only short-term relief with two sacroiliac (SI) injections using local anesthetics and steroids. Which of the following is the next treatment option?

   (A) SI joint fusion
   (B) S1, S2, S3, S4 radiofrequency denervation

(C) L5, S1, S2, S3 radiofrequency
denervation

(D) L4, L5, S1, S2, S3 radiofrequency
denervation

(E) None of the above

663. Which of the following includes published complications that may follow cervical transforaminal epidural steroid injection?

(A) Epidural abscess
(B) Neuropathic pain
(C) Quadriplegia and death
(D) All of the above
(E) None of the above

664. In order to minimize the risk for complications when cervical transforaminal epidural steroid injection is performed how should the needle be positioned in relation to the neural foramina?

(A) Anteriorly
(B) Posteriorly
(C) Superiorly
(D) Inferiorly
(E) None of the above

665. The single-needle approach to medial branch block diagnosis in comparison to standard multiple-needle approach

(A) causes less discomfort for the patient
(B) decreases the volume of local anesthetics used for the skin and subcutaneous tissues
(C) takes less time to perform
(D) all of the above
(E) none of the above

666. The incidental intrathecal overdose of intrathecal morphine while performing a pump refill should be treated by

(A) intrathecal and IV naloxone
(B) airway protection
(C) possible irrigation of the CSF with saline
(D) all of the above
(E) none of the above

667. While analyzing a malfunctioning SCS implanted device, a sign of lead breakage or disconnect is a measured impedance of

(A) < 1500 Ω
(B) > 1500 Ω
(C) < 4000 Ω
(D) > 4000 Ω
(E) < 500 Ω

668. Accurate placement of a stimulator lead for occipital nerve peripheral stimulation is

(A) posterior to the C3 spinous process
(B) lateral to the pedicles of C2 and C3
(C) 2 mm lateral to the odontoid process
(D) posterior to the C2 spinous process
(E) none of the above

669. Adequate SCS introducer needle epidural space at entry level for the desired coverage of the foot pain is

(A) L3-4 interspace
(B) L1-L2 interspace
(C) T12-L1 interspace
(D) T8-T9 interspace
(E) T10-T11 interspace

670. The placement of SCS electrodes for coverage of intractable chest pain caused by angina should be at the epidural level of

(A) T6
(B) C4-C5
(C) T1-T2
(D) C6-C7
(E) C3-C4

671. Most effective approach for performing lumbar epidural steroid injections is

(A) caudal
(B) interlaminar
(C) paramedian approach
(D) transforaminal
(E) Taylor approach

672. During interlaminar epidural steroid injections contrast should be

(A) used in the anteroposterior view
(B) used in the lateral view
(C) used in oblique view
(D) no contrast should be used
(E) A, B, and C

673. Which of the following is the most likely complication after successful SCS implant?

(A) Infection
(B) Persistent pain at the implant site
(C) Lead breakage or migration
(D) CSF leak requiring surgical intervention
(E) Paralysis or severe neurologic deficit

674. Which of the following is the most accurate statement regarding efficacy of SCS?

(A) For failed back surgery patients, SCS in addition to conventional medical management can provide better pain relief and improve health-related quality of life as compared to conventional medical management alone
(B) SCS is inefficacious for the indication of angina pectoris
(C) SCS for CRPS is efficacious for only about a year only then the efficacy diminishes
(D) SCS is not an effective treatment for sympathetically mediated pain
(E) Nociceptive pain is considered a better indication for SCS than neuropathic pain

675. Which of the following is not a relative contraindication to SCS?

(A) Unresolved major psychiatric comorbidity
(B) A predominance of nonorganic signs
(C) Spinal cord injury or lesion
(D) Alternative therapies with a risk to benefit ratio comparable to that of SCS remain to be tried
(E) Occupational risk

676. Which of the following statements is most accurate regarding cost-effectiveness of SCS?

(A) Nobody opines of its cost-effectiveness and the issue has not been addressed in literature
(B) The literature is clear and consistent; SCS is not cost-effective
(C) Although published conclusions may vary, a consensus of professionals has determined that SCS stimulation is not cost-effective
(D) Although published conclusions may vary, a consensus of professionals has determined that SCS is cost-effective for certain indications
(E) All published literature on the topic concludes that SCS is cost-effective

677. Which of the following are specifications for current SCS systems?

(A) Constant voltage, pulse width up to 2000 milliseconds
(B) Constant current, volume less 10 cm^3 (volume less than a standard matchbook)
(C) Constant resistance, pulse width up to 1000 milliseconds, cordless recharging
(D) Constant current, pulse width up to 1000 milliseconds, cordless recharging
(E) Constant current and constant resistance, cordless recharging, pulse width up to 1000 milliseconds

678. Which of the following is true?

(A) Dorsal column pathways do not play a role in visceral pain and therefore there is no role of SCS for visceral pain
(B) Pelvic pain has been demonstrated to consistently fail treatment with SCS
(C) The midline dorsal column pathway has been the proposed target for stimulation for chronic visceral pain
(D) Pelvic pain stimulation can best be achieved by first targeting the S2 foramen in a retrograde approach
(E) There is no therapeutic potential for treatment of chronic visceral pelvic pain with SCS

679. Which of the following is the best answer regarding lead geometry and spacing?

   (A) The goal of SCS in treatment of bilateral lower extremity neuropathy pain is most frequently to stimulate the dorsal roots rather than the dorsal columns

   (B) Tight lead spacing increases the ratio of dorsal column to dorsal root stimulation

   (C) Too much stimulation of the dorsal columns results in motor side effects

   (D) As the distance from the contact to the spinal cord increases, stimulation becomes more specific for the dorsal columns as opposed to the dorsal roots

   (E) Rostrocaudal contact size (contact length) is less important than lateral contact size (contact width)

680. The gate control theory is one postulated mechanism of action for SCS. Which of the following is the most accurate application of SCS to this postulated mechanism of action?

   (A) Activation of large-diameter afferents thereby "closing the gate"

   (B) Activation of large-diameter afferents thereby "opening the gate"

   (C) Activation of small-diameter afferents thereby "closing the gate"

   (D) Activation of small-diameter afferents thereby "opening the gate"

   (E) Activation of both large- and small-diameter afferents equally

681. Which of the following is most accurate regarding indications for SCS?

   (A) Nociceptive pain is traditionally considered a better indication than neuropathic pain

   (B) Receptor mediated pain is traditionally considered a better indication than neurogenic pain

   (C) SCS tends to more effectively treat sympathetically mediated pain than pain of the somatic nervous system

   (D) Intractable angina is not effectively treated with SCS

   (E) Persisting neuropathic extremity pain following spinal surgery is a better indication than pain of CRPS

682. Which of the following correctly arranges intraspinal elements from highest to lowest conductivity?

   (A) CSF, longitudinal white matter, gray matter, transverse white matter, dura

   (B) Longitudinal white matter, gray matter, CSF, transverse white matter, dura

   (C) Longitudinal white matter, transverse white matter, dura, gray matter, CSF

   (D) Gray matter, longitudinal white matter, transverse white matter, CSF, dura

   (E) Dura, transverse white matter, gray matter, longitudinal white matter, CSF

683. Which of the following is the most accurate explanation why thoracic level cord stimulator leads do not commonly stimulate intrathoracic structures such as the heart?

   (A) Thoracic placement of SCS leads is contraindicated and is therefore not a clinically used technique

   (B) The CSF is highly conductive and therefore diverts the stimulation into a different direction

   (C) The stimulation is very specific for neural tissues rather than visceral tissues

   (D) The dura has a very low conductivity and therefore insulates visceral structures from stimulation

   (E) The vertebral bone has a very low conductivity and therefore insulates visceral structures from stimulation

684. Which of the following best describes the proposed mechanism of action of SCS?

(A) There is evidence that during SCS large myelinated afferent fibers are activated in an antidromic manner

(B) There is a measurable increase in endogenous opioids in response to SCS

(C) Spinothalamic tract activation during SCS leads to an analgesic effect

(D) SCS causes an inhibition of ascending and descending inhibitory pathways

(E) SCS has no effect on abnormal A-β activity

685. Which of the following is true?

(A) Phenol theoretically carries a higher risk for neuroma formation than alcohol

(B) Radiofrequency ablation is particularly useful for field neurolysis

(C) Phenol is a particularly useful neurolytic agent for localized targets

(D) Alcohol is a particularly useful neurolytic agent because there is no pain upon injection

(E) Phenol causes wallerian degeneration

686. Which of the following is most painless upon delivery?

(A) Phenol

(B) Alcohol

(C) Radiofrequency

(D) Cryoanalgesia

(E) Cold knife excision of a nerve

687. Which of the following neurolytic techniques is most concerning for the side effect of arrhythmia?

(A) Laser neurolysis

(B) Cryoanalgesia

(C) Radiofrequency

(D) Alcohol

(E) Phenol

688. Which of the following statements is the most accurate comparison of radiofrequency ablation and cryoablation?

(A) Cryoanalgesia probes are generally smaller in diameter than the large-diameter probes used for radiofrequency procedures

(B) One disadvantage of cryoanalgesia technique is the operator must support a heavier instrument while maintaining the probe tip in accurate position

(C) The cryolesion and the radiofrequency lesion are similar in size

(D) Cryoanalgesia and radiofrequency lesion techniques have equal precision capability

(E) Cryoanalgesia is inferior to radiofrequency ablation because cryoanalgesia causes wallerian degeneration

689. Which of the following is most accurate regarding the electric field generated at the tip of a radiofrequency electrode?

(A) Flat conductors generate larger, stronger electric fields than round conductors

(B) With round conductors, the charge density is directly proportional to the radius of the circle

(C) The electric field around a radiofrequency cannula is more dense around the exposed shaft and becomes less dense at the tip

(D) Voltage, current, and power are the three basic variables governing formation of heat surrounding a radiofrequency cannula tip

(E) The heat lesion formed around the radiofrequency cannula is slightly pear-shaped with the base of the pear around the proximal end of the active tip and less projection of the heat at the needle tip

690. Which of the following is the most accurate statement regarding neuraxial neurolysis?

(A) Phenol has significant proven benefit over alcohol

(B) The technique is 100% efficacious

(C) The average pain relief is less than 6 months

(D) Bladder paresis and motor weakness occurs in close to 100% of those treated with neuraxial neurolysis

(E) Epidural neurolysis has a proven favorable risk to benefit ratio compared to subarachnoid neurolysis

691. While performing an intradiscal radiofrequency procedure using a posterior-oblique approach, the needle tip is advanced into the annulus fibrosus using fluoroscopic guidance. Impedance is noted. The needle tip is then advanced a little further. A drop in impedance is noted. Which of the following is the most likely explanation?

(A) Malfunction of radiofrequency machine
(B) Needle-tip entry into CSF
(C) Needle-tip entry into spinal cord
(D) Needle-tip has dry blood on it
(E) Needle-tip entry into nucleus pulposus

692. Which of the following is appropriate safety consideration when performing a radiofrequency ablation procedure?

(A) Motor stimulation is not needed if meticulous fluoroscopic technique is used
(B) A radiofrequency probe should be the length of the cannula or shorter, but never longer than the cannula
(C) The pain physician should always turn off a patient's sensing pacemaker prior to a radiofrequency procedure
(D) Complications during radiofrequency ablation are rare and need not be considered prior to the procedure
(E) A SCS should be turned off prior to a radiofrequency procedure

693. Coulomb per kilogram (C/kg) is

(A) the unit used to measure electrical charge produced by x- or γ-radiation similar to previous roentgen unit
(B) used to measure dose equivalent
(C) the daily radiation exposure per kilogram of body weight

(D) the intensity of radiation
(E) used to measure the amount of radiation absorbed

694. Gray (Gy) is used to measure

(A) yearly background exposure
(B) absorbed dose
(C) dose equivalent
(D) daily radiation exposure
(E) yearly radiation exposure

695. Maximum total permissible dose equivalents (in mSv) for a year is

(A) 75 mSv
(B) 100 mSv
(C) 150 mSv
(D) 50 mSv
(E) 25 mSv

696. How low should a clinician's hourly radiation exposure be?

(A) Less than 0.01 mSv/h
(B) Less than 0.05 mSv/h
(C) Less than 0.15 mSv/h
(D) As low as reasonably achievable
(E) Less than 0.25 mSv/h

697. Most operator exposure during fluoroscopically guided blocks is when

(A) the lateral views are taken
(B) the x-ray tube is above the patient
(C) the patient is obese
(D) the anteroposterior views are taken
(E) none of the above

698. The intensity of scattered beam is greater at the radiation entrance on the skin than exit site

(A) 3 times
(B) 10 times
(C) 30 times
(D) 985 times
(E) 1000 times

699. Average patient radiation exposure dose during pain procedures is

(A) 10 times less than during angiography

(B) same as during angiography

(C) 10 times more than during angiography

(D) less than computed tomographic (CT) scanning

(E) 20 times more than during angiography

700. Radiation dose to the patients and medical personnel can be reduced by

(A) decreasing the distance between the image intensifier and the patient

(B) increasing the distance between the image intensifier and the patient

(C) using continuous fluoroscopy

(D) oblique views

(E) none of the above

701. Personnel radiation protection can be achieved by

(A) lead aprons

(B) glasses

(C) increased distance from the x-ray

(D) all of the above

(E) none of the above

702. Lead aprons should be always hung:

(A) So that space is saved

(B) As the lead can be broken if folded

(C) They can be safely folded as well

(D) So they can be conveniently available

(E) None of the above

DIRECTIONS: For Question 703 through 742, ONE or MORE of the numbered options is correct. Choose answer

(A) if only answer 1, 2, and 3 are correct

(B) if only 1 and 3 are correct

(C) if only 2 and 4 are correct

(D) if only 4 is correct

(E) if all are correct

703. A patient with severe spasticity is a candidate for an intrathecal baclofen pump. He and his family have heard that "these pumps get infected." How do you respond?

(1) Device-related infection is the most common, potentially reducible, serious adverse event associated with intrathecal pumps

(2) The majority of infections occur at the lumbar site

(3) Management of infections associated with drug-delivery systems usually involves the administration of antibiotics and explantation of the device

(4) The chances of the pump getting infected are minimal and the family should only focus on the benefits that the device provides

704. When trialing intrathecal medication and placing intrathecal pumps, which of the following is considered good technique?

(1) Antibiotics are given during the course of the trial, and for 7 to 10 days after permanent implant

(2) If the entry point is above L2, the patient should be conversant, and the angle of entry should be as shallow as possible

(3) Placing the patient in the lateral decubitus position with the hips flexed, and the knees bent

(4) Electrocautery is now considered the gold standard for controlling bleeding

705. Which of the following is (are) disease state(s) that are amenable to treatment by intrathecal drug-delivery system?

(1) Intractable spasticity related to cerebral palsy and spinal cord injuries

(2) Interstitial cystitis

(3) Cancer-related syndromes

(4) Rheumatoid arthritis

706. A 56-year-old female who had an intrathecal pump placed secondary to metastatic renal cell carcinoma is having pain equivalent to a 6 on the visual analog scale (VAS). What is the proper titration regimen?

(1) Increase dose 10% to 25% over 3 to 4 days

(2) Increase dose 25% to 50% daily

(3) Hourly rates should be adjusted 35% to 50% twice daily until pain relief is achieved

(4) A therapeutic bolus should be considered

707. A 52-year-old female with pancreatic cancer and her family are trying to decide between continued medical management for pain versus an intrathecal drug-delivery system. Believing that this patient would most benefit from an intrathecal pump, you tell them that studies have shown that

(1) overall toxicity is better with intrathecal pumps

(2) pain relief is better with intrathecal pumps

(3) intrathecal pumps improve fatigue and level of consciousness in patients versus medical management

(4) there is a trend to increased survival in patients who have intrathecal pumps versus those continuing with medical management

708. Third occipital nerve

(1) innervates C2-3 facet joint

(2) curves around superior articular process of the C2 vertebrae

(3) curves around superior articular process of the C3 vertebrae

(4) innervates C3-4 facet joint

709. For the peripheral stimulation of the occipital nerve

(1) the electrode should be parallel to the occipital nerve in the occipital area of the scull

(2) only a "paddle-" type electrode should be used

(3) the entry site of the introducer needle should be at T1-T2 level

(4) the electrode should be placed subcutaneously at the C1-C2 level

710. T2 and T3 sympathetic block

(1) is used for treatment of upper extremity complex regional pain syndrome (CRPS)

(2) will help by denervating the Kuntz nerves

(3) can lead to pneumothorax

(4) should avoid radiofrequency of T2 and T3 sympathetic ganglia

711. Vertebroplasty may be indicated for

(1) multiple myeloma

(2) chronic compression fractures of vertebral body

(3) osteolytic metastatic tumors

(4) facet arthropathy

712. Complications from vertebroplasty include

(1) pulmonary embolus

(2) intradiscal leak of polymethyl methacrylate

(3) paraplegia

(4) psoas muscle leak of polymethyl methacrylate and femoral neuropathy

713. Which of the following is (are) correct with regards to piriformis muscle injection?

(1) Should be done at medial part of a muscle

(2) Botox can be used

(3) Nerve stimulation may aid in muscle location

(4) Identification of the muscle can be done through rectal examination

714. SI joint pain

(1) is transmitted by the S1-S4 levels of spinal nerves

(2) has been treated by the SI joint fusion

(3) can be relieved by blind steroid injections

(4) is transmitted by L4 medial branch, L5 dorsal ramus, and S1-3 lateral branches

715. Celiac plexus block can be performed by

(1) anterior approach

(2) retrocrural approach

(3) anterocrural approach

(4) lateral approach

716. Ganglion impar block

(1) is indicated for testicular pain

(2) is indicated for sympathetically maintained pain in perineal area

(3) is best performed by anococcygeal approach

(4) can be complicated by perforation of rectum

717. With cervical interlaminar epidural steroid injection

(1) loss of resistance technique can be inaccurate in up to 50% cases

(2) unilateral medication spread can be achieved in 50% cases

(3) contrast spread should be checked in lateral views

(4) transforaminal approach is safer than interlaminar

718. Which of the following includes complication(s) of intrathecal pump?

(1) Granuloma formation

(2) CSF leak

(3) Pump rotation

(4) Hormonal imbalance

719. In relation to increased pain in patient with intrathecal opioid delivery which of the following is (are) true?

(1) It can mean progression of disease

(2) Catheter kink should be considered

(3) One should look for withdrawal symptoms

(4) Opioids should be increased first

720. Which of the following is (are) drug(s) used in decompressive neuroplasty?

(1) Hyaluronidase

(2) Hypertonic saline

(3) Steroids

(4) Local anesthetics

721. SCS been used for the treatment of

(1) interstitial cystitis

(2) postlaminectomy syndrome

(3) CRPS

(4) sympathetically mediated pain

722. Spinal cord stimulation

(1) should be used early in the course of the postherpetic neuralgia pain syndrome

(2) has been found efficacious for the failed back surgery syndrome

(3) has been used for peripheral vascular disease and ischemic disease

(4) has a proven and elucidated mechanism of action

723. The transverse tripolar SCS arrangement

(1) involves a central anode surrounded by cathodes

(2) contributes maximum dorsal column stimulation with minimal dorsal root stimulation

(3) is most frequently used to improve stimulation of the feet

(4) usually involves an octapolar spinal midline lead and two adjacent quadripolar leads

724. Which of the following is (are) true for SCS for the indication of angina pectoris?

(1) Improves exercise capacity

(2) Probably only helps for a year and then the stimulator should be removed

(3) In addition to providing antianginal effects it also provides a reduction in ischemia

(4) Is contraindicated because it masks significant ischemic events

725. Which of the following is (are) the risk(s) associated with SCS?

(1) Epidural hematoma
(2) Spinal cord injury
(3) Implanted pulse generator failure
(4) Electromechanical failure of lead or extension cable

726. Which of the following is (are) true regarding SCS for visceral pain?

(1) SCS suppresses visceral response to colon distention in animal models
(2) SCS is a first-line treatment for visceral pain
(3) Case studies have indicated SCS may be helpful for visceral pain but at this time there is a lack of supporting randomized controlled trials
(4) A good lead placement for stimulation of chronic pancreatitis would logically be around T12 or L1

727. Which of the following is (are) the best answer(s) regarding lead spacing and electrical fields created by a dual-lead stimulation system as pictured?

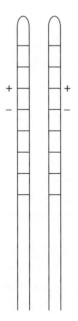

(1) With larger distances between anodes and cathodes, the electric field tends to form a sphere
(2) With tighter lead spacing and smaller distances between anodes and cathodes, the electric field is pulled towards the anode
(3) Tight lead spacing increases the ratio of dorsal column to dorsal root stimulation
(4) The anode is the positive contact and the cathode is the negative contact

728. Which of the following should be considered when selecting patients for SCS?

(1) Disease pathology
(2) Untreated drug addiction
(3) Patient comorbidities
(4) Physician's monthly case quota

729. Which of the following is (are) considered indication(s) for SCS?

(1) Phantom limb pain
(2) Spinal cord injury pain
(3) Intractable abdominal or visceral pain
(4) Neurogenic thoracic outlet syndrome

730. Which of the following is (are) true regarding the history of electrical stimulation for the treatment of pain?

(1) Electrical stimulation for the treatment of pain dates back to the first century ad when electrical fish were documented to be used in the treatment of gout
(2) Implantable SCS were used for treatment of pain for a decade prior to the published gate control theory of pain
(3) Early stimulation case reports were of peripheral nerve stimulation; later emphasis turned toward SCS
(4) Psychiatric and/or psychologic screening evaluation prior to implants was a new idea imposed upon physicians by health maintenance organizations in the 1990s

731. Which of the following is (are) accurate statement(s) regarding neuromodulation of the sacral nerves?

(1) Sacral neuromodulation is not effective for idiopathic urinary frequency
(2) Both percutaneous and surgical lead placement techniques have been described
(3) Must be performed by a surgeon because only a surgical technique is available
(4) Urgency and urge incontinence are indications

732. Which of the following is (are) true regarding radiofrequency procedures?

(1) Pulsed radiofrequency lesioning temperature goal is generally around 42°C to 43°C
(2) Prior to application of the radiofrequency lesion, sensory testing should be applied at 2 Hz
(3) The standard pulsed radiofrequency lesion is 500,000 Hz for 20 milliseconds pulses once every 0.5 second for 90 to 240 seconds
(4) Prior to application of the radiofrequency lesion, motor testing should be applied at 50 Hz

733. Which of the following element(s) is (are) necessary to complete a radiofrequency circuit?

(1) The radiofrequency generator
(2) Insulated needle cannula with radiofrequency probe
(3) Dispersive electrode (grounding pad)
(4) The patient

734. Which of the following is (are) the possible mechanism(s) of action of radiofrequency ablation?

(1) Vascular injury causing endoneural edema
(2) Formation of a static electric field
(3) Lipid extraction with protein precipitation
(4) Generation of heat

735. Which of the following is (are) the most accurate answer(s) regarding radiofrequency treatment of the SI joint?

(1) Evidence is strong for efficacy of radiofrequency ablation techniques for SI joint pain
(2) The universally accepted screening protocol prior to SI joint injection involves SI tenderness, positive SI provocative maneuvers, and two positive local anesthetic–only SI joint injection procedures
(3) There is no evidence for the role of pulsed radiofrequency treatment of SI joint pain
(4) Radiofrequency treatment of sacral lateral branches have been proposed for efficacious treatment of SI joint pain

736. Purported advantages of percutaneous radiofrequency lesions over other neuroablative techniques include

(1) predictable and quantifiable lesions
(2) avoids the extensive soft tissue damage of surgical techniques
(3) ability to confirm needle-tip proximity to sensory and motor nerves
(4) ability to cover a wide field

737. Which of the following is (are) accurate regarding the history of ablation techniques?

(1) Norman Shealy reported the first use of radiofrequency lesioning for treatment of facet pain in 1975
(2) The first report of percutaneous radiofrequency lesioning for treatment of pain came in 1981
(3) Slappendel reported the first clinical use of pulsed radiofrequency lesioning in 1997
(4) Although a modern cryoneuroablation device was developed and refined in the 1960s, the application for pain management gained popularity in the 1980s

738. Which of the following is (are) accurate regarding lesion size?

   (1) The size of a continuous radiofrequency lesion depends on temperature induced

   (2) The size of a continuous radiofrequency lesion depends on the width of the needle

   (3) A 2 mm cryoanalgesia probe forms an ice ball about 5.5 mm thick

   (4) A 1.4 mm cryoanalgesia probe forms an ice ball about 3.5 mm thick

739. Which of the following is (are) components of a cryoanalgesia system?

   (1) Outer tube with smaller inner tube

   (2) Pressurized gas in inner tube

   (3) Fine aperture in tip of inner tube which allows gas to rapidly expand in tip of outer tube

   (4) Fine aperture in tip of outer tube which allows gas to escape the tube system

740. Which of the following is (are) potential neuroablative procedure treatment options?

   (1) Radiofrequency ablation of the L2 ramus communicans for treatment of L4-L5 discogenic pain

   (2) Phenol neurolysis for treatment of the lumbar sympathetic plexus for treatment of CRPS of the lower extremity

   (3) Radiofrequency ablation for treatment of the lumbar sympathetic plexus for treatment of CRPS of the lower extremity

   (4) Cryoablation for the treatment of pain owing to superior gluteal nerve entrapment

741. Which of the following is (are) potential advantage(s) of pulsed radiofrequency procedure over continuous radiofrequency ablation?

   (1) Pulsed radiofrequency procedure is virtually painless as compared to continuous radiofrequency ablation during which patients often complain of pain

   (2) Overwhelming evidence of greater efficacy with pulsed radiofrequency procedure over continuous radiofrequency ablation

   (3) As compared to pulsed radiofrequency ablation, continuous radiofrequency ablation of lumbar medial branches carries a higher risk of inducing spinal instability secondary to multifidus muscle denervation

   (4) Complications caused by needle injury of tissues is less with pulsed radiofrequency procedure compared to continuous radiofrequency ablation

742. Which of the following is (are) correct regarding impedance measurement during radiofrequency procedures?

   (1) While performing a radiofrequency procedure, the lower the impedance value the better the expected outcome

   (2) Impedance measurement can detect needle-tip entry into different mediums such as vascular structures or periosteum

   (3) Impedance values are neither customary nor necessary when using fluoroscopic guidance

   (4) Impedance measurement can detect breaks or short circuits in the electrical circuit

Answers and Explanations

626. (D)

A. *Pseudomonas* species grew in 3% of infected wound cultures.

B. *Escherichia coli* is probably among the unknown or not reported 20% or the multiple or other species (7%).

C. and D. *Staphylococcus* species grew in cultures of infected sites 59% of the time. Most reports did not specify whether the cultured *Staphylococcus* organisms were *S aureus* or *S epidermidis*. However one study specifically emphasized *S epidermidis*, which arises from the skin of the patient or operating room personnel, as the most likely culprit. No growth took place in 9% of the infected-wound cultures. No positive fungal cultures were reported.

627. (E)

A. Subtle prodromal signs and symptoms during early growth of a catheter-tip mass include decreasing analgesic effects (loss of previously satisfactory pain relief) and unusual increase in the patient's underlying pain. Another occurrence was that patient required unusually frequent or high dose escalations to obtain analgesia. In certain instances, dose increases and large drug boluses reduced the patient's pain only temporarily or to a lesser degree than previous experiences predicted.

B. Catheter-tip masses in the lumbar region sometimes simulated nerve root compression from a herniated intervertebral disc or spinal stenosis.

C. When the catheter tip is located in the thoracic region, early signs and symptoms of an extra-axial inflammatory mass sometimes included thoracic radicular pain that stimulated intercostal neuralgia or cholecystitis.

Gradual, insidious neurologic deterioration weeks or months after the appearance of subjective symptoms was the most common clinical course before the onset of myelopathy or cauda equina syndrome.

Myelopathy is a term that means that there is something wrong with the spinal cord itself. This is usually a later stage of cervical spine disease, and is often first detected as difficulty while walking because of generalized weakness or problems with balance and coordination. This type of process occurs most commonly in the elderly, who can have many reasons for troubled walking or problems with gait and balance. However, one of the more worrisome reasons that these symptoms are occurring is that bone spurs and other degenerative changes in the cervical spine are squeezing the spinal cord. Myelopathy affects the entire spinal cord, and is very different from isolated points of pressure on the individual nerve roots. Myelopathy is most commonly caused by spinal stenosis, which is a progressive narrowing of the spinal canal. In the later stages of spinal degeneration, bone spurs, and arthritic changes make the space available for the spinal cord within the spinal canal much smaller. The bone spurs may begin to press on the spinal cord and the nerve roots, and that pressure starts to interfere with how the nerves function normally. Myelopathy can be difficult to detect, because this disease usually develops gradually and also occurs at a time in life when people are beginning to slow down a little bit anyway. Many people who have myelopathy will begin to have difficulty with activities that require a fair amount of coordination, like walking up and down the stairs or fastening the buttons on clothing. If a patient has had a long history of neck pain, changes in coordination, recent weakness, and difficulty doing tasks that used to be easier because your body seemed more responsive in the past, are definite warning signs that they should see a doctor. Surgery is usually offered as an early option for people with myelopathy who have evidence of muscle weakness that is being caused by nerve root or spinal cord compression. This is because muscle weakness is a definite sign that the spinal cord and nerves are being injured (more seriously than when pain is the only symptom) and relieving the pressure on the nerves is more of an urgent priority. However, the benefits of nerve and spinal cord decompression have to be weighed against the risks of surgery. Many people who have myelopathy caused by degenerative cervical disorders are older and often a bit frail. Spine surgery can be a difficult stress for someone who is old or who has many different medical problems. However, a surgeon will be able to discuss the risks and benefits of surgery, and what the likely results are of operative versus nonoperative treatment.

Cauda equina syndrome is a serious neurologic condition in which there is acute loss of function of the neurologic elements (nerve roots) of the spinal canal below the termination (conus) of the spinal cord. After the conus the canal contains a mass of nerves (the cauda equina—horse tail—branches off the lower end of the spinal cord and contains the nerve roots from L1-5 and S1-5. The nerve roots from L4-S4 join in the sacral plexus which affects the sciatic nerve which travels caudally (toward the feet). Any lesion which compresses or disturbs the function of the cauda equina may disable the nerves although the most common is a central disc prolapse. Other causes include protrusion of the vertebra into the canal if weakened by infection or tumor and an epidural abscess or hematoma. Signs include weakness of the muscles innervated by the compressed roots (often paraplegia), sphincter weaknesses causing urinary retention and postvoid residual incontinence. Also, there may be decreased rectal tone; sexual dysfunction; saddle anesthesia; bilateral leg pain and weakness; and absence of bilateral ankle reflexes. Pain may, however, be completely absent; the patient may complain only of lack of bladder control and of saddle-anesthesia, and may walk into the consulting-room. Diagnosis is usually confirmed by an MRI scan or a CT scan, depending on availability. If cauda equina syndrome exists, early surgery is an option depending on the etiology discovered and the patient's candidacy for major spine surgery.

Awareness of these two phenomena and maintenance of an index of suspicion are important factors to help physicians detect such inflammatory masses early in the clinical course.

An inflammatory mass or granuloma is resulted from a buildup of inflammatory material at the tip of the catheter. Signs and symptoms that warrant prompt diagnosis to rule out the presence of a catheter-tip mass include changes in the patient's neurologic condition, including motor weakness, such as gait difficulties; sensory loss, including proprioceptive loss; hyper- or hypoactive lower extremity reflexes; and any evidence of bowel or bladder sphincter dysfunction. The practitioner should also be suspicious of new or different reports of numbness, tingling, burning, hyperesthesia, hyperalgesia, or the occurrence of pain (especially radicular pain that corresponds to the level of the catheter tip) during catheter access port injections or programmed pump boluses. The latter finding should alert the physician to discontinue the procedure and perform a diagnostic imaging study as soon as possible.

If signs and symptoms suggestive of a catheter-tip mass are detected, the practitioner should first review the patient's current issues, history, and neurologic examination. Then, a nonsurgical pain practitioner should review imaging studies with a neurosurgeon. Third, the physician should arrange the performance of a definitive diagnostic imaging procedure to confirm or rule out the suspected diagnosis. Treatment should be started in a timely fashion. Laboratory tests and electromyography or nerve conduction studies are not apparently useful in this situation.

628. (E)

A. The premise behind intrathecal drug delivery is that by directly depositing drugs into the CSF, the first-pass effect is avoided.

B. Intrathecal morphine is 300 times as effective as oral morphine for equipotent pain treatment. From spinal to epidural morphine the conversion is in the ratio of 1:10. From epidural to IV morphine the conversion is in the ratio of 1:10. From IV to oral morphine the conversion is in the ratio of 1:3, hence $10 \times 10 \times 3 = 300$.

C. By the direct action of the medication, the number of CNS-derived side effects can be reduced.

629. (D) In choosing the right patient for an intrathecal drug-delivery system, several important questions must be asked, like

A. Does the patient have an adequate physiologic explanation for the pain syndrome? Does the diagnosis require aggressive pain treatment?

B. Does the patient have a life expectancy of 3 months or longer (required for both cancer and noncancer patients)?

C. Is the patient psychologically stable? A psychologist should assess the patient's mental status and stability prior to the procedure. Outcomes have been shown to deteriorate with the presence of untreated depression, untreated anxiety disorders, and suicidal or homicidal ideation. Results have also been negatively influenced by the presence of untreated illicit substance dependence. The presence of a personality disorder such as borderline, antisocial, or multiple personality disorder should cause extreme caution, with these patient receiving implants only in extenuating circumstances. Psychologic clearance is not needed in the patient with cancer pain, but many of these patients may benefit from counseling to better cope with the disease process.

E. Has the patient been reasonably compliant with past treatments? Has the patient failed other, less invasive therapies? What were they? Were they documented? Do they include physical therapy and oral medications? Are more conservative therapies unacceptable, not desired, or contraindicated? Do the symptoms of pain affect the patient's ability to function? Does the patient have a contraindication, such as a bleeding diathesis, or a localized or systemic infection? Has the patient had a successful intrathecal medication trial? The physician should write a detailed note regarding symptom relief, side effects, and overall patient acceptance. Does the patient have a realistic view of expectations? Does the patient accept the risks of the procedure/device and future medications?

630. (D)

A. and B. There is a definite justification for a trial that mimics the conditions that will be achieved by the implanted system. Important parameters include

- Site of medication delivery (intrathecal versus epidural, and spinal level)
- Whether the medication is delivered as a bolus or an infusion
- Infusion rate
- Dose/concentration range
- Length of trial
- Medication selected for trial

C. The patient should always be admitted and observed after an intrathecal medication trial. There was a comparison of trial methods in pain patients (nociceptive, neuropathic, or mixed) selected to have intrathecal pump placement. In the final analysis at 12 months after implantation, it was determined that there was no significant difference in trial method (single-shot intrathecal, continuous intrathecal, or continuous epidural) in outcomes with nociceptive pain. However, in neuropathic pain syndromes, the initial success of trial was significantly better if a continuous method was used. There was no difference noted in trial through the epidural route versus trial through the intrathecal route. The main difference between successful trials in patients with neuropathic pain and mixed pain syndromes was the inclusion of more than one medication to improve the success of the trial.

Morphine has been approved by the FDA for intrathecal drug-delivery systems, and is often the first choice of drug for trial. Local anesthetics or α-receptor–acting drugs are sometimes added to the trial in patients with burning or lancinating extremity pain with hopes of improving the success of the trial.

To be considered a success, the trial should induce significant pain relief, with minimal side effects, and noncancer patients should obtain purposeful improvement of function.

631. (D)

A. Bleeding at the wound site will be obvious with seepage into the dressing. Associated signs include edema, discoloration, and rubor. It can usually be treated with ice and compression; however, surgical exploration may be necessary. The presence of an active bleed does not necessitate the explantation of the intrathecal drug-delivery system.

B. A seroma is a collection of noninfectious fluid. It is usually treated with pressure dressings and conservatively allowing for resorption. If conservative treatment is not efficacious, sterile aspiration may be necessary. Its presence does not require the removal of the intrathecal pump.

C. A hygroma is a collection of CSF. Its most common cause is leakage of fluid around the catheter entry point and into the pocket. It can be treated with abdominal pressure, caffeine, and increased fluid intake.

D. Infection of the wound may be minor and superficial, or it may be severe enough to warrant the removal of the pump. An infection may present with fever, redness, frank pus, or purulent wound drainage. Incision and drainage, qualification of pathogenic culprit, and antibiotic therapy must be undertaken immediately. The decision to excise the pump is made based on the presence of necrotic tissue, the overall condition of the wound, and the condition of the patient.

The two most disastrous complications are epidural hematoma and neuraxial infection. An epidural hematoma may result in paralysis and should be suspected with any change in neurologic status postoperatively. This is an emergency and an immediate MRI and neurosurgical consultation should be obtained. The presence of an intrathecal pump is not a contraindication to MRI, and should not delay its use. A neuraxial infection can include meningitis or an epidural abscess and they must both be diagnosed immediately so that treatment can be started expeditiously.

632. (C) For the 2007 Polyanalgesic Consensus Guidelines, baclofen and midazolam were moved to special consideration categories. Midazolam may be used in end of life situations but only minimal/anecdotal evidence exists. Baclofen is to be used in patients that have spasticity-related pain, diseases associated with dystonia, or unrelenting spasms in muscle. It works via blockade of $GABA_B$ receptors in the spinal cord. Indications for intrathecal baclofen therapy: patient is intolerant of oral agents, pain is inadequately treated with oral agents, need exact control of dosing that only intrathecal delivery allows. Efficacy in neuropathic pain has been noted through case reports at doses of 100 to 460 µg/d (maximum FDA dosing is 900 µg/d). If significant dose increases are taking place, consider mechanical problems. Very good for exceptional long-term tolerability is expected. However, baclofen is not without complications. Withdrawal can occur secondary to catheter disruption, battery failure, or human error. There is a very wide spectrum of presentation ranging from asymptomatic to death. Granulomas are very rare. Overdose is usually results from human error and can be reversed with physostigmine, and flumazenil.

633. (C)

A. Numerous medications work by blocking sodium channels. Ziconotide is not one of them.

B. Pregabalin and gabapentin work by acting on $\alpha2\delta$ voltage-gated calcium channels. Their exact mechanism of action is unknown, but their therapeutic action on neuropathic pain is thought to involve voltage-gated N-type calcium ion channels. They are thought to bind to the $\alpha2\delta$ subunit of the voltage-dependent calcium channel in the CNS.

C. Ziconotide is a nonopioid, non-NSAID (nonsteroidal anti-inflammatory drug), nonlocal anesthetic used for the amelioration of chronic pain. Derived from the cone snail *Conus magus*, it is the synthetic form of the cone snail peptide ω-conotoxin M-VII-A. Previously known as SNX-111, it is a neuronal-specific calcium-channel blocker that acts by blocking N-type, voltage-sensitive calcium channels.

Scientists have been intrigued by the effects of the thousands of chemicals in marine snail toxins since the initial investigations in the late 1960s by Baldomero Olivera, who remembered the deadly effects from his childhood in the Philippines. Ziconotide was discovered in the early 1980s by Michael McIntosh, at the time barely out of high school and working with Olivera. It was developed into an artificially manufactured drug by

Elan Corporation. It was approved for sale under the name Prialt by the FDA in the United States on December 28, 2004, and by the European Commission on February 22, 2005.

The mechanism of ziconotide has not yet been discovered in humans. Results in animal studies suggest that ziconotide blocks the N-type calcium channels on the primary nociceptive nerves in the spinal cord.

As a result of the profound side effects or lack of efficacy when delivered through more common routes, such as orally or intravenously, ziconotide must be administered intrathecally (directly into the spine). As this is by far the most expensive and invasive method of drug delivery and involves additional risks of its own, ziconotide therapy is generally considered appropriate (as evidenced by the range of use approved by the FDA in United States) only for management of severe chronic pain in patients for whom intrathecal (IT) therapy is warranted and who are intolerant of or refractory to other treatment, such as systemic analgesics, adjunctive therapies or IT morphine.

The most common side effects are dizziness, nausea, confusion, and headache. Others may include weakness, hypertonia, ataxia, abnormal vision, anorexia, somnolence, unsteadiness on feet, and memory problems. The most severe, but rare side effects are hallucinations, suicidal ideation, new or worsening depression, seizures, and meningitis. Therefore, it is contraindicated in people with a history of psychosis, schizophrenia, clinical depression, and bipolar disorder.

D. Baclofen's proposed mechanism of action is by blocking the $GABA_B$ receptors in the spinal cord.

634. (C)

A. The diagnosis of aseptic or viral meningitis in the cancer patient with an intrathecal pump should not be an automatic reason for explantation of the device. Supportive care and neurologic monitoring should be provided until the symptoms resolve, but the pump and catheter do not need to be removed. If the meningitis is of a bacterial etiology, risk assessment, pain stratification, and life expectancy should be considered. Removal of the pump is suggested, but is not required because there is a potential for severe, uncontrolled pain.

B. Parenteral (IV) *not* enteral (via the GI tract) antibiotics should be started immediately if bacterial meningitis is suspected. More specific antibiotics should be administered after cerebrospinal bacterial cultures and sensitivities are obtained.

C. If the infection is vancomycin sensitive, and the patient refuses pump explantation, intrathecal vancomycin may be administered at 10 mg/d. Intrathecal vancomycin has been used successfully for 6 months in such patients.

D. The same group found that IV vancomycin combined with epidural vancomycin (150 mg/d for 3 weeks) abolished infection.

635.   **(C)**

B. and C. Morphine or hydromorphone should be used for nociceptive pain. Bupivacaine should be used for neuropathic pain. Morphine or hydromorphone plus bupivacaine should be used for mixed pain. Droperidol is 95% efficacious in the treatment of nausea and vomiting secondary to opioid intolerance, abdominal tumors, and/or chemotherapy/radiation therapy, and can be added at this point (dose: 25-250 µg/d).

Morphine, hydromorphone, or fentanyl/sufentanil with bupivacaine and clonidine for nociceptive or mixed pain. Morphine, hydromorphone, or fentanyl/sufentanil with bupivacaine for neuropathic pain.

Morphine, hydromorphone, or fentanyl/sufentanil with more than two adjuvants: the physician should use opiate plus local anesthetic plus clonidine and

- Baclofen for spasticity, myoclonus, or neuropathic pain

- Bupivacaine for neuropathic pain
- Second opioid (lipophilic/hydrophilic) as an adjuvant

Morphine, hydromorphone, or fentanyl/sufentanil with more than three adjuvants: in addition to second-line adjuvants, the physician should add

- Ketamine for neuropathic pain secondary to cord compression
- Midazolam for neuropathic pain
- Droperidol for neuropathic pain

Tetracaine may be used for chemical paralysis for inoperable cord compression, tachyphylaxis, or emergency hyperalgesia rescue.

Some cases may necessitate six adjuvants to control pain at the end of life with minimal side effects.

636.   **(B)** The 2007 Polyanalgesic Consensus Guideline panelists have addressed this topic fully. All panelists felt that catheter-related granulomas still remains one of the most grave adverse effects and risks of intrathecal pain management and impediments to the widespread use of the therapy. Several factors contribute to the development of granuloma, including the agent used, catheter position (majority of granulomas occur in thoracic area—where CSF volume and flow are reduced), CSF volume (especially if low), and the dose and concentration of the drug (low CSF volume means higher concentrations of drug). With morphine, the preponderance of cases have been described in patients receiving concentrations of 40 mg/mL or greater. In cases where hydromorphone was implicated, the majority of cases received concentrations of 10 mg/mL or greater. Even though some panelists felt that positioning the catheter into the larger CSF volume of the dorsal intrathecal space of the low thoracic cord, granulomas do occur even in cases where catheters have been inserted into that space. However, concentration of the agent used appears to be the major causal factor of intrathecal, catheter-related granulomas.

A., B., C., and D. Inflammatory masses have been reported to be associated with all medications administered in the intraspinal space except for sufentanil and rarely for fentanyl. As of this writing, there have been at least three reports published in the literature of baclofen-related granulomas. Even though the literature suggests a granuloma protective effect of clonidine, there have been reports of patients with intrathecal clonidine, alone, or in combination with other intrathecal agents developing granulomas.

637 to 643. 637 (A and B); 638 (E); 639 (B and D); 640 (C); 641 (A, D, and G); 642 (A); 643 (D)

Opioids can cause sedation, edema, constipation, nausea, and urinary retention.

Bupivacaine can cause urinary retention, weakness, and hypotension.

Baclofen can cause loss of balance, and auditory disturbances.

Clonidine can cause orthostatic hypotension, worsening of depression, edema, and sedation.

Droperidol can cause extrapyramidal side effects such as tremor, slurred speech, akathisia, dystonia, anxiety, distress, and paranoia.

Ketamine can cause increased anxiety and irritability, delusional ideation, and facial flushing.

Midazolam can cause sedation.

If a medication is not therapeutic for a patient or is causing significant adverse effects, it should be properly weaned, and the patient should be informed of likely withdrawal symptoms and arrange for outpatient interventions. Acute baclofen or clonidine termination can result in hemodynamic derangements, seizures, or death. To avoid these untoward effects, physicians should introduce oral replacement therapy on the stoppage of intrathecal medications and provide an appropriate weaning schedule to the patient.

644. (D)

A. The epidural steroid injections (ESI) and SCS are treatment choices for radicular pain caused in particular by disc herniation

causing mechanical and chemical irritation of the nerve root.

B. Presence of axial low back pain even in absence of MRI changes can indicate possible facet arthropathy. Facet and medial branch diagnostic blocks are likely the most sensitive and specific diagnostic test for facet pain. Facet radiofrequency (RF) denervation seems to be the best treatment choice for patients with short-term relief with facet blocks.

C. The SCS trial may be an excellent choice for radiating pain down the leg.

645. (D)

A. SI joint injection with local anesthetics and steroids may have good diagnostic and possibly therapeutic value if the pain is located in the SI joints.

B. Internal disc disruption or discogenic pain can be diagnosed with provocative discography.

C. Quadratus lumborum and psoas muscle pain represent a form of myofascial pain that can be a cause of low back pain. Diagnostic blocks may have a value in diagnosis of this type of myofascial pain.

646. (D) Diagnostic medial branch blocks have a very high false-positive rate as reported in studies. This can potentially decrease the success rate of RF denervation of facet joints since this procedure is based on good short-term results with diagnostic medial branch blocks. For this reason repeated confirmatory diagnostic block and use of small dose of local anesthetics (0.3-0.5 mL) is recommended by many.

647. (B) Placebo effect is responsible for pain relief in up to 35.2% interventional procedures. Despite the high rates of placebo response it is not recommended for routine clinical use.

648. (D)

A. Infection is a rare complication that can be difficult to treat.

B. It seems that the epistaxis is more common than thought and can occur if too much pressure is applied to the RF cannula. Hematoma can occur if maxillary artery of venous plexus is punctured.

   C. Bradycardia is likely caused by reflex similar to the oculocardiac reflex.

649. (B)

   A. Change in taste would more likely be associated with glossopharyngeal nerve, lingual nerve, and chorda tympani.

   B. Ataxia can occur in up to 95% cases of RF denervation of the TON, numbness in 97%, dysesthesia in 55%, hypersensitivity in 15%, and itching in 10% of cases. Third occipital neurotomy almost always partially denervates semispinalis capitis muscle and so interferes with tonic neck reflexes and causes ataxia in particular on looking downward. The sensation is readily overcome by relying on visual cues such as fixing on the horizon.

   C. Dysphagia is not associated with TON thermocoagulation.

650. (D)

   A. Provocative discography is best done while pressure of contrast has been continuously measured. Reproduction of pain at < 30 psi above the opening pressure may represent chemical sensitization of the disc.

   B. Pressures between 50 and 100 psi mean inconclusive results.

   C. Pressures of 10 to 15 psi are more consistent with the opening pressure. It represents the pressure at which the contrast is first seen in the nucleus pulposus.

   D. Reproduction of pain at < 50 psi above the opening pressure may represent mechanical sensitization of the disc. During provocative discography, besides pressure measurements, pain levels should be > 6/10 and pain location and quality should be similar to the chronic low back pain.

651. (A) Cervical discography is performed with patient in supine position, using oblique approach, similar to the stellate ganglion block. The esophagus is normally positioned slightly toward the left side of the neck. To prevent puncturing it, the best technique for needle insertion for cervical discography is anterior right-sided approach.

652. (D) The ligamentum flavum is discontinuous in cervical levels, therefore allowing for very high chances of false loss of resistance technique and therefore mandates the use of fluoroscopy and contrast administration. The use of fluoroscopy may improve the safety of this procedure, medication delivery to the site of pathology, and potential outcomes. In lumbar levels it seems that the false loss of resistance in nonfluoroscopically performed epidural steroid injections occurs in up to 30% of cases.

653. (A)

   A. Although there is no median septum of fat in cervical epidural levels the unilateral medication spread is common. Therefore injections should be performed toward the laterality of pathology.

   B. False loss of resistance technique when not performed under fluoroscopy is 30% in lumbar levels and 50% in cervical levels.

   C. Ventral epidural spread in cervical levels is close to 25%.

   D. Too low.

   E. Unilateral contrast spread in intralaminar cervical epidural injections may occur in roughly 50% of all cases.

654. (D)

   A. Genitofemoral neuralgia is very rare complication of lumbar sympathetic block but can occur since the genitofemoral nerve originates from L1 and L2 nerve root.

   B. In retrograde ejaculation, the bladder sphincter does not contract and the sperm goes to the bladder instead of penis. This can lead to infertility.

   C. Intravascular injection of large dose of local anesthetics can lead to seizures.

655. (D) Any temperature change in comparison to preprocedure temperatures is adequate enough to assess the adequacy of successful block.

656. (B) The stellate ganglion is formed by fusion of inferior cervical ganglion resting over the anterior tubercle of C7 and first thoracic ganglion resting over the first rib.

657. (A) In relation to stellate ganglion the subclavian artery is located anteriorly. For this reason, care should be taken not to inject the medication into the subclavian artery.

658. (D)

A. C5 nerve root injection may provide analgesia by sensory block.

B. Inferior cervical ganglion is part of the stellate ganglion.

C. First thoracic ganglion is part of the stellate ganglion.

D. The T2 and T3 gray rami do not pass through the stellate ganglion but join the brachial plexus and innervate the upper extremity. Failure to block these structures may result in inadequate block (Kuntz nerves).

659. (A)

A. The opening pressure is always subtracted from pressure reproducing pain in final calculations (eg, positive discography means: pressure with pain reproduction— opening pressure < 50 psi).

B. First appearance of contrast in annular tear usually coincides with the reproduction of pain.

C. Reproduction of concordant pain means positive discography at tested level.

D. Resting pressure measurements is not used for interpretation of provocative discography.

660. (B)

A. Discs are usually dark (dehydrated) on T2-weighted MRI images and this can only suggest discogenic pain.

B. Morbid obesity can decrease the success rate and increase the risks of IDET.

C. There are no studies proving that age influences outcomes of IDET but it seems that advanced age may decrease the rate of success of IDET treatment.

D. Radicular pain directly does not predict the outcome of IDET. Discogenic pain (referred pattern) can sometimes mimic radicular pain.

661. (C) It does not seem that the outcomes of discography are affected by laterality of needle insertion site.

662. (D) SI joint fusion has been used in the past as a treatment of SI pain with unfavorable results. The L4, L5, S1, S2, and S3 radiofrequency denervation is shown to be beneficial long-term treatment option in patients with SI pain.

663. (D)

A. Epidural abscess should be suspected if increased pain and new neurologic symptoms occur after the cervical epidural steroid injection.

B. Neuropathic pain may occur following epidural steroid injection.

C. If the steroid solution is injected intravascularly serious complications including possible spinal cord infarction may occur. The digital subtraction fluoroscopy and blunt needle use may help to minimize its occurrence if this procedure is performed.

664. (B) Placing needle posteriorly may minimize the risk of intravascular injection.

665. (D)

A. The use of single-needle technique may decrease procedural discomfort during medial branch blocks.

B. By minimizing the amount of local anesthetics for the skin and subcutaneous tissues the rate of false-positive blocks caused by treatment of myofascial pain may be diminished.

C. This approach may take less time to perform than the traditional multiple-needle technique.

666. **(D)**

   A. If IV naloxone is inadequate, intrathecal naloxone may be considered.

   B. Airway protection may be needed because of respiratory depression.

   C. Possible irrigation of CSF with saline may be necessary.

667. **(D)** Increased impedance may mean that there is lead fracture, disconnect, fluid leakage causing short circuit. The exactly same impedance at multiple leads may mean that there is a communication and short circuit between the leads.

668. **(D)** The lead should be positioned subcutaneously posterior to the C2 spinous process and perpendicular to the cervical spine.

669. **(A)** For the coverage of the foot, the SCS electrode position should be at the T11-T12 level. The more caudal entry level is desired in order to leave enough of the SCS lead in the epidural space and prevent dislodgement.

670. **(C)** In order to position the lead at T1-T2 level commonly the entry site may be at lower thoracic levels owing to the narrow space in between the laminae in thoracic spine.

671. **(D)** Although there is insufficient evidence, one study reported that transforaminal approach has better outcomes in comparison to interlaminar approach for epidural steroid injections. The caudal approach requires diluted solution and may not reach the area of pathology in some cases.

672. **(A)** Contrast media should be administered in anteroposterior view in order to rule out intravascular uptake.

673. **(C)**

   A. Infection rate of implanted hardware has been estimated at 3% to 5%.

   B. Persistent pain at the implant site has been estimated at approximately 5%.

   C. Lead breakage or migration has been estimated at 11% to 45%.

   D. CSF leak requiring surgical intervention has been reported.

   E. Paralysis or severe neurologic deficit is possible as with any type of spine surgery, but is not cited as a frequent occurrence.

674. **(A)**

   A. One study which validates this statement was published in the journal *Pain* in 2007. A randomized, crossover study was performed with intent-to-treat analysis for more than 12 months. One hundred patients were randomized to either SCS and conventional medical management or conventional medical management only. More patients in the SCS group achieved the primary outcome of 50% or more pain relief in the legs. Other secondary measures were also improved in the SCS group. [Kumar K, Taylor RS, Jacques L, et al. Spinal cord stimulation versus conventional medical management for neuropathic pain: a multicenter randomized controlled trial in patients with failed back surgery syndrome. *Pain.* 2007;132(1-2):179-188.]

   B. In a 2009 review article it was determined that SCS decreases use of short-acting nitrates, improves quality of life, and increases exercise capacity. [Deer TR. Spinal cord stimulation for the treatment of angina and peripheral vascular disease. *Curr Pain Headache Rep.* 2009;13(1):18-23.]

   C. Many follow-up studies have been published showing efficacy with short-term follow-ups such as 6 months. A recent 5 year follow-up of a randomized, controlled trial of SCS for CRPS revealed that 95% of patients would repeat the treatment for the same result. A retrospective telephone questionnaire study was performed in 21 CRPS patients with average follow-up at 2.7 years. Reduced pain and improved quality of life was sustained at long-term follow-up. [Kemler MA, de Vet HC, Barendse GA, et al. Effect of spinal cord stimulation for chronic complex regional pain syndromes type I: five-year final follow-up of patients in a randomized controlled trial. *J Neurosurg.* 2008;108(2):292-298.]

D. SCS is effective for the treatment of sympathetically mediated pain.

E. This is a false statement. Neuropathic pain has traditionally been considered an indication for SCS. Nociceptive pain is considered not amenable to treatment with SCS.

675. **(C)** In 2007, an article published an evidence-based literature review and consensus statement which addressed over 60 questions relating to clinical use of SCS. Spinal cord injury or lesion, is an etiology of neuropathic pain and is an indication for SCS. Certain occupations such as an electrician's are considered a relative contraindication to SCS therapy.

676. **(D)** Some published articles concluded that SCS is cost-effective. Some have concluded that SCS is not cost-effective, at least in certain patient populations. Variation may relate to specific parameters and patient inclusions in the study. Recent practice parameters concluded that SCS is cost-effective in the treatment of failed back surgery syndrome and CRPS and might be cost-effective in the treatment of other neuropathic pain indications. Furthermore it was concluded that cost-effectiveness can be optimized by adjusting stimulation parameters to prolong battery life, by minimizing complications, and by improving equipment design. [Mekhail NA, Aeschbach A, Stanton-Hicks M. Cost benefit of neurostimulation for chronic pain. *Clin J Pain* 2004;20(6):462-468.

Klomp HM, Steyerberg EW, van Urk H, et al. Spinal cord stimulation is not cost-effective for non-surgical management of critical limb ischemia. *Eur J Vasc Endovasc Surg.* 2006;31(5): 500-508.

North R, Shipley J, Prager J, et al. Practice parameters for the use of spinal cord stimulation in the treatment of chronic neuropathic pain. *Pain Med* 2007;8(suppl 4):S200-S275.]

677. **(D)**

A. One of the three commonly used manufacturers does use a constant voltage technology. None of the three manufacturers have

a system allowing pulse width much over 1000 milliseconds.

B. Two of the three commonly used manufacturers do use a constant current technology. Although battery sizes as small as 22 cm^3 are available with two companies, no company currently has a battery smaller than that in current clinical usage. This may change in the near future.

C. No SCS system relies on maintaining constant resistance. Resistance is not in the physician's control and varies with factors such as scar tissue formation. Cordless recharging is available with several manufacturers' systems.

D. This is a specification set that is currently available. A constant voltage system is also now available with pulse widths up to 1000 milliseconds.

E. Maintaining both constant current and constant resistance would not be achievable because resistance is not a controllable factor. Voltage, current, and resistance vary according to Ohm's law: voltage = current × resistance.

New batteries have reached the market including ones with constant voltage, pulse width of 1000 milliseconds, and battery size of about 22 cm^3.

678. **(C)**

A. Dorsal column pathways have been demonstrated to play a role in transmission of visceral pain.

B. Case reports have been published showing successful treatment of pelvic pain with SCS. One such report was a case series of six patients with pelvic pain of multiple diagnoses all treated successfully with SCS. Diagnoses included vulvar vestibulitis, endometriosis, pelvic adhesions, uterovaginal prolapsed, and vulvodynia.

C. Midline myelotomy may relieve visceral cancer pain. This is a deep pathway and therefore a tightly spaced lead which can drive the stimulation deeper would be advantageous for attempted SCS for visceral pain.

D. The stimulation "sweet spot" for pelvic pain has been reported to be around T12.

E. Case study evidence supports the role for SCS for chronic visceral pelvic pain. Further well-designed studies are needed.

679. (B)

A. The dorsal columns contain the primary cutaneous afferents which are the usual targets. Stimulation of a nerve root will lead to segmental paresthesia and will not be likely to encompass the entire area of the bilateral lower extremity neuropathic pain.

B. This is a correct statement and was supported by computer-modeled analysis.

C. To the contrary, motor side effects usually indicates stimulation of dorsal roots rather than the dorsal column.

D. This statement is incorrect because as the contact to spinal cord distance increases, stimulation becomes less specific and there is an increased chance of dorsal root stimulation.

E. This is a false statement because fiber type preference is more sensitive to rostrocaudal contact size then to lateral contact size.

680. (A) Ronald Melzack and Patrick Wall published the landmark gate control theory in the journal *Science* in 1965. According to this theory as published in 1965, large and small fibers project to the substantia gelatinosa. The substantia gelatinosa exerts an inhibitory effect on afferent fibers. Large fibers increase the inhibitory effect, "close the gate," and decrease the afferent pain signal. Small fibers decrease the inhibitory effect, "open the gate," and increase the afferent pain signal.

This gate control theory is commonly cited as the mechanism of action of SCS, but a 2002 review concludes that other mechanisms must also play a role. [Oakley JC, Prager JP. Spinal cord stimulation: mechanisms of action. *Spine.* 2002;27(22):2574-2583.

Melzack R, Wall PD. Pain Mechanisms: a new theory. A gate control system modulates sensory input from the skin before it evokes pain perception and response. *Science.* 1965;150(3699)]

681. (C)

A. The opposite of the given statement would be more accurate (ie neuropathic pain is traditionally considered a better indication than nociceptive pain).

B. This is a restatement of (A). The term "receptor mediated" is substituted for and synonymous with nociceptive. The term "neurogenic" is substituted for and synonymous with neuropathic.

C. Multiple authors have described beneficial results of SCS for sympathetic-mediated pain [Stanton-Hicks M. Complex regional pain syndrome: manifestations and the role of neurostimulation in its management. *J Pain Symptom Manage.* 2006;31(suppl 4): S20-S24.

Kumar K, Nath RK, Toth C. Spinal cord stimulation is effective in the management of reflex sympathetic dystrophy. *Neurosurgery.* 1997;40(3):503-508.

Harke H, Gretenkort P, Ladlef HU, et al. Spinal cord stimulation in sympathetically maintained complex regional pain syndrome type I with severe disability. A prospective clinical study. *Eur J Pain.* 2005;9(4):363-373.]

D. This is a false statement as some consider intractable angina to be the pain most effectively treated with SCS, with up to 90% effectiveness.

E. Both persisting neuropathic pain of the extremity following spinal surgery and pain of CRPS are indications for SCS. However, persisting neuropathic extremity pain following spinal surgery is not *a better* indication. In fact, SCS is considered by some to be a more effective treatment of CRPS than persisting neuropathic pain of the extremity following spinal surgery.

682. (A) The conductivity of intraspinal elements has clinical significance. While some tissues have sufficient conductivity to allow stimulation to reach afferent fibers and initiate a depolarization, other tissues provide an insulation-like effect to protect visceral organs. One would not have to know the actual conductivities of intraspinal elements to answer this question.

683. (E)

A. Thoracic placement of SCS leads is very common. Contacts are often placed at the T8 level for instance for treatment of lower extremity pain.

B. While it is true that CSF is highly conductive, it does not divert the stimulation away from thoracic structures.

C. While it is true that various fibers have differing thresholds for recruitment, a negatively charged electrode (a cathode) will cause a neuron to become more electrically charged and depolarized, regardless of the tissue of origin.

D. It is true that dura has a very low conductivity similar to vertebral bone. However, because the dura is so thin, it does not present significant resistance. This should also be instinctively false because if the dura insulated structures from stimulation, then it would not be possible to stimulate the neural structures of the spinal cord.

E. This is a true statement. The conductivity of vertebral bone is very low compared to other intraspinal tissues.

684. (A)

A. Antidromic responses can be measured at the sural nerve during SCS. This was described in a 2002 review of SCS mechanisms and also demonstrated in 21 measurements in 16 patients in another study in 2008. [Oakley JC, Prager JP. Spinal cord stimulation: mechanisms of action. *Spine.* 2002;27(22):2574-2583.

Buonocore M, Bonezzi C, Barolet G. Neurophysiological evidence of antidromic activation of large myelinated fibers in lower limbs during spinal cord stimulation. *Spine.* 2008;33(4):E90-E93.]

B. SCS efficacy is not reversed by naloxone and there is no relation of SCS to endogenous opioid levels.

C. This would be a mechanism of algesic effect. In fact, one of the proposed mechanisms

of action of SCS is spinothalamic tract inhibition.

D. This would be a mechanism of algesic effect. In fact, one of the proposed mechanisms of action of SCS is activation of ascending and descending inhibitory pathways. On review of the mechanisms of action of SCS, one possible mechanism of action was cited as activation of supraspinal loops relayed by the brain stem or thalamocortical systems resulting in ascending and descending inhibition. [Oakley JC, Prager JP. Spinal cord stimulation: mechanisms of action. *Spine.* 2002;27(22):2574-2583.]

E. According to a 2002 review, the predominant effect of SCS is on abnormal activity in A-β neurons related to the perception of pain. [Oakley JC, Prager JP. Spinal cord stimulation: mechanisms of action. *Spine.* 2002;27(22):2574-2583.]

685. (A) Because phenol destroys the basal neurolemma, wallerian degeneration does not occur and there is a higher risk for neuroma formation. Lesion size is more difficult to precisely control with a liquid neurolytic injectate as compared to radiofrequency ablation in which the lesion size occurs in a known distance around the needle tip. On the other hand, when a field lesion is needed, a liquid neurolytic may be a more practical approach.

686. (A) Phenol is not painful upon injection whereas the other listed techniques are painful.

687. (E) Phenol is concerning for arrhythmias, seizure, destruction of Dacron grafts, vasospasm, and vascular proteins. Alcohol is more concerning for vasospasm than phenol. Caution when considering radiofrequency neurolysis includes interference with electrical implants. Risks of cryoneurolysis include frostbite to adjacent tissues.

688. (B)

A. Cryoanalgesia probes are generally larger in diameter than radiofrequency probes. Current cryoanalgesia probes range in size from 1.4 to 2 mm. The 1.4-mm cryoprobe is used with a 14- or 16-gauge catheter. A 2-mm cryoprobe is inserted into a 12-gauge catheter. Radiofrequency procedures are commonly performed using a 22-gauge needle. A 22-gauge needle has an outside diameter of about 0.7 or 0.72 mm.

B. The cryoanalgesia instrument may be cumbersome to support while simultaneously maintaining accurate needle-tip position. The smaller and lighter probes used with radiofrequency lesioning machines are less cumbersome to manage.

C. The ice ball formed at the tip of the cryoprobe is larger in size than what can be obtained with radiofrequency lesions.

D. Because of the smaller obtainable lesion size with the radiofrequency techniques, a more precise target lesion can be achieved.

E. Both cryoanalgesia and radiofrequency techniques cause wallerian degeneration and therefore less risk for neuroma formation compared to phenol.

689. **(E)**

A. Round conductors generate larger, stronger electric fields than flat conductors.

B. With round conductors, the charge density is inversely proportional to the radius of the circle.

C. The electric field around the exposed shaft of a radiofrequency cannula is less dense and becomes more dense at the tip.

D. The three basic variables of electric current are voltage, current, and resistance. These are the three factors in Ohm's law.

E. Although the electric field is less dense around the shaft but more dense around the tip of the cannula, the shape of the heat lesion is different. The heat lesion is slightly larger around the proximal end of the active tip and smaller at the needle tip.

690. **(C)**

A. While phenol may be useful for its hyperbaric property, there is no clear benefit versus alcohol.

B. Excellent results are reported in 50% to 75% of patients.

C. The average duration of pain relief after neuraxial neurolysis has been reported at 4 months.

D. Bladder paresis and motor paresis occurs in approximately 5% of treated patients. Bowel paresis occurs in approximately 1% of treated patients.

E. There is no evidence for greater efficacy or lower risk for epidural neurolysis compared to subarachnoid neurolysis.

691. **(E)** From the described approach, further advancement of the needle tip should either remain in annulus fibrosis or enter the next tissue layer, nucleus pulposus. CSF and spinal cord are not expected in the described trajectory.

692. **(E)**

A. Motor stimulation can detect and prevent unexpected improper heat lesioning. For example, a break in the insulation of the needle shaft can allow current to leak into unexpected tissues.

B. The radiofrequency probe should extend to the tip of the cannula. Too short of a radiofrequency probe will result in temperature measurements that are lower than the actual tissue temperature. This is especially concerning as a radiofrequency unit with automatic temperature control would increase the output in this situation, leading to even higher tissue temperatures.

C. It is usually best to consult a cardiologist prior to radiofrequency procedures when the patient has a pacemaker. If the pacemaker is a sensing pacemaker, then changing the setting to a fixed rate is suggested.

D. It is best to prevent complications rather than treat complications.

E. The SCS should be turned off prior to radiofrequency procedures.

693. **(A)** Coulomb per kilogram is used to measure electrical charge produced by x- or γ-radiation similar to previous roentgen unit in a standard volume of air by ionization. Sievert (Sv) is used to measure dose equivalent.

694. (B) Gray (Gy) measures absorbed dose (energy deposited per unit mass). One gray is equal to 1 J/kg.

695. (D) Individual doses may vary (eg, eye 12.5 mSv).

696. (D) As low as reasonably achievable is also known as ALARA (As low as reasonably achievable).

697. (B) The x-ray tube above the patient provides most operator exposure because the scattered beam is greater at the entrance site of the skin compared to exit site.

698. (D) As the intensity of scattered beam is greater at the radiation entrance on the skin than exit site the radiation exposure to the operator is significantly increased when the x-ray tube is above the patient.

699. (C) The patient radiation doses of angiography are on the other hand 10 times higher than gastrointestinal fluoroscopy and CT imaging.

700. (A) Oblique views can also increase the radiation to the patients and operators.

701. (D) Lead aprons contain equivalent of 0.5 mm of lead and can reduce the radiation exposure by 90% from scatter.

702. (B) Broken lead in aprons can provide suboptimal radiation protection.

703. (B) The diagnosis of an implantable device-related surgical-site infection is definitively made by identification or culture of microorganisms (most commonly bacteria) or both on specimens from a clinically suspected surgical wound or implant site. Signs of wound infection include fever, erythema, edema, pain, wound exudates, poor healing, or skin erosion at the implant site. Meningismus indicates CSF involvement.

    1. Infections related to the implantation of a SCS or an intrathecal drug-delivery system is the most common, potentially reducible, serious adverse events associated with these devices.

    2. In the comparison of drug-delivery device-related infections in multicenter studies the pump pocket was the site of infection between 57.1% and 80% of the time, the lumbar site was the infection location between 13% and 33% of the time, and meningitis was the infection between 10% and 14.3% of the time.

    3. Management of infections associated with drug-delivery and SCS systems typically involves administration of antibiotics and explantation of the devices.

    4. You should always worry about potential complications.

The infection rates, based on the number of infections that occurred and the number of patients that were evaluated have varied from 2.5% to 9.0% of implanted patients. The highest infection rate (9%), occurred in the 10-mL SynchroMed pump that was used in pediatric patients with spasticity of cerebral origin (n = 100), predominantly spastic cerebral palsy. The lowest infection rate, (2.5%), occurred in the group that received intrathecal recombinant methionyl human brain-derived neurotrophic factor (BDNF) to treat amyotrophic lateral sclerosis. 36 infections in 35 patients were described in a total of 700 patients (5% overall infection rate).

704. (A)

    1. The most common antibiotics used are a third-generation cephalosporin or vancomycin. Intraoperatively, many physicians irrigate the wound with antibiotic solution. Adjustments to antibiotic regimens should be made based on the most common pathogens seen in the community and medical center.

    2. In most instances the needle entry point into the intrathecal space is below L2. Sometimes, although rare, the entry point is at the level of the cord. If the entry point is above L2, the patient should be communicating with the physicians and nurses, and the angle of entry should be as small as possible. If any paresthesia is experienced, the needle should be removed and

repositioned. Once the catheter is properly positioned, a purse-string suture should be fashioned to secure the tissue around the catheter. Then, an anchor should be used to fasten the catheter to fascia. Given recent studies on inflammatory masses at catheter tips, whether the distal end of the catheter should be placed near the supposed pain generator or not is still up for debate.

3. While the patient may be positioned prone for catheter placement, placing them in the lateral decubitus position precludes having to reposition them for pocket creation. The usual site for pump placement is the lateral anterior abdominal wall at the level of the umbilicus. The pump should be anchored in a manner to prevent flipping.

4. The physician should meticulously obtain proper hemostasis during the case. Small venous and arterial bleeders can be recognized by retracting the wound after antibiotic irrigation. Numerous techniques exist to obtain hemostasis:

- Simple pressure
- Sponges soaked in 3% hydrogen peroxide solution may be packed into the wound for 3 to 5 minutes (may be very helpful with small vessels)
- Electrocautery for more pronounced bleeding [*Note:* overheating tissue can cause trauma or seroma formation, which can lead to delayed healing, dehiscence, or infection of the wound]
- Suturing a vessel is still the gold standard

A large sterile pressure dressing should be applied over the wound plus/minus an abdominal binder to reduce the risk of seroma formation and bleeding. Antibiotic ointment is also frequently used immediately over the incision; it may help in preventing the spread of infection. When considering dressing changes, the physician should be judicious—they can take place daily or only if the dressing is excessively saturated.

705. (E) In the early 1980s intrathecal drug-delivery was initiated for the treatment of intractable spasticity related to cerebral palsy and spinal cord injuries. This therapy eventually evolved to use in implacable cancer pain. Intrathecal preservative-free baclofen and morphine are FDA approved for the treatment of moderate to severe spasticity and moderate to severe pain, respectively. A study in oncology patients showed a major improvement using intrathecal medication delivery in cancer pain versus thorough medical management in the areas of tiredness, level of consciousness, and survival. [Smith TJ, Staats PS, Deer T et al. Randomized clinical trial of an implantable drug delivery system compared with comprehensive medical management for refractory cancer pain: impact on pain, drug-related toxicity, and survival. *J Cli.* 2002;20(19):4040-4049.]

Other disease states found to be responsive to intrathecal drug-delivery systems are

- Spinal stenosis
- Radiculitis
- Compression fractures
- Spondylosis
- Spondylolisthesis
- Foraminal stenosis
- Arachnoiditis
- Syrinx
- Ankylosing spondylitis
- Spinal cord trauma
- Spinal infarction
- Paraplegia
- Cauda equina syndrome
- Peripheral neuropathy
- Phantom limb pain
- Rheumatoid arthritis
- Radiation neuritis
- Postherpetic neuralgia
- Postthoracotomy syndrome
- Interstitial cystitis
- Chronic pain of the abdomen and pelvis

706. **(C)** Patients with a VAS pain scale of 7 to 10 may necessitate inpatient/hospice care for pain treatment. For those who wish to remain in a home environment, a 50% to 100% increase in their medication dose may be in order. Therapeutic boluses should be administered to an end point

of pain relief, as well as daily medication adjustments to the same end point. Significant, abrupt increase in medication may cause severe side effects, and physicians should be available in the first 12 hours following the modification, to manage potential complications.

707. **(E)** A multicenter, randomized, prospective study compared intrathecal drug delivery to comprehensive medical management. The results showed a statistically significant advantage of intrathecal pumps on

- Overall toxicity
- Pain relief
- Fatigue and level of consciousness
- Improved survivability

The study hinted that more patients with moderate to severe cancer pain should be considered for intrathecal pumps. [Smith TJ, Staats PS, Deer T et al. Randomized clinical trial of an implantable drug delivery system compared with comprehensive medical management for refractory cancer pain: impact on pain, drug-related toxicity, and survival. *J Clin.* 2002;20(19):4040-4049.]

708. **(B)** The third occipital headache is caused by third occipital neuralgia. The TON innervates the C2-3 zygapophysial joint and curves around the superior articular process of the C3 vertebral body. Among patients with whiplash injuries, third occipital headache is common, with a prevalence of 27%.

709. **(D)** The occipital nerve stimulator is a useful tool in managing occipital neuralgia. Although paddle electrodes are not necessary they may provide better coverage than the regular electrode.

710. **(A)** T2 and T3 sympathetic blocks are a useful tool in conjunction with stellate ganglion block for upper extremity CRPS. By blocking them, Kuntz nerves will be blocked that bypass the stellate ganglion. RF denervation of these nerves may lead to prolonged pain relief.

711. **(A)** Vertebroplasty is best used for acute vertebral fracture where bone cement is percutaneously injected into a fractured vertebra in order to stabilize it. Alternatively, kyphoplasty involves placement of a balloon into a collapsed vertebra, followed by injection of bone cement to stabilize the fracture. It is not clear if one procedure has an advantage over the other. Both procedures may obtain almost immediate pain relief. And they are indicated for painful compression fractures because of osteoporosis and metastatic tumors.

712. **(E)** Complications from vertebroplasty can be serious. Intravascular injection of polymethyl methacrylate can lead to pulmonary embolus and spinal cord damage and leak into intrathecal space can cause spinal cord injury. Lumbar procedures may lead to leak into psoas muscle and femoral neuropathy.

713. **(E)** Piriformis injection should be done in the medial part of a muscle since the lateral part contains more ligaments. If injection of local anesthetics and steroids provides short-term pain relief only, the injection of botulinum toxin type A may provide longer pain relief. The use of nerve stimulator, fluoroscopy, and contrast administration may help to assure proper needle placement. Tenderness over the piriformis muscle, positive Pace and Freiberg signs and rectal examination can be helpful in examining the piriformis muscle.

714. **(D)**

1. The innervation of the SI joint is from L4 medial branch, L5 dorsal ramus, S1, S2, and S3 lateral branches. Some authors also state that the L3 medial branch may be involved.
2. SI joint fusion is used only in cases where serious anatomical problems (eg, fracture) are present in addition to pain.
3. SI joint injection should be done under fluoroscopic guidance to assure accuracy of needle placement.

715. **(B)**

1. Anterior approach was initial approach described for blocking celiac plexus. Its advantage is that patient can be in more comfortable, supine position.

2. Although the retrocrural block may partially block the nerve supply to the celiac plexus actually blocks the splanchnic plexus.

3. Anterocrural approach is done with patient in prone position using one or two needles. Transaortic and transdiscal variation of this approach has been published as well.

4. Lateral approach is not used for celiac plexus block.

716. (C)

1. Testicular pain is treated by ilioinguinal block or lumbar sympathetic block.

2. Ganglion impar is the most caudal sympathetic ganglion.

3. The ganglion impar is located at the level of the sacrococcygeal junction that marks the termination of the paired paravertebral sympathetic chains. Initial approach described was through anococcygeal ligament. However, the trans-sacrococcygeal approach seems much safer way to perform this procedure.

4. Perforation of rectum may occur in particular if anococcygeal approach is used.

717. (A)

1. As a result of discontinuous ligamentum flavum the loss of resistance is often inaccurate in cervical levels and more often in comparison to lumbar levels (30%).

2. The fluoroscopic guidance should be used and medication should be deposited ipsilateral to the pathology.

3. Final needle advancement and contrast spread should be first checked in lateral fluoroscopic views.

4. Transforaminal approach (most likely because of intravascular particulate steroid uptake) can lead to serious complications such as spinal cord infarction, quadriplegia, and death.

718. (E)

1. Granuloma formation can occur at the tip of the intrathecal catheter and can lead to serious complications including spinal cord injury.

2. CSF leak is a relatively common complication of intrathecal pump placement.

3. Pump rotation can cause kinking of the catheter and symptoms of increased pain and withdrawal.

4. Intrathecal opioids can lead to serious hormonal changes including weight gain.

719. (A) Increased pain, in particular with withdrawal symptoms should be considered as a pump failure and treated promptly.

720. (E) Combination of hyaluronidase and hypertonic saline seems to increase the duration of procedure effect. Intrathecal injection of hypertonic saline can lead to serious complications and should be performed carefully.

721. (E) Traditional indications for SCS include postlaminectomy syndrome and CRPS. Indications have been expanding. Intestinal cystitis is now a commonly accepted indication. SCS is an accepted method for effective treatment of sympathetically mediated pain.

722. (A) According to a review in 2008, SCS should be considered early in the course of postherpetic neuralgia and peripheral nerve stimulation should be considered if SCS fails. SCS is about 50% effective for failed back surgery syndrome and more so effective for peripheral vascular disease and ischemic disease. Although the gate control theory is a commonly cited mechanism of action for SCS, literature reflects that this one mechanism alone is not sufficient to explain the mechanism of action. According to a 2002 review article, there are 10 proposed mechanisms of action found in literature. [Oakley JC, Prager JP. Spinal cord stimulation: mechanisms of action. *Spine*. 2002; 27(22): 2574-2583.]

723. (C) Transverse tripolar SCS on involves a central *cathode* surrounded by *anodes*. This is proposed to drive current deeper and thus stimulate fibers innervating the *back*. Therefore is it used to cover back pain, not foot pain. Statement (4) is also correct as most current SCS systems allow up to a total of 16 leads.

724. **(B)** In a 2006 review article SCS was concluded to increase exercise capacity as well as decrease use of short-acting nitrates and improve quality of life. The review also found that at 5 years 60% of patients still had beneficial effects. Exercise stress testing and electrocardiogram (ECG) monitoring evidence showed reduced ischemia in addition to the antianginal effects. Pain perception remains intact and patients were still able to detect significant ischemic events. [Deer TR, Raso LJ. Spinal cord stimulation for refractory angina pectoris and peripheral vascular disease. *Pain Physician* 2006;9(4): 347-352.]

725. **(E)** All listed factors are risks of SCS. Other risks include nerve injury, dural puncture, infection, and electrode migration.

726. **(B)** In animal models, SCS has been shown to suppress visceral responses. There have been multiple case reports of SCS being used successfully for visceral pain; however, current practice parameters do not address treatment of such pain. Since the pancreas is innervated by spinal segments around T5-T11, a lead placement would be much too low of a logical starting place. One case study reported placing the lead at T6 resulting in appropriate stimulation for treatment of chronic pancreatitis.

727. **(E)** Anode is the correct designation for a positive contact and cathode is the correct designation for a negative contact. With a dual-lead system as pictured, the electric field would be pulled toward the anode if lead spacing were tight. With larger lead spacing, the electric field would tend to be more spherical and positioned around the cathode. Tight lead spacing increases the dorsal column to dorsal root stimulation ratio because the less spherical electric field would stimulate less laterally and therefore would have less stimulation in the areas of the nerve roots.

728. **(A)** According to a review article on selection criteria for SCS, selection criteria may relate to the patient's disease state or to other important patient characteristics. Current randomized controlled trials or prospective trials

support efficacy of SCS for certain disease states such as failed back surgery syndrome, CRPS, axial back pain, postherpetic neuralgia, neuropathy, and pelvic pain. Current case report evidence exists for SCS in the treatment of ischemic limb pain, and visceral pain. Anginal pain has also been investigated. Patient characteristics of concern include systemic disease such as diabetes, immunocompromised, degree of stenosis especially for cervical placed leads, anticoagulation, psychologic comorbidities, unrealistic outcome expectations, and, untreated drug addictions. [Oakley JC. Spinal cord stimulation: patient selection, technique, and outcomes. *Neurosurg Clin N Am.* 2003;14(3):365-380.]

729. **(E)** The indications for SCS are expanding. All of the listed etiologies are now considered indications for SCS.

730. **(B)**

1. Scribonius Largus documented application of the live black torpedo fish under the foot for treatment of the pain of gout. *"For any type of gout a live black torpedo should, when the pain begins, be placed under the feet. The patient must stand on a moist shore washed by the sea and he should stay like this until his whole foot and leg up to the knee is numb. This takes away present pain and prevents pain from coming on if it has not already arisen. In this way Anteros, a freedman of Tiberius, was cured."*

2. The gate control theory of pain was published in 1965. This laid the theoretical foundation for electrical stimulation for pain. The first modern case report of electrical stimulators for treatment of pain was 2 years later. It described eight cases in which sensory nerves or roots were stimulated resulting in relief of pain. [Melzack R, Wall PD. Mechanisms: a new theory. A gate control system modulates sensory input from the skin before it evokes pain perception and response. *Science.* 1965;150(3699).

    Wall PD, Sweet WH. Temporary abolition of pain in man. *Science.* 1967;155(758):108-109.]

3. In the peripheral nerves, motor and sensory fibers are within closer vicinity. The window

of amplitude available to provide analgesia without excessive motor stimulation is therefore much less than in the spinal cord where sensory and motor fibers run in more discrete and separate pathways. This played a role in switching emphasis from peripheral nerve stimulation toward SCS.

4. The first documented cases of modern day stimulation for pain was a case series of eight patients published in 1967. This case series reported three of the eight patients received psychiatric evaluation prior to the procedures. The psychiatric/psychologic evaluation gives the patient an opportunity to belay anxiety, ask questions, address body image issues, and communicate expectations. [Wall PD, Sweet WH. Temporary abolition of pain in man. *Science.* 1967;155(758):108-109.]

731. **(C)** Sacral neuromodulation has been reported as effective for idiopathic urinary frequency, urgency, and urge incontinence. Both percutaneous and surgical sacral neuromodulation procedures have been described. Percutaneous techniques include (1) placement of a lead directly into the sacral nerve root foramen and (2) a percutaneous retrograde approach. Surgical techniques include (1) performing a sacral laminectomy and attaching the electrodes directly to the sacral nerve roots and (2) dissection to sacral periosteum where a plastic anchor is used to affix a transforaminal lead. Techniques that are limited to one lead placement may have limitations in terms of efficacy for certain indications. While a single lead has been generally efficacious for voiding dysfunctions, chronic neuropathic pain syndromes may benefit from a more extensive field of neuromodulation with additional electrodes.

732. **(B)**

1. Temperatures above 45°C cause irreversible neural tissue damage. If temperatures of 45°C are reached, then the voltage should be decreased to compensate.

2. Sensory testing is applied at 50 Hz.

3. The pulsed technique allows tissues to cool somewhat between cycles. A voltage

of 45 V generally corresponds to a 43°C tip temperature. If the tip temperature exceeds 43°C, then the voltage should be reduced.

4. Motor testing is applied at 2 Hz.

733. **(E)** All the options mentioned in the question are required elements to complete the circuit. The current goes from the probe tip, through the patient and to the grounding pad which carries the current back to the radiofrequency generator.

734. **(C)** Formation of a static electric field and generation of heat are two phenonemon that have been postulated as possible mechanisms of action of radiofrequency ablation. The mechanism of action of cryoablation involves vascular injury which causes severe endoneural edema. The mechanism of action of alcohol ablative techniques is lipid extraction with protein precipitation.

735. **(D)**

1. Although there are several studies looking at radiofrequency neuroablation for the SI joint, according to a recent systematic review evidence is still limited for its therapeutic value.

2. Although there are guidelines such as those posed by International Association for the Study of Pain (IASP), evidence and universal acceptance are still lacking. Some studies have refuted SI provocative maneuvers as predictive at all while others found that three of five positive provocative maneuvers provide predictive value. The role of adding steroids to diagnostic SI injections is similarly debated.

3. Pulsed radiofrequency treatment was given to 22 patients with injection evidence of SI pain. Sixteen patients (73.9%) had 50% or better relief for more than 3 months.

4. In a 2003 pilot study, 8 of 9 patients experienced 50% or better pain relief after radiofrequency lesioning at L4 primary dorsal rami and S1-S3 lateral branches. Relief persisted at 9 month follow-up.

736. **(A)** Other advantages of radiofrequency lesions include avoids sticking and charring (in contrast to direct current electrical lesions), no gas formation (in contrast to direct current electrical lesions), impedance monitoring, and amenable to fluoroscopic and CT guidance. Ability to identify needle-tip proximity to motor and sensory nerves is a characteristic of radiofrequency procedures, although cryoanalgesia probes are also available with built-in nerve stimulators. Ability to cover a wide field is not an advantage of percutaneous radiofrequency lesion. Percutaneous radiofrequency techniques deliver relatively smaller, more defined treatment areas and therefore a great deal of lesions would be needed in order to cover a wide field target.

737. **(E)** These are all accurate historical events as described and cited in current literature reviews. Pulsed radiofrequency techniques have received growing interest since 1997, when treatment of the cervical spinal dorsal root ganglions with pulsed radiofrequency suggested efficacy and safety. In 1961, Cooper described a device which used liquid nitrogen in a hollow tube that was insulated at the tip and achieved temperatures as low as −190°C. He published his description in a hospital bulletin. Six years later an ophthalmic surgeon by the name of Amoils improved on the device. Lloyd coined the term "cryoanalgesia" in 1976. The technique was popularized in the 1980s, but publications have declined since. [Cooper IS, Lee AS. Cryostatic congelation: a system for producing a limited, controlled region of cooling or freezing of biologic tissues. *J Nerv Ment Dis.* 1961;133:259-263.]

Amoils SP. The Joule Thomson cryoprobe. *Arch Opthalmol.* 1967:78(2):201-207.

Lloyd JW, Barnard JD, Glynn CJ. Cryoanalgesia. A new approach to pain relief. *Lancet.* 1976;2(7992):932-934.]

738. **(E)** The size of a continuous radiofrequency lesion depends on temperature, width of needle, and length of exposed (uninsulated) cannula. The 1.4-mm cryoanalgesia probe forms an ice ball about 3.5 mm thick, while the larger 2-mm probe forms and ice ball about 5.5 mm thick. Thus the ice ball is about 2.5 to 2.75 times larger than the probe for these size probes.

739. **(A)** A cryoprobe is comprised of a tube within a tube. The inner tube is pressurized with a gas such as nitrous oxide or carbon dioxide at 600 to 800 psi. As the gas escapes through a narrow aperture at the tip of the inner tube, it (the gas) abruptly expands in the larger outer tube at a lower pressure of about 10 to 15 psi. As the gas expands, it (the gas) cools. This is known as the Joule-Thompson effect. An ice ball then forms at the tip of the probe. The gas does not escape out through a fine aperture in the tip of the outer tube. This would allow the gas to enter the patient's tissues. Instead, gas escapes back up the larger outer tube in a closed system design.

740. **(E)**

1. It has been postulated that the sinuvertebral nerves at each lumbar level transmit sensory information from the intervertebral discs to the paravertebral chain on each side. The rami communicans then communicate this sensory information to the dorsal root ganglia at L1 and L2.

2. and 3. Both radiofrequency and phenol lumbar sympathetic neurolytic techniques have been described for the treatment of lower extremity CRPS.

4. Cryoablation has been utilized for pain of the superior gluteal nerve. (Trescot, Pain Physician, 2003, v. 6, p. 345-360, Cryoanalgesia in interventional pain management)

741. **(B)**

1. Pulsed radiofrequency procedure is virtually painless. Continuous radiofrequency ablation is painful with application.

2. There is debate in literature as to whether pulsed radiofrequency procedure is as efficacious as radiofrequency ablation.

3. In addition to innervating the zygapophysial joint, the medial branch of the dorsal ramus also innervates the multifidus, interspinales,

and intertransversarii mediales muscles, the interspinous ligament, and, possibly, the ligamentum flavum.

4. In both cases a cannula and radiofrequency probe of similar size are inserted.

742. (C)

1. Too low an impedance may indicate the needle tip is in nontarget tissues such as vasculature, CSF, or nucleus pulposus.

2. This statement is correct.

3. It is traditional to use impedance information in assisting needle-tip placement even during fluoroscopically guided procedures.

4. This statement is correct. Superior gluteal nerve entrapment is amenable to cryoablation.

CHAPTER 9

Complementary and Alternative Medicine
Questions

DIRECTIONS (Questions 743 through 755): Each of the numbered items or incomplete statements in this section is followed by answers or by completions of the statement. Select the ONE lettered answer or completion that is BEST in each case.

743. Acupuncture needles used in current practice

   (A) are under same marketing rules as syringes
   (B) are under same standard control like medical needles
   (C) have same quality control as surgical scalpels
   (D) are used once only
   (E) all of the above

744. Which of the following statements is incorrect?

   (A) Acupuncture was widely practiced by thousands of physicians, dentists, acupuncturists, and other practitioners
   (B) Acupuncture can be used to relive pain and in various other health conditions
   (C) The National Institutes of Health (NIH) have funded many research projects relating to acupuncture
   (D) In a national survey, the number of visits to alternative medicine was nearly twice of the visits to primary care physician
   (E) Few medical schools in the United States have included subjects on integrated medicine

745. Which of the following statements is correct?

   (A) There are 600 to 2000 acupuncture points on the human body
   (B) Acupuncture points are mostly located along the meridians
   (C) Acupuncturist could use points on the ears, scalp, hands, and feet to treat diseases
   (D) Each treatment may use different acupuncture points even with the same disease
   (E) All of the above

746. In the acupuncture theory

   (A) "qi" is the life force or energy that flows through the body
   (B) "qi" influences our health at physical, mental, emotional, and spiritual levels
   (C) any excess or deficiency of "qi" will contribute to our health problems
   (D) blockage of "qi" may cause pain
   (E) all of the above

747. Which of the following statements is incorrect?

(A) Electroacupuncture (EA) can be used through needles to enhance the stimulation of acupuncture points

(B) Percutaneous electric nerve stimulation (PENS) is a modified form of acupuncture treatment

(C) "Deqi" sensation is a side effect of acupuncture

(D) Moxibustion can be used with or without insertion of acupuncture needles

(E) Acupressure and cupping are also helpful in treating different diseases

748. Which one of the following complications associated with acupuncture is mostly reported?

(A) Infection

(B) Bruising or bleeding

(C) Transient vasovagal response

(D) Pneumothorax

(E) Intra-abdominal abscess

749. With regard to the scientific basis of acupuncture's effects, which of the following statements is incorrect?

(A) Electric acupuncture can activate the central nervous system (CNS) to release endogenous opioids into blood or cerebrospinal fluid (CSF)

(B) The analgesic effects of acupuncture may occur after 20 to 30 minutes of treatment

(C) Naloxone and other opioid antagonists can inhibit the acupuncture analgesia

(D) Acupuncture analgesia can not be passed from one animal to another animal via CSF transfer or blood transfer

(E) Substances that inhibit endorphin enzymatic degradation enhance the analgesic effects of acupuncture treatment

750. Which of the following is not involved in the analgesic effect of acupuncture?

(A) Nicotine

(B) Serotonin

(C) Norepinephrine

(D) Nitric oxide

(E) β-Endorphin

751. Which of the following is the condition/disease that acupuncture has not shown to be an effective treatment modality?

(A) Allergies

(B) Dysmenorrhea

(C) Leukemia

(D) Biliary colic

(E) Leukopenia

752. Complementary and alternative medicine includes all of the following EXCEPT

(A) herbs

(B) mind-body therapy

(C) massage

(D) aspirin

(E) homeopathic therapy

753. Mind-body interventions have been used in all the following conditions EXCEPT

(A) headache

(B) low back pain

(C) arthritis

(D) chemotherapy-induced nausea and vomiting

(E) none of the above

754. The following statements regarding *Ginkgo biloba* are true EXCEPT

(A) *Ginkgo biloba* has been used to treat multiple conditions such as asthma, bronchitis, fatigue and tinnitus

(B) *Ginkgo biloba* has also been tried to improve Alzheimer disease and dementia

(C) patients with intermittent claudicating, multiple sclerosis have tried *Ginkgo biloba* supplement

(D) *Ginkgo biloba* has side effects including headache, nausea, diarrhea, dizziness, and allergic skin reactions

(E) *Ginkgo biloba* does not increase bleeding risk so it can be safely taken with other anticoagulant drugs

755. The evidence from research supports the following effects of ginseng EXCEPT

(A) ginseng supports overall health and boost immune system

(B) ginseng does not cause allergic reactions

(C) ginseng can increase both mental and physical performance

(D) some studies have shown that ginseng lowers the blood glucose level

(E) most common side effects of ginseng are headache, sleep disturbances, and gastrointestinal (GI) problems

DIRECTIONS: For Question 756 through 762, ONE or MORE of the numbered options is correct. Choose answer

(A) if only answer 1, 2, and 3 are correct

(B) if only 1 and 3 are correct

(C) if only 2 and 4 are correct

(D) if only 4 is correct

(E) if all are correct

756. The biologically based practice is a domain of complementary and alternative medicine. It includes

(1) vitamins

(2) fatty acids

(3) proteins

(4) prebiotics

757. Naturopathy is a system of healing. Its principles include the following:

(1) The healing power of nature

(2) Identification and treatment of the cause of disease

(3) Treatment of the whole person

(4) The doctor as a teacher

758. Which of the following statement(s) is (are) correct for homeopathy?

(1) It stimulates the body's ability to heal by itself

(2) Remedy contains giving small doses of highly diluted substance that can cause similar symptoms

(3) Same substance if given in a larger dose would produce illness or symptoms

(4) "Principle of similar" is not the theory of homeopathy

759. Glucosamine and chondroitin are used to treat knee osteoarthritis, which of the following statements is (are) correct?

(1) In the United States, glucosamine and chondroitin are considered dietary supplements

(2) It may cause serious adverse events such as congestive heart failure and chest pain

(3) It may have more substantial treatment effects in a subgroup of patients with moderate to severe pain

(4) Overall, glucosamine and chondroitin sulfate alone or in combination reduces the pain effectively in patients with knee osteoarthritis

760. Which of the following is (are) true about mind-body interventions?

(1) May have impact on health by the mechanism of the brain and CNS influencing immune, endocrine, and autonomic function

(2) Multicomponent mind-body interventions may be useful adjunctive treatment for coronary artery disease and certain pain-related disorders

(3) Cognitive behavioral therapy, combined with educational/informational component can be effectively used as adjuncts in the management of variety of chronic conditions

(4) When applied presurgically, a group of mind-body therapies (imaginary, hypnosis, relaxation) may improve recovery time and reduce pain following surgical procedures

761. Which of the following is (are) true about *Echinacea*?

  (1) Studies indicate that *Echinacea* does not prevent colds or other infections

  (2) Studies have not proven that *Echinacea* shortens the course of colds or flu

  (3) *Echinacea* can cause allergic reactions including rash, asthma, and anaphylaxis

  (4) GI side effects are most common

762. Which of the following is (are) true about chiropractic practice?

  (1) It is an alternative medical system and takes a different approach from conventional medicine in diagnosing, classifying, and treating medical problems

  (2) The chiropractic theories consider that the body has a powerful self-healing ability and the body structure and its function are closely related and this relation affects our health

  (3) The goal of this therapy is to normalize the relation of structure and function

  (4) There have been serious reported adverse effects such as stroke, caudal equine syndrome associated with chiropractic therapy

Answers and Explanations

743. **(E)** In 1996, the US Food and Drug Administration (FDA) changed the classification of acupuncture needles from experimental to medical equipment. So acupuncture needles are under the same strict quality control standards demanded for medical needles, syringes, or surgical scalpels. It includes manufacture, marketing, and use.

744. **(E)** Acupuncture is being "widely" practiced by thousands of physicians, dentists, acupuncturists, and other practitioners for relief or prevention of pain and for various other health conditions. The majority of medical schools in the United States have already added courses on integrated medicine. In a 1998 survey, the number of visits to alternative medicine was almost twice that of visits to primary care physician.

745. **(E)** There are between 600 and 2000 acupuncture points on the human body in 12 major meridians named after organ systems, and 8 minor meridians. There are also points on the ears, hands, feet, and scalp corresponding to organs throughout the body, and extra points outside the traditional meridians. Acupuncture points are usually chosen based on the practitioner's assessment of the particular imbalance that needs to be restored. Even with the same patient and medical condition, acupuncture points used in each acupuncture treatment may be different.

746. **(E)** According to traditional Chinese medicine, "qi" (pronounced "chee") is the life force or energy that flows through all living things. "Qi" affects our body at physical, mental, emotional, and spiritual levels. Any imbalance (deficiency or excess) or blockage of "qi" may result in disease or pain. Acupuncture treats disorders by influencing the flow of "qi," thus restoring the normal balance of organ systems.

747. **(C)** EA uses electrical impulses conducted through needles for enhanced stimulation of acupuncture points. Different frequencies of electrical stimulation have showed distinctive effects and mechanisms of action. PENS is an adapted form of acupuncture that is widely practiced. Other techniques include moxibustion (burning of herbs to apply heat near acupuncture points), acupressure and reflexology (stimulation of points without penetration of the skin with needles), and cupping (heat creates a partial vacuum in small jars, which are used to stimulate points with suction). The sensations of "deqi" at the insertion site noted by the patient include aching, tingling, numbness, warmness, or heavy pressure feeling. It usually corresponds to the acupuncturist's feeling of the needle "catching" in the muscle. deqi is thought to be necessary for achieving the acupuncture therapeutic effect.

748. **(B)** In the hands of a skilled practitioner, complications associated with acupuncture are actually quite rare, and usually very mild. The most commonly reported complication is bruising or bleeding. A second, less common side effect is a transient vasovagal response. Severe complications and fatal reactions such as pneumothorax, abdominal abscess, or pericardial effusion associated with acupuncture are rare.

749. **(D)** In the most widely accepted acupuncture model, needling of nerve fibers in the muscle sends impulses that activate the spinal cord, midbrain, and hypothalamus-pituitary system.

Subsequently, it releases β-endorphin into the blood and CSF to cause analgesia at a distance. The effects of acupuncture are not immediate; rather analgesia occurs after a 20- to 30-minute induction period. Analgesia persists for 1 to 2 hours after cessation of acupuncture. Naloxone and other opiate antagonists inhibit acupuncture analgesia. Substances that inhibit endorphin enzymatic degradation enhance acupuncture effects. Acupuncture analgesia can be passed from one animal to another via CSF transfer or via cross-circulation of blood between two animals.

750. **(A)** EA induces upregulation of neuronal nitric oxide/nicotinamide adenine diphosphate (NADPH) diaphorase expression in the gracile nucleus in rats, and then mediates acupuncture signals through dorsal medulla-thalamic pathways. This may play a significant role in central autonomic regulation of somatosympathetic reflexes that contribute to acupuncture effects in somatic and visceral pain processing, and cardiovascular regulation. Other evidence also supports the notion that those neurotransmitters (eg, serotonin and norepinephrine) as well as β-endorphin all act as mediators.

751. **(C)** In 2002, the World Health Organization (WHO) published a summary and review of all clinical trials through the year 1999, and determined four categories of disorders treated by acupuncture. Allergies, dysmenorrhea, biliary colic, and leukopenia are disorders among many others in the category of proven efficacy of acupuncture through controlled trials.

752. **(D)** Complementary and alternative medicine include following practices: mind-body medicine, biologically based practices, manipulative and body-based practices, energy medicine, and whole medical systems. Whole medical systems include homeopathic medicine, naturopathic medicine, traditional Chinese medicine (herb, acupuncture, massage, meditation, etc), and ayurveda (herb, massage, and yoga).

753. **(E)** Mind-body interventions have also been applied to various types of pain. Clinical trials indicate that these interventions may be a particularly effective adjunct in the management of arthritis, with reductions in chronic pain for up to 4 years and reductions in the number of physician visits. When applied to more general acute and chronic pain management, headache, and low back pain, mind-body interventions show some evidence of effects, although results vary based on the patient population and type of intervention involved. Evidence from multiple studies with various populations of cancer patients suggests that mind-body interventions can improve mood, quality of life, and coping as well as ameliorate disease- and treatment-related symptoms, such as chemotherapy-induced nausea, vomiting, and pain.

754. **(E)** Recently, *Ginkgo biloba* has been used to treat a variety of health conditions, including asthma, bronchitis, fatigue, and tinnitus. Some encouraging results have been seen from the studies of Alzheimer disease/dementia, intermittent claudication, and tinnitus. But a trial of more than 200 healthy adults older than 60 years found that *Ginkgo biloba* taken for 6 weeks did not improve memory. Side effects of *Ginkgo biloba* include headache, nausea, GI upset, diarrhea, dizziness, or allergic skin reactions. More severe allergic reactions have occasionally been reported. There are some data to suggest that *Ginkgo biloba* can increase bleeding risk, so people who take anticoagulant drugs, have bleeding disorders, or have scheduled surgery or dental procedures should use caution.

755. **(B)** Ginseng has numerous potential benefits which include: supporting overall health and boosting the immune system; improving recovery from illness; increasing a sense of well-being and stamina; improving both mental and physical performance; treating erectile dysfunction, hepatitis C; reducing symptoms related to menopause; lowering blood glucose; and controlling blood pressure. The most common side effects are headaches and sleep disturbance and GI problems. Ginseng can cause allergic reactions. There have been reports of breast tenderness, menstrual irregularities, and high blood pressure associated with ginseng products. Ginseng may lower the level of blood glucose; this effect may be seen more often in patients

with diabetes. Therefore, diabetic patients should use extra caution with Asian ginseng, especially if they are taking medicines to lower blood sugar or taking other herbs.

756. **(E)** The biologically based practice is a branch of complementary and alternative medicine. It includes, but is not limited to, botanicals, animal-derived extracts, vitamins, minerals, fatty acids, amino acids, proteins, prebiotics and probiotics, whole diets, and functional foods.

757. **(E)** Naturopathy is a system originating from Europe. It considers that a disease is a manifestation of alterations in the processes by which the body naturally heals itself. It emphasizes health restoration as well as disease treatment. There are six principles that form the basis of naturopathic practice in North America: (1) the healing power of nature; (2) identification and treatment of the cause of disease; (3) the concept of "first do no harm"; (4) the doctor as teacher; (5) treatment of the whole person; and (6) prevention.

758. **(A)** Homeopathy is a complete system of medical theory and practice that is founded by the German physician Samuel Christian Hahnemann. He hypothesized that one can select therapies on the basis of how closely symptoms produced by a remedy match the symptoms of the patient's disease. He called this the "Principle of similar." Hahnemann proceeded to give repeated doses of many common remedies to healthy volunteers and carefully record the symptoms they produced. As a result of this experience, Hahnemann developed his treatments for sick patients by matching the symptoms produced by a drug to symptoms in sick patients.

759. **(A)** In the United States, glucosamine and chondroitin sulfate are considered dietary supplements and are not held to the stringent standards of pharmaceutical manufacture. Treatment effects were more substantial in the subgroup of patients with moderate to severe pain. Overall, glucosamine and chondroitin sulfate were not significantly better than placebo in reducing knee pain by only 20%. Adverse events were generally mild, but some serious adverse events were judged by the investigator to be related to

the study treatment: congestive heart failure (in a patient receiving combined treatment) and chest pain (in a patient receiving glucosamine).

760. **(E)** Recent evidence from randomized controlled trials, case reports, and systematic reviews of the literature suggest that the mechanism of mind-body therapy may rely on the brain and CNS influence immune, endocrine, and autonomic functioning, which is known to have an impact on health. Mind-body interventions can be effective in the treatment of coronary artery disease. In a study, mind-body intervention enhanced the effect of standard cardiac rehabilitation in reducing all-cause mortality and cardiac event recurrences for up to 2 years. This treatment modality has also been used to treat various types of pain. Clinical trials indicate that these interventions may be a particularly effective adjunct in the management of arthritis, with reductions in chronic pain for up to 4 years and reductions in the number of physician visits. When applied to more general acute and chronic pain management, headache, and low back pain, mind-body interventions show some evidence of effects, although results vary based on the patient population and type of intervention involved. In multiple studies with different types of cancer patients, it is suggested that mind-body interventions can improve mood, quality of life, and coping, as well as ameliorate disease- and treatment-related symptoms, such as cancer-related pain, nausea, or vomiting from chemotherapy. Other studies have shown that this behavioral therapy has effects of reducing discomfort and adverse effects during percutaneous vascular and renal procedures, reducing self-administration of analgesic drugs and improving hemodynamic stability in the perioperative period.

761. **(E)** *Echinacea* has been used to treat or prevent colds, flu, and other infections that are believed to stimulate the immune system to help fight infections. Less commonly, *Echinacea* has been used for wounds and skin problems, such as acne or boils. With recent evidence, it is indicated that *Echinacea* does not appear to prevent colds or other infections, shortens the course of colds or flu. For example, two studies did not

find any benefit from Echinacea, either as *Echinacea purpurea* fresh-pressed juice for treating colds in children, or as an unrefined mixture of *Echinacea angustifolia* root and *E purpurea* root and herb in adults. Other studies have shown that *Echinacea* may be beneficial in treating upper respiratory infections. When taken by mouth, *Echinacea* usually does not cause side effects other than mild GI side effects. However, some people have experienced allergic reactions, including rashes, worsening asthma, and life threatening anaphylaxis. People are more likely to experience allergic reactions to *Echinacea* if they are allergic to related plants in the daisy family, which includes ragweed, chrysanthemums, marigolds, and daisies. Also, people with asthma or atopy may be more likely to have an allergic reaction when taking *Echinacea*.

762. **(E)** Chiropractic focuses on the relationship between the body's structure, primarily of the spine, and its functions. The basic concepts of chiropractic can be summarized as follows: the body has a powerful self-healing ability; the body's structure, essentially the spine, and its function are closely related and this relationship affects health. Chiropractic therapy practices with the goals of normalizing the relationship between spine and its function, and assisting the body as it heals. Conditions commonly treated by chiropractors include neck pain, back pain, sports injuries, repetitive strains, and headaches. Patients with pain associated with other conditions, such as arthritis, also seek this treatment. In the United States, chiropractors perform more than 90% of manipulative treatments. With current data, the risk appears to be very low. The serious complication appears to be more associated with neck manipulation. Stroke has been reported with cervical spine manipulation and rarely, cauda equina syndrome with low back adjustment. Such risk was estimated to be one in one million treatments.

CHAPTER 10

Interdisciplinary Pain Management
Questions

DIRECTIONS (Questions 763 through 832): Each of the numbered items or incomplete statements in this section is followed by answers or by completions of the statement. Select the ONE lettered answer or completion that is BEST in each case.

763. The second most common cause of pain in the elderly is

    (A) musculoskeletal
    (B) cancer
    (C) temporal arteritis
    (D) postherpetic neuralgia
    (E) diabetic neuropathy

764. Pain assessment in the elderly is usually more difficult than in the young because it is often complicated by

    (A) good health status which may confuse the physician
    (B) poor memory
    (C) depression, which is only seen in cancer pain patients
    (D) most complains are psychiatric as opposed to organic
    (E) none of the above

765. Which of the following includes recommendations by the American Geriatric Society for pain patients?

    (A) Pain and its response to treatment do not necessarily need to be measured
    (B) Nonsteroidal anti-inflammatory drugs (NSAIDs) are contraindicated in older patients
    (C) Acetaminophen is the drug of choice for relieving mild to moderate pain

    (D) Nonopioid analgesic medications may be appropriate for some patients with neuropathic pain and other chronic pain syndromes
    (E) Nonpharmacologic approaches (eg, patient and caregiver education, cognitive-behavioral therapy, exercise) have no role in the management of geriatric pain

766. The functional pain scale has been standardized for the older population. Which of the following includes levels of assessment in this scale?

    (A) Rating pain as tolerable or intolerable
    (B) A functional component that adjusts the score depending on whether a person can respond verbally
    (C) A 0 to 5 scale that allows rapid comparison with previous pain levels
    (D) Only A and C are correct
    (E) A, B, and C are correct

767. Which of the following is a major concern regarding antiepileptic agents when used to treat neuropathic pain in the elderly patient?

    (A) Propensity to interfere with vitamin D metabolism
    (B) Need to use higher doses than those used in the young adult
    (C) May disrupt balance
    (D) Only A and C are correct
    (E) A, B, and C are correct

768. Which of the following is true regarding opioid use in the geriatric patient?

(A) Use of long-acting opioids may facilitate tolerance and lead to higher opioid dosage requirements for adequate pain control

(B) μ-Receptor antagonists are less desirable in the elderly

(C) Meperidine is an excellent choice alone or in combination with adjuvant medications for intractable pain

(D) Moderate to severe pain responds well to agonists-antagonists agents

(E) The transdermal route of fentanyl should be used as the first choice in the elderly, in order to increase compliance with the treatment

769. Which of the following is true about the elderly and pain?

(A) Incidence of chronic pain in the community-dwelling elderly is the same as in nursing home residents

(B) The prevalence of pain in patients older than 60 years of age is twice the incidence of those younger than 60 years of age

(C) The geriatric population in the United States consumes more than 50% of all prescription drugs

(D) The elderly often report pain differently from other patients because of decreased pain threshold

(E) None of the above

770. When referring to pharmacokinetics in the elderly, which of the following variables is altered in the elderly?

(A) Volume of distribution (Vd)
(B) Clearance of drugs (Cl)
(C) Elimination half-life ($t_{1/2}\,\beta$)
(D) Receptor binding affinity
(E) All of the above

771. Which of the following is true regarding pharmacodynamics in the elderly?

(A) Pharmacodynamic changes in the elderly are closely associated with age-related decline in central nervous system (CNS) function

(B) Decreased sensitivity to benzodiazepines

(C) Increased sensitivity to β-blockers

(D) Decreased sensitivity to opioids

(E) When compared to the young adult, there are no changes in pharmacodynamics in the elderly

772. Which of the following includes factors with clear associations contributing to poor compliance in the elderly?

(A) Race
(B) Religious beliefs
(C) Physician-patient communication
(D) Only A and C are correct
(E) A, B, and C are correct

773. An 82-year-old male suffers from low back pain caused by facet arthropathy. His pain has been well under control with weak opioids for several years. Over the last year pain has increased in severity and current pain medications, although still make him slightly drowsy, do not provide adequate pain relief. The next step in the management of this patient's pain should be

(A) switching to strong opioids
(B) diagnostic lumbar facet blocks
(C) radiofrequency lesions to the lumbar medial branches
(D) using a combination of two different weak opioids
(E) intrathecal opioids

774. Chronic use of NSAIDs in the geriatric patient should be accompanied by

(A) monitoring liver function test when appropriate
(B) monitoring renal function
(C) concomitant use of medications such as misoprostol or histamine-2 (H_2)-blockers
(D) occasional testing for occult blood in stool
(E) all of the above

775. When opioid therapy is first begun in the geriatric patient which of the following should be considered?

  (A) It is desirable to use drugs with short half-life ($t_{1/2}$)
  (B) Close monitoring of side effects should occur for the first three $t_{1/2}$ while a therapeutic blood level is obtained
  (C) Meperidine would be a better choice as an initial opioid than hydromorphone
  (D) Methadone is an excellent choice owing to its $t_{1/2}$
  (E) If pain control with minimal side effects has been established with a short-acting opioid, it is never recommended to switch to a controlled-release formulation of the opioid

776. Which of the following is an important goal for the elderly patient undergoing physical therapy for pain management?

  (A) Obtaining a gainful employment
  (B) Live a more independent life with enhanced dignity
  (C) Improve sleeping pattern
  (D) Gain back the physical skills they had as a young adult
  (E) None of the above

777. Prior to a chemical neurolysis to be performed in an 80-year-old male for trigeminal neuralgia, potential risks must be explained to the patient. Which of the following is a potential hazard?

  (A) Motor weakness
  (B) Neuritis
  (C) Deafferentation pain
  (D) Persistent pain at the site of injection
  (E) All of the above

778. Which of the following best describes the definition of recurrent abdominal pain in childhood and adolescence?

  (A) Abdominal pain resulting from gastrointestinal disease occurring on at least three occasions over a 3-month period
  (B) Abdominal pain resulting from gastrointestinal disease, gynecologic conditions, or congenital anomalies, occurring on at least three occasions over a 3-month period
  (C) Abdominal pain with no organic cause occurring on at least three occasions over a 3-month period that is severe enough to alter the child's normal activity
  (D) Abdominal pain with an organic cause, such as metabolic disease, neurologic disorders, hematologic disease, gastrointestinal disease, gynecologic condition, or other, that occurs at least in three occasions over a 3-month period
  (E) Acute abdominal pain from intestinal, renal, and gynecologic disorders, which can be treated surgically

779. Which of the following is true regarding migraine headaches in the pediatric population?

  (A) Incidence of migraine is higher in prepubertal children when compared to those who have reached puberty
  (B) In children with common migraine, there is unilateral localization of pain which is mostly preceded by an aura
  (C) Classic migraine usually present in children with an aura, followed by a bifrontal or bitemporal pain
  (D) Most children with common migraine present with abdominal pain
  (E) Ophthalmoplegic migraine is fairly common in children younger than 4 years of age, and is usually accompanied by miosis

780. Which of the following best describes chest pain during childhood?

(A) Cardiac involvement is extremely rare; an electrocardiogram (ECG) is indicated but mainly for reassurance of the parents, since it will be normal in most cases

(B) It is seen more often in children younger than 10 years of age

(C) It is more common than abdominal pain or headaches

(D) Costochondritis ranks second to cardiac involvement in being the most common cause of chest pain in this population

(E) Muscle strain is the most common cause of chest pain in children

781. Which of the following is false regarding sickle cell anemia in children?

(A) Pain occurs when and where there is occlusion of small blood vessels by sickled erythrocytes, usually small bones of the extremities in smaller children and abdomen, chest, long bones, and lower back in older children

(B) Tricyclic antidepressants are recommended for analgesia during the acute phase of a vasoocclusive crisis

(C) Use of opioids is indicated in patients with severe pain

(D) Painful crisis can be triggered by hypoxemia, cold, infection, and hypovolemia

(E) In children with excruciating pain that does not respond to nonnarcotic analgesics, and inadequate treatment of the painful crisis can lead to drug-seeking behavior and profound psychosocial problems

782. Which of the following is the best choice for management of the painful hemarthroses in children suffering from hemophilia?

(A) Aspirin
(B) Pentazocine
(C) Cortisone
(D) Ibuprofen
(E) Acetaminophen

783. Which of the following is false regarding complex regional pain syndrome type I (CRPS I) in children?

(A) The affected area is usually the upper limb as opposed to the lower limb in adults

(B) Physical therapy is withheld for cases that do not respond to oral medication and/or sympathetic blocks in the first place

(C) Multidisciplinary treatment combining transcutaneous electrical nerve stimulation (TENS), physical therapy, psychotherapy using behavior modification techniques, and oral medications is effective in most children

(D) Typical children with CRPS I or CRPS II show a profile of being intelligent, driven overachievers who are involved in very competitive activities and who often react to the loss of this activity with depression

(E) Sympathetic blocks are indicated to permit more vigorous physical therapy if pain prevents the start of these therapies

784. Which of the following is true regarding sport injuries in the pediatric patient?

(A) The injuries encountered are overuse injuries similar to those found in the adult recreational athlete who does not train correctly, usually doing too much in too short a time

(B) Growth is not an important factor in these injuries

(C) Growth spurts in children cause tendon and muscle tightness, both of which minimize the chances of a sport injury

(D) Treatment options such as oral acetaminophen, NSAIDs and aspirin do not provide adequate pain relief and should not be used in these cases

(E) Sport injuries are responsible for less than 10% of the cases of low back pain in children

785. Which of the following statements is false regarding pediatric cancer pain?

(A) Phantom sensations and phantom limb pain are common among children following amputation for cancer in an extremity

(B) Phantom pain in children tends to increase with time

(C) Some patients have chronic lower extremity pain caused by avascular necrosis of multiple joints

(D) An example of a neuropathic pain syndrome in pediatric cancer patients is postherpetic neuralgia

(E) Children with cancer pain often present with longstanding myofascial pain

786. Which of the following statements is false regarding interventional approaches for pediatric cancer pain management?

(A) In the pediatric cancer population, many children and parents are reluctant to consider procedures with the potential for irreversible loss of somatic function

(B) Dose requirements vary dramatically for spinal infusions in children, and they require individualized attention

(C) For pediatric spinal infusions, the process of converting from systemic to spinal drug is often quite unpredictable, with the potential for either oversedation or withdrawal symptoms

(D) As opposed to the adult population, celiac plexus blockade barely produces pain relief for children with severe pain caused by massively enlarged upper abdominal viscera owing to tumor

(E) In pediatric patients, it is recommended to place catheters while patients are under general anesthesia or deep sedation, not awake

787. In the immediate postoperative period, why are parenteral pain medications best given by continuous infusion rather than intermittent intravenous (IV)/intramuscular (IM) boluses?

(A) Opioid infusions do not cause nausea or vomiting

(B) Continuous infusions are associated with higher serum concentrations of the drug

(C) Opioid infusions are not associated with somnolence or respiratory depression, as opposed to intermittent opioid dosing

(D) No need of monitoring pediatric patients with continuous opioid infusions as opposed to constant monitoring in patients with intermittent boluses

(E) Boluses are associated with frequent periods of inadequate pain relief

788. Which of the following is an acceptable alternative for postoperative pain management in children when able to tolerate the oral route?

(A) Codeine
(B) Acetaminophen
(C) Methadone
(D) Immediate-release morphine
(E) All of the above

789. Which of the following is true regarding pediatric regional anesthesia?

(A) Epidural catheters placed in the thoracic or lumbar spine should not be left in place for more than 2 days because of concerns about infection, displacement, or discomfort

(B) Caudal epidural catheters are contraindicated for postoperative pain management in small children because of the high incidence of infection

(C) Spinal anesthesia has had limited indications in children and adolescents because of the incidence of postspinal headache in this age group

(D) In newborns and infants, spinal anesthesia provides anesthesia with a profound motor block for a prolonged period of time, making it a useful alternative for postoperative pain relief

(E) All of the above

790. In pediatric patients taking high doses of opioids, it is advised that an opioid contract should be signed by all parties involved. Which of the following should be included in this contract?

    (A) Use of multiple prescriptions for all pain-related medications

    (B) Use of as many pharmacies as possible

    (C) A statement specifying that there is no need for monitoring compliance of treatment since this does not apply to pediatric patients

    (D) Need for random urine or serum medication levels screening, regardless that the patient is a child

    (E) None of the above

791. Which of the following includes common misconceptions regarding pediatric pain?

    (A) It appears that adults are more likely to be believed than children when they complain of pain or discomfort

    (B) Neonates and young children do not display learned pain behavior and therefore do not express pain in an adult fashion

    (C) Silence is interpreted as a sign of being comfortable

    (D) Immobility without facial grimace or focus on the pain source is interpreted as absence of pain

    (E) All of the above

792. Differences between opioid abuse and opioid physical dependence include

    (A) physical dependence involves loss of control and compulsive use regardless of the adverse consequences

    (B) opioid abuse is characterized by presence of withdrawal symptoms during abstinence

    (C) physical dependence is a physiologic state characterized by the presence of withdrawal symptoms during abstinence

    (D) physical dependence and addiction are synonymous

    (E) patients presenting opioid abuse are not likely to develop addiction in the future

793. The term "whiplash injury" that results in chronic neck pain describes the resultant injury caused by an abrupt

    (A) hyperflexion of the neck from a direct force

    (B) hyperextension of the neck from an indirect force

    (C) hyperflexion of the neck from an indirect force

    (D) hyperextension of the neck from a direct force

    (E) rotation of the neck from a direct force

794. After sustaining a rear-end collision in a car accident, a 25-year-old male patient complains of neck pain. Which of the following are the cervical structures involved in this whiplash injury?

    (A) Sternocleidomastoid muscle

    (B) Longus colli muscle

    (C) Scalene muscles

    (D) Only A and C are correct

    (E) A, B, and C are correct

795. Which of the following is a prognostic indicator of chronic symptoms after sustaining a whiplash injury?

    (A) Use if a cervical collar for more than 12 weeks

    (B) Physical therapy restarted more than once

    (C) Numbness and pain in the upper extremity

    (D) Requirement of home traction

    (E) All of the above

796. A 32-year-old male sustained a blunt trauma to the left supraorbital area of his face. The patient manifests burning pain, occasional tingling, and intermittent stabbing. Which of the following is true about this patient's pain?

    (A) This is a self-limiting condition that generally resolves spontaneously within several years

    (B) With trophic changes, edema, and redness, CRPS I should be suspected

(C) Sympathetic blockade of the stellate ganglion may be effective

(D) Amitriptyline may reduce pain

(E) All of the above

797. Which of the following variables may improve significantly in a patient with multiple rib fractures and an epidural infusion of epidural bupivacaine?

(A) Vital capacity (VC)

(B) Hematocrit

(C) Expiratory reserve volume (ERV)

(D) Platelet aggregation

(E) Hemoglobin oxygen saturation

798. Flail chest because of multiple rib fractures may result in

(A) changes in oxygenation, but not in ventilation status

(B) mild pain that usually does not results in splinting or atelectasis

(C) increase in shunt fraction

(D) increase in ventilation and hypocarbia

(E) shunt, but no ventilation and perfusion mismatch

799. When sustaining trauma to the spine, which of the following statements regarding elements injured is correct?

(A) Disc injuries are common in the thoracic spine

(B) Vertebral end-plate fractures are common in the cervical spine

(C) Injury to the thoracic facets is more common than to the cervical facets

(D) Disc injuries are predominant in the cervical spine

(E) The posterior elements of the vertebral fractures are never involved

800. Which of the following is true regarding the management of pain in the traumatic injury pain patients?

(A) Obtaining hemodynamic stability is one of the main goals

(B) It is important to sustain sympathetic hyperactivity

(C) Uncontrolled pain may contribute to the development of posttraumatic stress disorder

(D) When pain is adequately treated, these patients will always present with impairment of consciousness

(E) None of the above

801. Techniques in the management of pain in patients with spinal cord injury (SCI) include

(A) opioid analgesics via IV patient-controlled analgesia (PCA)

(B) bedside placement of epidural catheters for continuous infusion

(C) bedside placement of intrathecal catheters for continuous infusion

(D) no need for oral adjuvant medications besides opioids

(E) all of the above

802. Which of the following is a good alternative for pain control in the patient with post–burn injury pain?

(A) Scheduled around-the-clock opioid boluses

(B) Continuous IV infusion of hydromorphone

(C) Transdermal fentanyl

(D) Intramuscular morphine given only as needed

(E) None of the above

803. In the patient with trauma injuries involving an extremity it is important to monitor for compartment syndrome. When using a regional technique for pain control, methods that may help monitoring compartment syndrome include

(A) use of epidural infusion containing local anesthetics at doses where motor block is present

(B) continuous plexus catheter using high concentration of local anesthetics to avoid incidental pain with movement

(C) continuous peripheral nerve catheter using low-dose local anesthetic

(D) continuous IV local anesthetic infusion

(E) all of the above

804. In the trauma patient with chest injury, epidural analgesia has been proven to provide excellent pain control and to

(A) avoid endotracheal intubation is some cases

(B) shorten the stay at the intensive care unit (ICU)

(C) decrease ventilator dependence

(D) shorten hospital stay

(E) all of the above

805. Types of pain commonly treated after major abdominal surgery for patients with a well-known history SCI are

(A) musculoskeletal pain

(B) visceral pain

(C) at-level neuropathic pain

(D) below-level neuropathic pain

(E) all of the above

806. Characteristics of below-level neuropathic pain in patients with SCI include

(A) spontaneous pain cephalad to the level of SCI

(B) not related to position or activity

(C) only present in patients with partial injuries to the spinal cord

(D) associated to sensation of dull ache

(E) intermittent, but never constant

807. Which of the following medications have proven to be useful in the treatment of neuropathic pain of patients with SCI?

(A) IV propofol infusion

(B) IV ketamine infusion

(C) Intrathecal clonidine

(D) Only A and C are correct

(E) A, B, and C are correct

808. Drug exposure prior to organogenesis (before the fourth menstrual week) usually results in

(A) an all-or-none effect; either the embryo does not survive, or it develops without abnormalities

(B) single-organ abnormalities

(C) multiple-organ abnormalities

(D) developmental syndromes

(E) intrauterine growth retardation

809. The US Food and Drug Administration (FDA) have developed a five-category labeling system for all approved drugs in the United States. Which if the following is not a category in the mentioned system?

(A) Category A: controlled human studies indicate no apparent risk to fetus. The possibility of harm to the fetus seems remote (eg, multivitamins)

(B) Category B: Animal studies do not indicate a fetal risk or animal studies do indicate a teratogenic risk, but well-controlled human studies have failed to demonstrate a risk (eg, acetaminophen, caffeine, fentanyl, hydrocodone)

(C) Category C: studies indicate teratogenic or embryocidal risk in animals, but no controlled studies have been done in women or there are no controlled studies in animals or humans (eg, aspirin, ketorolac, codeine, gabapentin)

(D) Category D: there is positive evidence of human fetal risk, but in certain circumstances, the benefits of the drug may outweigh the risks involved (eg, amitriptyline, imipramine, diazepam, phenobarbital, phenytoin)

(E) Category E: there is positive evidence of significant fetal risk, and the risk clearly outweighs any possible benefit (eg, ergotamine)

810. Acetaminophen falls in which of the following FDA labeling categories regarding risk of teratogenic or embryotoxic effects?

(A) Category A
(B) Category B
(C) Category C
(D) Category D
(E) Category X

811. During pregnancy, NSAIDs may

(A) accelerate the onset of labor
(B) increase amniotic fluid volume
(C) decrease the newborn's risk for pulmonary hypertension
(D) increase the risk of renal injury
(E) all of the above

812. Which of the following is true regarding use of opioids during pregnancy?

(A) Mixed agonist-antagonist opioid analgesic agents are superior to pure opioid agonists in providing analgesia
(B) Opioids are excreted into breast milk in negligible amounts
(C) Methadone is not compatible with breast-feeding
(D) Significant accumulation of normeperidine is unlikely in the parturient who receives single or infrequent doses
(E) All of the above

813. A 25-year-old primigravida just gave birth to a healthy baby boy. She had an epidural infusion containing lidocaine for labor analgesia. She asks you how long does she has to wait

after the infusion is turned off in order to be able to breast-feed her son. Your answer is

(A) she should wait at least 24 hours since concentration of lidocaine in breast milk may be toxic at this time
(B) it is safe to breast-feed her son since concentration of lidocaine is minimal in breast milk after an epidural infusion
(C) it would be safer to breast-feed if the infusion had bupivacaine, but since lidocaine was used, she will need to wait 36 hours
(D) mothers who had an epidural infusion for labor should not be allowed to breast-feed until 1 week postpartum
(E) none of the above

814. A 23-year-old female patient with chronic low back pain as a result of a motor vehicle accident becomes pregnant. For the past 4 years she has been taking diazepam for muscle spasms and to help her sleep at night. She asks for your advice in terms of continuing or quitting diazepam during her pregnancy. Your answer should be

(A) second-trimester exposure to benzodiazepines may be associated with an increased risk of congenital malformations
(B) diazepam's association with cleft lip, cleft palate, and congenital inguinal hernia has been disregarded recently
(C) neonates who are exposed to benzodiazepines in utero usually do not experience withdrawal symptoms after birth since the amount that crosses the placenta is negligible
(D) it appears most prudent to avoid any use of benzodiazepines during organogenesis, near the time of delivery, and during lactation
(E) all of the above

815.   A 28-year-old female with myofascial pain is taking tricyclic antidepressants for pain control with good results. She is planning to become pregnant in the next few months. Which of the following is true regarding use of tricyclic antidepressants during pregnancy?

(A)   Amitriptyline, nortriptyline, and imipramine are all safe to use since they are rated risk Category D by the FDA

(B)   Amitriptyline, nortriptyline, and desipramine are found in high quantities in breast milk, and are not safe to use while breast-feeding

(C)   The selective serotonin reuptake inhibitors (SSRIs) fluoxetine and paroxetine are rated FDA risk Category B. These are safe to administer while breast-feeding

(D)   Withdrawal syndromes have not been reported in neonates born to mothers using nortriptyline, imipramine, and desipramine

(E)   All of the above

816.   Which of the following is true regarding the use of anticonvulsants for neuropathic pain during pregnancy?

(A)   In general, the use of anticonvulsants during lactation does not seem to be harmful to infants

(B)   Frequent monitoring of serum anticonvulsant levels and folate supplementation should be initiated, and maternal α-fetoprotein screening may be considered to detect fetal neural tube defects

(C)   Pregnant women taking anticonvulsants for chronic pain have a lower risk of fetal malformations than patients taking the same medications for seizure control

(D)   Women who are taking anticonvulsants for neuropathic pain should strongly consider discontinuation during pregnancy, particularly during the first trimester

(E)   All of the above

817.   Caffeine is found in many over-the-counter pain medications. Pregnant women should be careful because

(A)   caffeine ingestion of more than 300 mg/d is associated with decreased birth weight

(B)   caffeine ingestion combined with tobacco use increases the risk for delivery of a low-birth-weight infant

(C)   caffeine ingestion is associated with an increased incidence of tachyarrhythmias in the newborn

(D)   moderate caffeine ingestion during lactation does not appear to affect the infant

(E)   all of the above

818.   A 23-year-old female at 24 weeks of gestation shows to the clinic with low back pain of sudden onset. She describes her pain as originating lateral to the left lumbosacral junction. The pain radiates to the posterior part of the left thigh and does not extend below the knee. Which of the following is the most likely diagnosis?

(A)   Transient osteoporosis of the hip
(B)   Sacroiliac joint pain
(C)   Osteonecrosis of the hip
(D)   Sciatica
(E)   None of the above

819.   Which of the following is not a main cause of low back pain during pregnancy?

(A)   Increased incidence of herniated nucleus pulposus during pregnancy

(B)   The lumbar lordosis becomes markedly accentuated during pregnancy

(C)   Endocrine changes during pregnancy soften the ligaments around the pelvic joints and cervix

(D)   Direct pressure of the fetus on the lumbosacral nerves may cause radicular symptoms

(E)   Sacroiliac joint dysfunction is common during pregnancy

820. Which of the following is a true statement regarding headaches during pregnancy?

   (A) In pregnant women with a history of migraines prior to pregnancy, more than 50% will report worsening of migraine headaches during this period

   (B) In women of childbearing age, their first migraine headache will usually occur during pregnancy

   (C) Pregnant patients presenting with "the worst headache of my live" should have an immediate rule out of subarachnoid hemorrhage

   (D) Preeclampsia usually does not presents with headaches

   (E) Initial presentation of headaches during pregnancy should not precipitate thorough search for potential pathology unless the headaches continue after labor and delivery

821. A 22-year-old female patient presents to the office with sudden onset of abdominal pain. She has a 10-week pregnancy history and no other symptoms upon questioning. Pain is localized to the lower portion of the abdomen. The differential diagnosis should not include

   (A) miscarriage
   (B) ovarian torsion
   (C) ectopic pregnancy
   (D) myofascial pain
   (E) sacroiliac joint pain

822. Which of the following opioids is considered to be compatible with breast-feeding by the American Academy of Pediatrics?

   (A) Codeine
   (B) Methadone
   (C) Fentanyl
   (D) Propoxyphene
   (E) All of the

823. In the critically ill patient, true statements regarding pain assessment include all of the following, EXCEPT

   (A) pain assessment tools such as the visual analogue scale or numeric rating scale (NRS) are most useful

   (B) in noncommunicative patients, assessment of behavioral and physiologic indicators is necessary

   (C) the NRS may be preferable because it is applicable to many age groups and does not require verbal responses

   (D) patient self-reporting is not useful for the assessment of pain and the adequacy of analgesia

   (E) the patient and family should be advised of the potential for pain and strategies to communicate pain

824. A 27-year-old male patient is at the ICU after sustaining multiple body traumas in a motor vehicle accident. The patient is on a mechanical ventilator with mild sedation. He has acute renal insufficiency and vital signs show mild to moderate hypotension. Upon evaluation it is determined that he has moderate to severe pain in both upper extremities and in the chest area as a result of multiple fractures. Which of the following would be the best medication to provide by an IV infusion for pain control?

   (A) Fentanyl
   (B) Morphine sulfate
   (C) Ketorolac
   (D) Demerol
   (E) Hydromorphone

825. In the critically ill patient, which of the following supports that epidural analgesia is a good alternative for pain control?

   (A) It results in more stable hemodynamics
   (B) There is reduced blood loss during surgery
   (C) Better suppression of surgical stress
   (D) Improved peripheral circulation
   (E) All of the above

826. In certain populations of patients, epidural analgesia has been associated with

(A) prolonged intubation time
(B) fewer ICU stays
(C) respiratory failure after surgery
(D) poor pain relief if initiated prior to the surgery
(E) none of the above

827. Which of the following is a reason for poor symptom management in critically ill patients with pain?

(A) The majority of pain scales do not require patient self-report
(B) For these patients it is easy to titrate sedatives and analgesics to their desired level of consciousness, but they are not encouraged to do so
(C) Physicians and other caregivers feel uncomfortable about giving high doses of sedatives, analgesics, and other mood-altering agents
(D) No need for pain medications as long as patient is sedated
(E) None of the above

828. Which of the following is a nonpharmacologic intervention for pain relief in an ICU patient?

(A) Provoking encephalopathy that results from the hypercapnia and hypoxia in chronic obstructive pulmonary disease (COPD) patients if tolerated
(B) Ketosis in terminally ill patients that forgo nutrition and hydration
(C) Placing patients in a quiet environment where family and friends may visit
(D) Proper treatment of anxiety and depression
(E) All of the above

829. Which of the following is a known fact about opioid infusions?

(A) Fentanyl is about 10 times more potent than morphine
(B) Hydromorphone is more sedating than morphine and produces more euphoria
(C) Release of histamine during morphine administration may cause vasodilation and hypotension
(D) Sedation, respiratory depression, constipation, urinary retention, and nausea are side effects that are only seen after administration of morphine, but not with the administration of fentanyl or hydromorphone
(E) All of the above

830. A 37-year-old female is at the ICU recovering after major abdominal surgery. Patient is breathing spontaneously, has stable vital signs, and is not able to tolerate oral feedings at this time. Alternatives for administration of opioids for pain relief include

(A) IV morphine PCA
(B) oral controlled-release oxycodone
(C) transdermal hydromorphone
(D) oral immediate-release oxycodone
(E) all of the above

831. A 33-year-old male underwent major abdominal surgery and is transferred to the ICU for postoperative management. Which of the following would be the best choice for postoperative pain management?

(A) IV hydromorphone PCA
(B) IV fentanyl infusion
(C) Controlled-release oxycodone via nasogastric tube
(D) Bupivacaine and fentanyl mix via epidural catheter
(E) None of the above

832. In order to prevent atelectasis and pulmonary complications in patients at the ICU

(A) pain management is important in maintaining a balance between splinting and sedation with hypoventilation

(B) it is important to titrate opioids to the lowest possible since respiratory depression is detrimental in these patients

(C) hyperventilation from mild to moderate pain is beneficial for faster recovery; opioids should not be administered during this period of time

(D) epidural analgesia has no role in preventing pulmonary complications and minimizing intubation time in these patients

(E) none of the above

Answers and Explanations

763. **(B)** Many other studies have verified that the predominant cause of pain in the elderly is, by far, musculoskeletal. The second most common source of pain is caused by cancer. Rheumatologic diseases are, therefore, important to the pain practitioner because these diseases are usually amenable to various treatment modalities. Other types of pain found commonly in the elderly include herpes zoster, postherpetic neuralgia, temporal arteritis, polymyalgia rheumatica, atherosclerotic and diabetic peripheral vascular disease, cervical spondylosis, trigeminal neuralgia, sympathetic dystrophies, and neuropathies from diabetes mellitus, alcohol abuse, and malnutrition.

764. **(B)** Pain assessment in the elderly is usually more difficult than in the young because it is often complicated by poor health, poor memory, psychosocial concerns, depression, denial, and distress. Caution in not attributing new pain complaints to preexisting disease processes is mandatory. Most pain complaints in the elderly are of organic, not psychiatric, origin. Nonetheless, concomitant depression is also usually present among the elderly with chronic, nonmalignant pain.

765. **(C)** Recommendations from the American Geriatric Society for the management of patients with pain are

1. Pain should be an important part of each assessment of older patients; along with efforts to alleviate the underlying cause, pain itself should be aggressively treated.

2. Pain and its response to treatment should be objectively measured, preferably by a validated pain scale.

3. NSAIDs should be used with caution. In older patients, NSAIDs have significant side effects and are the most common cause of adverse drug reactions.

4. Acetaminophen is the drug of choice for relieving mild to moderate musculoskeletal pain.

5. Opioid analgesic drugs are effective for relieving moderate to severe pain.

6. Nonopioid analgesic medications may be appropriate for some patients with neuropathic pain and other chronic pain syndromes.

7. Nonpharmacologic approaches (eg, patient and caregiver education, cognitive-behavioral therapy, exercise), used alone or in combination with appropriate pharmacologic strategies, should be an integral part of care plans in most cases.

8. Referral to a multidisciplinary pain-management center should be considered when pain-management efforts do not meet the patients' needs. Regulatory agencies should review existing policies to enhance access to effective opioid analgesic drugs for older patients in pain.

9. Pain-management education should be improved at all levels for all health care professionals.

766. **(E)** The functional pain scale, which has been standardized in an older population for reliability, validity, and responsiveness, has three levels of assessment: first, the patient rates the pain as tolerable or intolerable. Second, a functional component adjusts the score depending on whether a person can respond verbally. Finally, the 0 to 5 scale allows rapid comparison with prior pain levels. Ideally all patients should reach a 0 to 2 level.

767. (D) Antiepileptic medications are used to manage certain painful conditions, including trigeminal neuralgia. Gabapentin is indicated for postherpetic neuralgia and may be effective when administered initially at 100 mg orally one to three times per day and increased by 300 mg/d as needed. Clonazepam, phenytoin, and carbamazepine are other alternatives. The greatest concern with antiepileptic agents is their propensity to disrupt balance and to interfere with vitamin D metabolism.

768. (B)

A. Use of short-acting opioids (not long-acting opioids) may facilitate tolerance and lead to higher opioid dosage requirements for adequate pain control.

B. Opioids that are antagonistic to the μ-receptor are less desirable, given the high prevalence of unrecognized and untreated depression in seniors who can benefit from the euphoric component that occurs with binding to the μ-receptor.

C. Meperidine has been associated with a host of adverse events in seniors and should be avoided either alone or in combination with a product such as hydroxyzine, which is anticholinergic and can be associated with orthostatic hypotension and confusion.

D. There is no role for the geriatric patient for agonist-antagonists.

E. Transdermal fentanyl patch may be useful when oral medications cannot be administered and subcutaneous and intrathecal routes are too cumbersome. In the older patient, these patches should be carefully considered before using as a first-line agent because age-related changes in body temperature and subcutaneous fat may cause fluctuations in absorption.

769. (B)

A. Of the community-dwelling elderly, 25% to 50% suffer from chronic pain. Of nursing home residents, 45% to 80% have chronic pain.

B. The prevalence of pain is twofold higher in those older than 60 years (250 per 1000) compared with those younger than 60 years (125 per 1000).

C. Older Americans make up approximately 13% of the US population, yet consume 30% of all prescription drugs (including pain medications) and about 50% of all over-the-counter medications purchased.

D. The elderly often report pain very differently from the younger people suffering from pain and are more stoic, consequently underreporting their pain.

770. (E)

A. Vd is a function of drug protein binding and its lipid solubility. Vd is altered significantly in the elderly, in that the lipid content increases from 14% to 30%, with a decrease in the lean body mass between ages 25 and 75 years. As a result of the increased lipid content in older people, lipid-soluble drugs (opioids, benzodiazepines, barbiturates) can therefore have dramatically altered elimination $t_{1/2}$ in this patient population.

B. The clearance of drugs from the body (Cl) is the rate at which drugs are removed from the blood (ie, $mL/min/m^2$). This elimination of drugs usually occurs in the liver and kidneys, but lungs and other organs may also contribute. In general, most drugs undergo somewhat slower biotransformation and demonstrate prolonged clinical effects if they require hepatic or renal degradation.

C. Aging adversely affects the elimination $t_{1/2}$ of drugs.

D. Receptor-binding affinity is a pharmacodynamic variable.

771. (A) Pharmacodynamic principles describe the responsiveness of cell receptors at the effector site. In general, the elderly usually have increased sensitivity to centrally acting drugs (ie, benzodiazepines and opioids), whereas the adrenergic and cholinergic autonomic nervous systems generally have decreased sensitivity to receptor-specific drugs (ie, β-blockers).

Pharmacodynamic changes in the elderly are closely associated with age-related decline in CNS function.

772. **(D)** The rate of compliance with long-term medication regimens is approximately 50% across most age groups. Many reasons have been cited for this low rate, but the major factor predicting compliance is because of simply the total number of different medications taken; the more the medications, the worse the compliance. Other factors with clear associations contributing to poor compliance in the elderly include race, drug and dosage form, cost, insurance coverage, and physician-patient communication. Alternatively, inconsistent findings regarding compliance and the following factors have also been noted: age, sex, comorbidity, socioeconomic status, living arrangement, number of physician visits, and knowledge, attitudes, and beliefs about one's health.

773. **(B)** In the elderly, if weak opioids are not efficacious in attenuating pain intensity, an analysis of the risk to benefit ratio would recommend that therapeutic nerve blocks or low-risk neuroablative pain procedures should be employed prior to strong opioids. For example, a geriatric patient with severe lower back pain resulting from facet arthropathy might significantly benefit from a facet rhizotomy after a diagnostic nerve block with local anesthetic proves efficacious. In this case, the risk to benefit ratio is tilted toward minimally invasive pain procedures, as opposed to opioid therapy, since opioid therapy has the potential to impair both cognitive and functional status in addition to its many other known side effects.

774. **(E)** Chronic use of NSAIDs in the elderly must be accompanied by vigilance in monitoring for the various side effects. This vigilance includes determining (when appropriate) liver function tests, hematocrit, renal function, and occult blood in stool. Long-term use should probably also include use of misoprostol, which can reduce the incidence of NSAID-induced ulcers; empirical data suggest that other drugs (H_2-blockers, sucralfate, antacids, H^+ pump blockers) may have similar effects.

775. **(A)** When opioid therapy is first begun, it is desirable to use drugs with short $t_{1/2}$ so that a therapeutic blood level of drug can be reached relatively quickly. It is during this initial trial of opioids that close monitoring for side effects must occur, especially during the first six $t_{1/2}$ while a therapeutic blood level of drug is being obtained. Consequently, drugs such as hydromorphone and oxycodone, which have minimal active metabolites and relatively short $t_{1/2}$ (ie, 2-3 hours), are more desirable than drugs with variable $t_{1/2}$, such as methadone (ie, 12-190 hours) or meperidine with its accumulation of metabolites toxic to both the kidneys and the CNS.

776. **(B)** Rehabilitation is an important treatment modality for the older patient in pain. By decreasing pain and improving function, rehabilitation allows the patient to live a more independent life with enhanced dignity. This is in contrast to the rehabilitation goals of persons younger than 65 years of age in whom the primary emphasis is on obtaining gainful employment. Rehabilitation among chronic geriatric pain patients involves adapting, in an optimal way, to the loss of physical, psychologic, or social skills they once possessed prior to complaints of chronic pain.

777. **(E)** Prior to a chemical neurolysis, patients must have had successful pain relief after a diagnostic local anesthetic block and no intolerable side effects. They must also be fully informed of the risks, benefits, and options available to them prior to consenting for the procedure. Many medicolegal issues have resulted from this technique because of its complications. Most of these complications result from the spread of the neurolytic solution to the surrounding anatomic structures. Frequent side effects (depending on location) can include persistent pain at the site of injection, paresthesias, hyperesthesia, systemic hypotension, bowel and bladder dysfunction, motor weakness, deafferentation pain, and neuritis.

778. **(C)**

A. and B. The definition of recurrent abdominal pain in childhood excludes abdominal pain resulting from known medical conditions such as pain from neurologic disorders, metabolic disease (diabetes, porphyria, hyperparathyroidism), hematologic disease (sickle cell anemia), gastrointestinal disease, gynecologic conditions, chronic infection, and pain related to congenital anomalies

C. The definition of recurrent abdominal pain in childhood and adolescence is pain with no organic cause occurring on at least three occasions over a 3-month period that is severe enough to alter the child's normal activity.

D. and E. The definition of recurrent abdominal pain in childhood excludes abdominal pain resulting from known medical conditions such as pain from neurologic disorders, metabolic disease (diabetes, porphyria, hyperparathyroidism), hematologic disease (sickle cell anemia), gastrointestinal disease, gynecologic conditions, chronic infection, and pain related to congenital anomalies. It also excludes acute pain from acute renal, intestinal, and gynecologic disorders, which can be treated surgically.

779. (D)

A. The incidence of migraine is about 3% to 5% of prepubertal children. After puberty, the incidence of migraine increases notably, reaching 10% to 20% of children by age 20 years.

B. Common migraine is the type seen in children before puberty. Most recurrent childhood migraine is of this type. There is no aura before the headache and no unilateral focal localization of the pain. The pain is usually bifrontal or bitemporal.

C. Classic migraine is different from common migraine; the former starts with a visual aura in 30% of children affected and a sensory, sensorimotor aura, or speech impairment in 10%. These auras are followed by severe, throbbing, hemicranial, well-localized headache.

D. Migraine in children can be defined as recurrent headache accompanied by three of the following symptoms:

- Recurrent abdominal pain with or without nausea or vomiting
- Throbbing pain on one side of the cranium
- Relief of the pain by rest
- A visual, sensory, or motor aura
- A family history of migraine

About 70% of children with common migraine have abdominal pain.

E. Ophthalmoplegic migraine is rare in children before 4 to 5 years of age, usually affects only one eye, and is often accompanied by mydriasis.

780. (A)

A. Identification of the origin of the pain and reassurance of the patient and family are often the most important elements of treatment provided that specific organic causes have been investigated. Since cardiac involvement is what worries the child and family most, it should be stressed that this cause is extremely rare. An ECG will be normal and is indicated only to reassure the parents.

B. and C. Chest pain is relatively common in children. It ranks third in frequency after headache and abdominal pain and may be as common as limb pain. It is seen most often between 10 and 21 years of age.

D. Costochondritis is the most common cause of chest pain in children. It often occurs after an upper respiratory infection, can radiate to the back, and can last from a few days to several months. The pain can be reproduced by palpating the painful area or by mobilizing the arm or shoulder.

E. Costochondritis is the most common cause of chest pain in children. Trauma, muscle strain, chest wall syndrome, rib anomalies, and hyperventilation have been cited as other causes of the pain.

781. (B)

A. Sickle cell anemia is the most common hemoglobinopathy in the United States. It occurs in 0.3% to 1.3% of the African American population. Pain occurs during vasoocclusive crisis, the frequency of which is unpredictable and ranges from less than one crisis a year to a crisis several times a year or several times a month. Pain occurs when and where there is occlusion of small blood vessels by sickled erythrocytes, usually small bones of the extremities in smaller children and abdomen, chest, long bones, and lower back in older children.

B. Tricyclic antidepressants are not recommended for analgesia during the acute phase of a vasoocclusive crisis because they do not act quickly enough. They can, however, be useful for long-term use in patients who have frequent crises.

C. and E. Although the use of narcotics can lead to complications such as respiratory depression as well as complications from atelectasis and focal pulmonary hypoxia, this issue alone should not preclude the use of potent analgesics for patients in severe pain. On the contrary, these children can have excruciating pain that does not respond to nonnarcotic analgesics, and inadequate treatment of the painful crisis can lead to drug-seeking behavior and profound psychosocial problems.

D. The painful crisis can be triggered by hypoxemia, cold, infection, and hypovolemia and evolves in three phases:

1. The *prodromal phase* occurs up to 2 days before the actual sickle crisis with paresthesias, numbness, and an increase in circulating sickle cells.

2. The following phase or *initial phase* lasts 1 to 2 days and includes pain, anorexia, and fear and anxiety.

3. During the *established phase*, pain that lasts 3 to 7 days, inflammation, swelling, and leukocytosis are present.

782. **(E)**

A. Analgesic therapy is an important part of the management of hemophilia, although it is secondary to replacement therapy. Aspirin and drugs that inhibit platelet function should be avoided, but acetaminophen, codeine, hydromorphone, and methadone can be given orally.

B. Pentazocine is never indicated in patients with painful hemarthroses secondary to hemophilia because it causes dysphoria.

C. and D. Steroids and NSAIDs can be used to relieve pain from arthritis, but caution should be exercised when these drugs are used because they inhibit platelet activity.

E. Acetaminophen, codeine, hydromorphone, and methadone can be given orally for the treatment of painful hemarthroses in these patients.

783. **(B)**

A. CRPS I has been reported in children as young as 3 years. It is characterized by severe pain, often burning in quality, persisting much longer than would be expected after the initial injury. The affected area, more often an upper limb than a lower limb in children (most common areas are hand or wrist, elbow, shoulder, or hip), is intermittently swollen, mottled, and alternately red or cyanotic.

B. Physical therapy is probably the most important intervention and combines cautious manipulation of the affected limb, hot and cold therapy, whirlpool massages, and a program of intense active exercise.

C. Multidisciplinary treatment combining TENS, physical therapy, psychotherapy using behavior modification techniques, and oral medications is effective in most children. The TENS unit is worn for a few hours every day or for 1 to 2 hours before going out for some activity or to school. TENS brings some degree of pain relief to many patients and produces spectacular results in a few. Behavior modification is an important part of the treatment and should be instituted from the beginning of the therapeutic plan. Patients are taught relaxation techniques and are given relaxation tapes to use at home. An NSAID and an antidepressant at a low analgesic dose are often given, as is an anticonvulsant.

D. Sometimes a particular psychologic profile can be seen in children with CRPS I or CRPS II. The children are intelligent, driven overachievers who are involved (usually with success) in very competitive activities and who often react to the loss of this activity with depression. Other psychologic issues such as family discord or divorce and enmeshment with one parent are found. School attendance is often an issue.

E. In patients with CRPS, if pain or dysfunction prevents the start of physiotherapy or persists despite these treatments, sympathetic blocks such as lumbar, stellate ganglion, or epidural with dilute solutions of local anesthetics are indicated. The goals of the sympathetic blockade are to

1. Ascertain the sympathetic origin of the disorder.
2. Break the vicious circle of sympathetically maintained pain.
3. Permit more vigorous physical therapy.

784. (A)

A. The sports injuries encountered in children are overuse injuries similar to those found in the adult recreational athlete who does not train correctly, usually doing too much in too short a time. The causes of these injuries also include muscle-tendon imbalance, anatomical malalignment, inadequate footwear, and growth.

B. and C. Growth is an important factor in sports injuries for two reasons:

1. Growth cartilage is less resistant to injury than the adult-type cartilage.
2. Growth spurts in children cause tendon and muscle tightness, leading to pain and sometimes stress fracture. These fractures are most often seen in the tibia or the fibula.

D. Treatment consists of immobilization of fractures, straight leg strengthening exercises with use of leg braces in cases of knee injuries, rest, and use of orthotic footwear. NSAIDs and minor pain medicine, such as aspirin and acetaminophen, are useful when pain is present. These injuries usually respond well to these conservative measures but are best avoided through primary prevention, because it is recognized that

they are bound to happen in young children involved in sports.

E. Low back pain is rare in children and shares neither the etiology nor the poor prognosis with the adult form. Most cases of low back pain in children and adolescents are sports-related and occur during the growth spurt phase. A tendency for lordosis of the spine to develop appears at that time. With overuse, low back pain may develop.

785. (B)

A. and B. Phantom sensations and phantom limb pain are common among children following amputation for cancer in an extremity. Phantom pain in children tends to decrease with time. Preamputation pain in the diseased extremity may be a predictor for subsequent phantom pain.

C., D., and E. Long-term survivors of childhood cancer occasionally experience chronic pain. Neuropathic pains include peripheral neuralgias of the lower extremity, phantom limb pain, postherpetic neuralgia, and central pain after spinal cord tumor resection. Some patients have chronic lower extremity pain caused by a mechanical problem with an internal prosthesis or a failure of bony union or avascular necrosis of multiple joints. Others have long-standing myofascial pains and chronic abdominal pain of uncertain etiology. Some patients treated with shunts for brain tumors have recurrent headaches that appear unrelated to intracranial pressure or changes in shunt functioning.

786. (D)

A. and D. As with adults, celiac plexus blockade can provide excellent pain relief for children with severe pain caused by massively enlarged upper abdominal viscera owing to a tumor. Many children and parents are reluctant to consider procedures with the potential for irreversible loss of somatic function. Decompressive operations on the spine can in occasional cases produce dramatic relief of pain.

B., C., and E. Spinal infusions can provide excellent analgesia in refractory cases, but they require individualized attention and should not be undertaken by inexperienced practitioners without guidance. Dose requirements vary dramatically, and the process of converting from systemic to spinal drug is often quite unpredictable, with the potential for either oversedation or withdrawal symptoms. If children with spinal infusions are to be treated at home, it is essential to have resources available to manage new symptoms, such as terminal dyspnea and air hunger. In pediatric patients, it is recommended to place catheters while patients are under general anesthesia or deep sedation, not awake.

787. **(E)**

A., B., C., and D. The most common side effects found with narcotic administration are nausea or vomiting and pruritus. The former usually respond to perphenazine or prochlorperazine and the latter to diphenhydramine or promethazine. Because somnolence and respiratory depression can also occur, patients receiving infusions of narcotics require close attention, especially when the pain is so well-controlled that the pain stimulus of respiration is no longer present.

E. Drugs can be given as boluses or continuous infusions. Boluses are easy to administer and provide rapid pain relief; however, they have the disadvantage of providing short periods of analgesia sometimes associated with side effects when serum drug concentration peaks, followed by inadequate pain relief while the level decreases until the next injection. Continuous infusions, conversely, avoid this roller coaster of pain relief followed by pain and provide continuous analgesia with low plasma levels of drugs even in newborns and infants.

788. **(E)** Postoperatively, when the oral route can again be used, methadone can be prescribed at a dose one- to twofold that of the IV route. Oral morphine sulfate can also provide adequate

pain relief for moderate to severe pain. Codeine can be given orally alone or in combination with acetaminophen or aspirin for moderate pain; mild pain is relieved by acetaminophen alone in most cases. In any case, the most important aspect of postoperative pain control is to assess pain repeatedly with simple pain and behavior scales and to adapt pain medication to the pain scores provided by these scales and physiological findings.

789. **(C)**

A. and B. These catheters can be left in place for as long as a week or more without concerns about infection, displacement, or discomfort. An alternate approach to the epidural space is catheter placement via the caudal route, but its proximity to the anus raises concern about puncture site infection in the postoperative period, especially in small children.

C. and D. Spinal anesthesia has had limited indications in children and adolescents because of the incidence of postspinal headache in this age group. In newborns and infants, it provides anesthesia with a profound motor block for a short time (45-100 minutes) and thus cannot be used for postoperative pain relief. It is indicated in infants born prematurely and are less than 45 to 60 weeks' postconceptual age in whom general anesthesia and sedation have been shown to induce postoperative apnea.

790. **(D)** Opioid contracts are used in many adult practices, but their use is not common in pediatrics. The opioid contract clearly defines the expectations and responsibilities of the patient, parent, and medical caregiver. Guidelines from the Medical Society of Virginia's special Pain Management Subcommittee have been employed by many pain physicians throughout the United States.

Written documentation of both physician and patient responsibilities must include

1. Risks and complications associated with treatment using opioids
2. Use of a single prescriber for all pain-related medications

3. Use of a single pharmacy, if possible
4. Monitoring compliance of treatment
    a. Urine or serum medication levels screening (including checks for nonprescribed medications and substances) when requested
    b   Number and frequency of all prescription refills
    c. Reasons for which opioid therapy may be discontinued

791. **(E)** There are several distinctions between pediatric pain concerns and adult pain concerns. Misconceptions about a child's inability to feel pain persists. The belief that children "tolerate pain well" still prevails. Children continue to receive fewer analgesics than adults do in comparable settings.

Adults indirectly require that children prove their pain to merit the administration of pain interventions. If a child does not act as if he or she is experiencing severe pain, the child is less likely to receive analgesic care. It appears that adults are more likely than children to be believed when they complain of pain or discomfort. Studies show that for similar surgeries in adult and pediatric patients, the adults receive more doses of analgesic medications.

Neonates and young children do not display learned pain behavior and therefore do not express pain in an adult fashion. Adult caregivers often miss pain cues that are developmentally appropriate. Silence is interpreted as a sign of being comfortable. Similarly, immobility without facial grimace or focus on the pain source is interpreted as absence of pain. Yet, on direct questioning about the existence of pain, many children do affirm that they are experiencing pain. Children may lie quietly and enjoy television; however, they do not want to move because of fear of increased pain.

792. **(C)** The term "addiction" is familiar to medical and private sectors, but both factions often misuse the term as describing both physical and psychologic dependence. Addiction is a disease process involving the use of opioids wherein there is a loss of control, compulsive use, and continued use despite adverse social, physical,

psychologic, occupational, or economic consequences. *Physical dependence* is a physiological state of adaptation to a specific opioid characterized by the emergence of a withdrawal syndrome during abstinence, which may be relieved totally or in part by readministration of the substance. Physical dependence is predictable sequelae of regular, legitimate opioid or benzodiazepine use and is not identical to addiction. The incidence of addiction in children receiving prescribed opioids is low.

The present climate of drug-abuse prevention has, in part, emphasized the predatory nature of drug addiction and heightens fear in children and adults. More education is needed by lay people and health care professionals in distinguishing addiction from physical dependence. Patients who receive analgesics for a recognized pain complaint are not more likely to become addicted than the general population. The incidence of addiction in children receiving prescribed opioids is low.

793. **(B)** Neck injuries often are a result of motor vehicle accidents. Some studies have shown that up to 60% of patients injured in car accidents present to the hospital with neck pain. The term "whiplash" describes the resultant injury caused by an abrupt hyperextension of the neck from an indirect force.

794. **(E)** After a whiplash injury, symptoms may occur 12 to 24 hours later. This is because of the fact that muscular hemorrhage and edema may need to evolve prior to inciting a nociceptive response. The cervical flexors, specifically the sternocleidomastoid, scalene, and the longus colli undergo acute stretch reflex. Some fibers are torn.

795. **(E)** A substantial number of patients with whiplash have chronic symptoms. Prognostic indicators for chronic symptoms include numbness and pain in the upper extremity, use of a cervical collar for more than 12 weeks, requirement of home traction, physical therapy restarted more than once.

796. **(E)** Facial pain may occur after trauma. Examples include bullet wounds, maxillofacial surgery, and dental procedures. Some patients manifest constant burning pain, occasionally with tingling and intermittent stabbing. With trophic changes, edema, and redness, CRPS I should be suspected. In patients with burning pain, sympathetic blockade of the stellate ganglion may be effective. Amitriptyline may reduce pain.

797.   **(A)** Rib fracture pain may cause a decrease in ventilatory function and increase in incidence of pulmonary morbidity. It has been found that epidural analgesia is an independent predictor of decreased mortality and incidence of pulmonary complications. Significant improvements in VC and FEV_1 (forced expiratory volume) occur in patients with rib fractures who receive thoracic epidural bupivacaine compared with those that receive lumbar epidural morphine. There are no changes in hematocrit, oxygen saturation, platelet aggregation, or expiratory reserve volume.

798.   **(C)** Trauma to the chest is a significant cause of morbidity and mortality. The pathophysiologic sequelae of multiple rib fractures, especially with flail chest, are pain and hypoxia. Hypoxia results from the ventilation and perfusion mismatch in the underlying contused lung. Uncontrolled pain can result in splinting and muscle spasms, which lead to decreased ventilation and atelectasis. The compromise in pulmonary function causes hypoxemia, an increase in shunt fraction, or infection.

799.   **(D)** When comparing injuries in the thoracic and cervical spine areas after sustained trauma, it is observed that there are similar incidences of facet injuries in the upper thoracic spine and the cervical spine. By contrast, in the anterior elements, vertebral end-plate fracture and bone bruising are more common in the thoracic spine, whereas disc injuries predominate in the cervical spine. This raises the question whether interscapular pain is referred from the neck or arises locally. Investigations of pathology, to be correlated with the effect of local anesthetic blocks, should enable the clinician to distinguish the true pain source.

800.   **(C)** Hemodynamic stability, minimal impairment of the patient's level of consciousness and responsiveness, and adequate analgesia to reduce sympathetic hyperactivity and to allow patient rehabilitation efforts are the primary goals in the management of the patient with pain after traumatic injury. Uncontrolled pain following traumatic injury compounds the anxiety and posttraumatic sympathetic nervous system hyperactivity. Uncontrolled pain following traumatic injury has been associated with the development of posttraumatic stress disorder.

801.   **(A)** Patients with spine injury are usually managed with systemic analgesic techniques because of the risk of SCI or obscuring ongoing neurologic assessment with epidural analgesic techniques. Systemic opioid analgesic techniques, such as intravenous PCA, allow patient titration of analgesia and ongoing neurologic evaluation. Adjuvant analgesics, such as acetaminophen, may improve pain relief while reducing opioid requirements and opioid-related side effects. Intraoperative administration of epidural or intrathecal opioid analgesics with epidural catheter placement and maintenance of continuous postoperative epidural opioid analgesia is an excellent technique for postsurgical analgesia. The percutaneous exit site for the epidural catheter can be made some distance lateral to the surgical incision, minimizing the effects on wound healing or infection.

802.   **(B)** Post–burn injury pain has two primary components: a relatively constant background pain and an intermittent procedure-related pain. Continuous IV infusion of opioid analgesics is an effective method of managing the background pain component. Morphine and fentanyl have been extensively used in this setting although rapid escalation of opioid dose requirement and hemodynamic instability are not uncommonly seen. Hydromorphone is another alternative. A continuous IV titration paradigm for methadone has been described which produces effective and stable analgesia with minimal hemodynamic effects. Patients receive an IV loading dose by IV infusion of

methadone over an initial period of 2 hours at 0.1 mg/kg/h. The infusion is terminated prior to the end of the initial 2-hour period if the patient develops signs of excessive somnolence or respiratory depression. This initial loading dose infusion is followed by a maintenance infusion of 0.01 mg/kg/h of methadone. Transdermal preparations are not appropriate.

803. **(C)** Trauma patients with extremity injuries can be managed with a variety of techniques, including peripheral neural blockade, epidural analgesia, and systemic opioid analgesia. Adjuvant analgesics, such as acetaminophen and NSAIDs, are particularly effective in providing supplemental analgesia for orthopedic injuries, reducing opioid requirements and opioid-related side effects. Brachial plexus or peripheral neural blockade is effective for upper extremity injuries, whereas lumbar plexus or sciatic or femoral neural blockade techniques are effective for many lower extremity injuries. Continuous analgesia can be maintained with continuous plexus or peripheral nerve catheter techniques or continuous epidural analgesia. Monitoring for compartment syndrome may be necessary in some patients with extremity trauma, although low concentrations of local anesthetics (bupivacaine 0.125% or ropivacaine 0.2%) and opioids allow continued monitoring of compartment pressures and subjective changes in pain report in most patients. Intermittent interruption in continuous local anesthetic infusions may provide a greater margin of safety in patients at high risk for development of compartment syndrome.

804. **(E)** Effective analgesia is especially important in the postinjury rehabilitation of the patient with a chest injury such as rib fractures, flail chest, sternal fractures, or thoracostomy drainage tubes because of the risk of chest wall splinting and inadequate lung expansion and clearance of pulmonary secretions secondary to pain. Several studies have demonstrated a significant benefit in avoidance of endotracheal intubation, earlier postinjury extubation, decreased ventilator dependence, shorter stay in the ICU, shorter hospital stay, and improved postinjury rehabilitation with the use of continuous epidural analgesia with local anesthetic and opioid or intercostal neural blockade for pain management following chest injury.

805. **(E)**

A. Most patients who sustain an injury to the spinal cord have also received massive trauma to the vertebral column and its supporting structures, and will have acute nociceptive pain arising from damage to structures such as bones, ligaments, muscles, intervertebral discs, and facet joints. Some acute musculoskeletal pain is also related to structural spinal damage and instability without necessarily having spinal cord damage.

B. Pathology in visceral structures, such as urinary tract infections, bowel impaction, and renal calculi, will generally give rise to nociceptive pain, although the level of the injury will affect the quality of the pain. Therefore paraplegic patients may experience visceral pain that is identical to that in patients who have no spinal cord damage. However, tetraplegic patients may experience more vague generalized symptoms of unpleasantness that are difficult to interpret.

C. The diagnosis of neuropathic pain is largely based on descriptors (sharp, shooting, electric, burning, and stabbing), and the pain is located in a region of sensory disturbance. Neuropathic at-level pain refers to pain with these features, and present in a segmental or dermatomal pattern within two segments above or below the level of injury. This type of pain is also referred to as segmental, transitional zone, border zone, end zone, and girdle zone pain, names that reflect its characteristic location in the dermatomes close to the level of injury. It is often associated with allodynia or hyperesthesia of the affected dermatomes.

D. This type of pain, which is also referred to as central dysesthesia syndrome, central pain, phantom pain, or deafferentation pain, presents with spontaneous and/or evoked pain that is present often diffusely caudal to the level of SCI. It is characterized by sensations of burning, aching, stabbing, or electric shocks, often with hyperalgesia, and it often develops sometime after the initial injury. It is constant but may fluctuate with mood, activity, infections, or other factors, and is not related to position or activity. Sudden noises or jarring movements may trigger this type of pain. Differences in the nature of below-level neuropathic pain may be apparent between those with complete and incomplete lesions. Both complete and partial injuries may be associated with the diffuse, burning pain that appears to be associated with spinothalamic tract damage. However, incomplete injuries are more likely to have an allodynia component because of sparing of tracts conveying touch sensations.

806. (B)

807. (E)

A. IV administration of propofol, a $GABA_A$ receptor agonist, has been reported to be more effective than placebo in relieving neuropathic SCI pain.

B. The efficacy of IV ketamine infusion in the management of neuropathic SCI pain has been evaluated. IV infusion of ketamine (bolus 60 µg followed by 6 µg/kg/min) results in a significant reduction in the evoked and spontaneous neuropathic pains associated with SCI.

C. Clonidine administered spinally either alone or in combination with morphine may also be effective for the control of neuropathic SCI pain. Clonidine has been found to be more effective than morphine for pain relief in patients with SCI. Combinations of clonidine with other agents may also be effective.

808. (A) Drug exposure before organogenesis (before the fourth menstrual week) usually causes an all-or-none effect; either the embryo does not survive, or it develops without abnormalities. Drug effects later in pregnancy typically lead to single- or multiple-organ involvement, developmental syndromes, or intrauterine growth retardation.

809. (E)

A. The FDA has developed a five-category labeling system for all approved drugs in the United States. This labeling system rates the potential risk for teratogenic or embryotoxic effects, according to available scientific and clinical evidence. Category A: controlled human studies indicate no apparent risk to fetus. The possibility of harm to the fetus seems remote (eg, multivitamins).

B. Category B: animal studies do not indicate a fetal risk or animal studies do indicate a teratogenic risk, but well-controlled human studies have failed to demonstrate a risk (eg, acetaminophen, butorphanol, nalbuphine, caffeine, fentanyl, hydrocodone, methadone, meperidine, morphine, oxycodone, oxymorphone, ibuprofen, naproxen, indomethacin, metoprolol, paroxetine, fluoxetine, and prednisolone).

C. Category C: studies indicate teratogenic or embryocidal risk in animals, but no controlled studies have been done in women or there are no controlled studies in animals or humans. (eg, aspirin, ketorolac, codeine, propoxyphene, gabapentin, lidocaine, mexiletine, nifedipine, propranolol, sumatriptan).

D. Category D: there is positive evidence of human fetal risk, but in certain circumstances, the benefits of the drug may outweigh the risks involved (eg, amitriptyline, imipramine, diazepam, phenobarbital, phenytoin, valproic acid).

E. Category E is not part of the FDA labeling system. Category X is part of the FDA labeling system and includes drugs were there is positive evidence of significant fetal risk, and the risk clearly outweighs any possible benefit (eg, ergotamine).

810. (B)

A. The FDA has developed a five-category labeling system for all approved drugs in the United States. This labeling system rates the potential risk for teratogenic or embryotoxic effects, according to available scientific and clinical evidence. Category

A: Controlled human studies indicate no apparent risk to fetus. The possibility of harm to the fetus seems remote (eg, multivitamins).

B. Category B Animal studies do not indicate a fetal risk or animal studies do indicate a teratogenic risk, but well-controlled human studies have failed to demonstrate a risk. (eg, acetaminophen, butorphanol, nalbuphine, caffeine, fentanyl, hydrocodone, methadone, meperidine, morphine, oxycodone, oxymorphone, ibuprofen, naproxen, indomethacin, metoprolol, paroxetine, fluoxetine, prednisolone).

C. Category C: studies indicate teratogenic or embryocidal risk in animals, but no controlled studies have been done in women or there are no controlled studies in animals or humans. (eg, aspirin, ketorolac, codeine, propoxyphene, gabapentin, lidocaine, mexiletine, nifedipine, propranolol, sumatriptan).

D. Category D: there is positive evidence of human fetal risk, but in certain circumstances, the benefits of the drug may outweigh the risks involved. (eg, amitriptyline, imipramine, diazepam, phenobarbital, phenytoin, valproic acid).

E. Category X is part of the FDA labeling system and includes drugs were there is positive evidence of significant fetal risk, and the risk clearly outweighs any possible benefit. (eg, ergotamine).

811. (D)

A. Aspirin remains the prototypical NSAID and is the most thoroughly studied of this class of medications. Prostaglandins appear to trigger labor, and the aspirin-induced inhibition of prostaglandin synthesis may result in prolonged gestation and protracted labor.

B. and D. The use of ibuprofen during pregnancy may result in reversible oligohydramnios (reflecting diminished fetal urine output) and mild constriction of the fetal ductus arteriosus. Similarly, no data exist to support any association between naproxen administration and congenital defects. Because it shares the renal and vascular effects of ibuprofen, naproxen should be considered to have the potential to diminish ductus arteriosus diameter and to cause oligohydramnios.

C. Circulating prostaglandins modulate the patency of the fetal ductus arteriosus. NSAIDs have been used therapeutically in neonates with persistent fetal circulation to induce closure of the ductus arteriosus via inhibition of prostaglandin synthesis. Patency of the ductus arteriosus in utero is essential for normal fetal circulation. Indomethacin has shown promise for the treatment of premature labor, but its use has been linked to antenatal narrowing and closure of the fetal ductus arteriosus.

812. (D)

A. Although mixed agonist-antagonist opioid analgesic agents are widely used to provide analgesia during labor, they do not appear to offer any advantage when compared to pure opioid agonists. When compared, meperidine and nalbuphine provide comparable labor analgesia as well as similar neonatal Apgar and neurobehavioral scores. Use of either nalbuphine or pentazocine during pregnancy can lead to neonatal abstinence syndrome.

B. Opioids are excreted into breast milk. Pharmacokinetic analysis has demonstrated that breast milk concentrations of codeine and morphine are equal to or somewhat greater than maternal plasma concentrations. Meperidine use in breast-feeding mothers via PCA resulted in significantly greater neurobehavioral depression of the breast-feeding newborn than equianalgesic doses of morphine

C. Methadone levels in breast milk appear sufficient to prevent opioid withdrawal symptoms in the breast-fed infant. The American Academy of Pediatrics considers methadone doses of up to 20 mg/d to be compatible with breast-feeding. Recognition of infants at risk for neonatal abstinence syndrome and institution of appropriate supportive and medical therapy typically results in little short-term consequence to the infant. The long-term effects of in utero opioid exposure are unknown.

D. Meperidine undergoes extensive hepatic metabolism to normeperidine, which has a long elimination $t_{1/2}$ (18 hours). Repeated dosing can lead to accumulation, especially in patients with renal insufficiency. Normeperidine causes excitation of the CNS, manifested as tremors, myoclonus, and generalized seizures. Significant accumulation of normeperidine is unlikely in the parturient who receives single or infrequent doses; however, meperidine offers no advantages over other parenteral opioids.

813. **(B)** Few studies have focused on the potential teratogenicity of local anesthetic agents. Lidocaine and bupivacaine do not appear to pose significant developmental risk to the fetus. Only mepivacaine had a suggestion of teratogenicity in one study. However, the number of patient exposures was inadequate to draw conclusions. Animal studies have found that continuous exposure to lidocaine throughout pregnancy does not cause congenital anomalies but may decrease neonatal birth weight. Neither lidocaine nor bupivacaine appears in measurable quantities in the breast milk after epidural local anesthetic administration during labor. IV infusion of high doses (2-4 mg/min) of lidocaine for suppression of cardiac arrhythmias led to minimal levels in breast milk. Based on these observations, continuous epidural infusion of dilute local anesthetic solutions for postoperative analgesia should result in only small quantities of drug actually reaching the fetus. The American Academy of Pediatrics considers local anesthetics to be safe for use in the nursing mother.

814. **(D)**

A. and B. Benzodiazepines are among the most frequently prescribed of all drugs and are often used as anxiolytic agents, as an aid to sleep in patients with insomnia, and as skeletal muscle relaxants in patients with chronic pain. First-trimester exposure to benzodiazepines may be associated with an increased risk of congenital malformations.

Diazepam may be associated with cleft lip and cleft palate as well as congenital inguinal hernia. However, epidemiologic evidence has not confirmed the association of diazepam with cleft abnormalities; the incidence of cleft lip and palate remained stable after the introduction and widespread use of diazepam. Epidemiologic studies have confirmed the association of diazepam use during pregnancy with congenital inguinal hernia.

C. and D. Aside from the risks of teratogenesis, neonates who are exposed to benzodiazepines in utero may experience withdrawal symptoms immediately after birth. In the breast-feeding mother, diazepam and its metabolite desmethyldiazepam can be detected in infant serum for up to 10 days after a single maternal dose. This is caused by the slower metabolism in neonates than in adults. Clinically, infants who are nursing from mothers receiving diazepam may show sedation and poor feeding. It appears most prudent to avoid any use of benzodiazepines during organogenesis, near the time of delivery, and during lactation.

815. **(C)**

A. and C. Antidepressants are often employed in the management of migraine headaches as well as for analgesic and antidepressant purposes in chronic pain states. Amitriptyline, nortriptyline, and imipramine are all rated risk Category D by the FDA. The SSRIs, fluoxetine and paroxetine, are rated FDA risk Category B. Desipramine and all other conventional antidepressant medications are Category C.

B. Amitriptyline, nortriptyline, and desipramine are all excreted into human milk. Pharmacokinetic modeling suggests that infants are exposed to about 1% of the maternal dose. Amitriptyline, nortriptyline, desipramine, clomipramine, and sertraline were not found in quantifiable amounts in nurslings and that no adverse effects were reported.

D. Withdrawal syndromes have been reported in neonates born to mothers using nortriptyline, imipramine, and desipramine, with symptoms that include irritability, colic, tachypnea, and urinary retention.

816. (A)

A. The use of anticonvulsants during lactation does not seem to be harmful to infants. Phenytoin, carbamazepine, and valproic acid appear in small amounts in breast milk, but no adverse effects have been noted.

B. and D. For patients contemplating childbearing who are receiving anticonvulsants, their pharmacologic therapy should be critically evaluated. Women who are taking anticonvulsants for neuropathic pain should strongly consider discontinuation during pregnancy, particularly during the first trimester. Consultation with a perinatologist is recommended if continued use of anticonvulsants during pregnancy is being considered. Frequent monitoring of serum anticonvulsant levels and folate supplementation should be initiated, and maternal α-fetoprotein screening may be considered to detect fetal neural tube defects.

C. While anticonvulsants have teratogenic risk, epilepsy itself may be partially responsible for fetal malformations. Perhaps pregnant women taking anticonvulsants for chronic pain have a lower risk of fetal malformations than patients taking the same medications for seizure control.

817. (E)

A. and B. Early studies of caffeine ingestion during pregnancy suggested an increased risk of intrauterine growth retardation, fetal demise, and premature labor. However, these early studies did not control for concomitant alcohol and tobacco use. Subsequent work that controlled for these confounding factors found no added risks with moderate caffeine ingestion, although ingestion of more than 300 mg/d was associated with decreased birth weight. Caffeine ingestion combined with tobacco use increases the risk for delivery of a low-birth-weight infant.

C. Ingestion of modest doses of caffeine (100 mg/d) in caffeine-naïve subjects produces modest cardiovascular changes in both mother and fetus, including increased maternal heart rate and mean arterial pressure, increased peak aortic flow velocities, and decreased fetal heart rate. The modest decrease in fetal heart rate and increased frequency of fetal heart rate accelerations may confound the interpretation of fetal heart tracings. Caffeine ingestion is also associated with an increased incidence of tachyarrhythmias in the newborn, including supraventricular tachyarrhythmias, atrial flutter, and premature atrial contractions.

D. Many over-the-counter analgesic formulations contain caffeine (typically in amounts between 30 and 65 mg per dose), and one must consider the use of these preparations when determining total caffeine exposure. Moderate ingestion of caffeine during lactation does not appear to affect the infant. Breast milk usually contains less than 1% of the maternal dose of caffeine, with peak breast milk levels appearing 1 hour after maternal ingestion. Excessive caffeine use may cause increased wakefulness and irritability in the infant.

818. (B)

A. and C. Two relatively rare conditions—osteonecrosis and transient osteoporosis of the hip—both occur with somewhat greater frequency during pregnancy. Whereas the exact etiology is not known, high levels of estrogen and progesterone in the maternal circulation and increased interosseous pressure may contribute to the development of osteonecrosis. Transient osteoporosis of the hip is a rare disorder characterized by pain and limitation of motion of the hip and osteopenia of the femoral head. Both conditions present during the third trimester with hip pain that may be either sudden or gradual in onset.

Osteoporosis is easily identified by plain radiography, which demonstrates osteopenia of the femoral head with preservation of the joint space. Osteonecrosis is best evaluated with magnetic resonance imaging (MRI), which shows changes before they appear on plain radiographs.

B. and D. The hormonal changes that occur during pregnancy lead to widening and increased mobility of the sacroiliac synchondroses and the symphysis pubis as early as the 10th to 12th weeks of pregnancy. This type of pain is often described by pregnant women and is located in the posterior part of the pelvis distal and lateral to the lumbosacral junction. Many terms have been used in the literature to describe this type of pain, including "sacroiliac dysfunction," "pelvic girdle relaxation," and even "sacroiliac joint pain." The pain radiates to the posterior part of the thigh and may extend below the knee, often resulting in misinterpretation as sciatica. The pain is less specific than sciatica in distribution and does not extend to the ankle or foot.

819. (A)

A. and D. Although radicular symptoms often accompany low back pain during pregnancy, the incidence of herniated nucleus pulposus is only 1:10,000. The prevalence of lumbar intervertebral disk abnormalities is not increased in pregnant women. Direct pressure of the fetus on the lumbosacral nerves has been postulated as the cause of radicular symptoms.

B. Back pain occurs at some time in about 50% of pregnant women and is so common that it is often looked on as a normal part of pregnancy. The lumbar lordosis becomes markedly accentuated during pregnancy and may contribute to the development of low back pain.

C. Endocrine changes during pregnancy may also play a role in the development of back pain. Relaxin, a polypeptide secreted by the corpus luteum, softens the ligaments around the pelvic joints and cervix, allowing accommodation of the developing fetus and facilitating vaginal delivery. This laxity may cause pain by producing an exaggerated range of motion.

E. The hormonal changes that occur during pregnancy lead to widening and increased mobility of the sacroiliac synchondroses and the symphysis pubis as early as the 10th to 12th weeks of pregnancy.

820. (C)

A. Migraines occur more often during menstruation, because of decreased estrogen levels. During pregnancy, 70% of women report improvement or remission of migraines.

B. and E. Migraine headaches rarely begin during pregnancy. Headaches that initially present during pregnancy should initiate a thorough search for potentially serious causes. Examples may include strokes, pseudotumor cerebri, tumors, aneurysms, atrioventricular malformations, and others.

C. Patients presenting with their first severe headache should receive a complete neurologic examination, toxicology screen, serum coagulation profiles, and an MRI should be encouraged. In the patient who presents with "worst headache of my life," subarachnoid hemorrhage should be ruled out.

D. Progressively worsening of headaches in the setting of weight gain may be secondary to preeclampsia or pseudotumor cerebri. Preeclampsia has the triad of elevated blood pressure, proteinuria, and peripheral edema.

821. (E)

A., B., C., and D. One of the most common causes of abdominal pain early in pregnancy is miscarriage, presenting with abdominal pain and vaginal bleeding. Ectopic pregnancy and ovarian torsion may present with hypogastric pain and suprapubic tenderness. Once these conditions have been ruled out, myofascial causes of abdominal pain should be considered.

E. Sacroiliac joint pain or sacroiliac dysfunction usually does not presents with abdominal pain, but with low back pain that may radiate to the hip and thigh area.

822. (E) Opioids are excreted into breast milk. It has been shown that concentrations of morphine and codeine are equal to or greater than maternal plasma concentrations. The American Academy of Pediatrics considers use of many opioid analgesics including codeine, fentanyl, methadone, morphine, and propoxyphene to be compatible with breast-feeding.

823. (D) Perception of pain is influenced by prior experiences, expectations, and the cognitive capacity of the patient. The patient and family should be advised of the potential for pain and strategies to communicate pain. Patient self-reporting is the gold standard for the assessment of pain and the adequacy of analgesia. Pain assessment tools such as the visual analogue scale or numeric rating scale are most useful. The numeric rating scale may be preferable because it is applicable to many age groups and does not require verbal responses. In non-communicative patients, assessment of behavioral (movements, facial expressions, posturing) and physiologic (heart rate, blood pressure, respiratory rate) indicators is necessary.

824. (A)

A. Opioids are the mainstay of pain management in the ICU. Desired properties of an opiate include rapid onset of action, ease of titration, lack of accumulation of parent drug or active metabolites, and low cost. The most commonly prescribed opioids are fentanyl, morphine, and hydromorphone. Fentanyl has a rapid onset of action and short $t_{1/2}$ and generates no active metabolites. It is ideal for use in hemodynamically unstable patients or in combination with benzodiazepines for short procedures. Continuous infusion may result in prolonged effect owing to accumulation in lipid stores, and high dosing has been linked to muscle rigidity syndromes.

B., D., and E. Morphine has a slower onset of action (compared to fentanyl) and longer $t_{1/2}$. It may not be suitable for hemodynamically unstable patients because associated histamine release may lead to vasodilatation and hypotension. An active metabolite can accumulate in renal insufficiency. Morphine can also cause spasm of the sphincter of Oddi, which may discourage its use in patients with biliary disease. Hydromorphone has a $t_{1/2}$ similar to morphine but generates no active metabolites and no histamine release. All opioid analgesics are associated with varying degrees of respiratory depression, hypotension, and ileus.

C. Alternatives to opioids include acetaminophen and NSAIDs. Ketorolac is the only available intravenous NSAID. It is an effective analgesic agent used alone or in combination with an opioid. It is primarily eliminated by renal excretion, so it is relatively contraindicated in patients with renal insufficiency. Prolonged (> 5 days) use has been associated with bleeding complications.

825. (E) Many benefits of epidural anesthesia have been reported, including better suppression of surgical stress, more stable hemodynamics, better peripheral circulation, and reduced blood loss. A prospective, randomized study of 1021 abdominal surgery patients demonstrated that epidural opioid analgesia provides better postoperative pain relief compared with parenteral opioids. Furthermore, in patients undergoing abdominal aortic operations, overall morbidity and mortality were improved and intubation time and ICU length of stay were shorter.

826. (B) A large, multicenter, randomized investigation of epidural narcotics compared to parenteral narcotics performed in veterans affairs hospitals found that patients receiving epidural analgesia had better pain relief, shorter durations of intubation, and fewer ICU stays. In contrast, a multicenter trial in Australia that included both, men and women as well as very high-risk patients found that epidural analgesia had no effect on mortality or length of stay. Postoperative respiratory failure occurred significantly less frequently, however, in the patients receiving epidural analgesia. At a minimum, it appears that epidural analgesia can produce superior pain relief, particularly if it is initiated prior to the surgical incision, and it may be associated with fewer complications and a lower incidence of respiratory failure than parenteral narcotics in selected patients.

827. (C)

A. Pain and other symptoms also may be poorly managed because they are subjective experiences that are not easily assessed by objective methods. Pain and sedation scales have been developed to quantify the levels of pain and anxiety among patients who can self-report. Nevertheless, some patients cannot adequately communicate these sensations, either because they cannot find the words or because they are intubated and sedated. To detect pain in these patients, physicians and other caregivers must attend to patient grimacing and other admittedly nonspecific manifestations of pain, including tachycardia and hypertension.

B. Some patients value symptom relief highly and would prefer to be rendered unconscious rather than to experience pain, anxiety, or dyspnea, especially at the end of life. Others, however, would be willing to tolerate these symptoms or have them mitigated only slightly in order to stay awake. Dying patients may find it difficult to titrate sedatives and analgesics to their desired level of consciousness, although they should be encouraged to do so. Physicians and caregivers may find it even more difficult to achieve the ideal level of sedation and analgesia for patients who cannot communicate or administer drugs to themselves.

C., D., and E. Symptoms may be inadequately managed because physicians and other caregivers feel uncomfortable about giving high doses of sedatives, analgesics, and other mood-altering agents. In some instances, this discomfort stems from a reluctance to cause drug addiction in dying patients, a phenomenon irrelevant to the patients' condition.

828. (E) Pain can be managed indirectly by non-pharmacologic means. For example, placing patients in a quiet environment where friends and family can visit may diminish the sense of pain, as may the proper treatment of anxiety and depression. Although respiratory depression caused by drugs or underlying disease usually is undesirable in patients with COPD,

the encephalopathy that results from the hypercapnia and hypoxia may be tolerated, if not favored, in terminal patients because it attenuates pain. Similarly, patients who forgo nutrition and hydration at the end of life may develop a euphoria that has been attributed to the release of endogenous opioids or the analgesic effects of ketosis.

829. (C) A direct approach to pain control generally centers on the use of opioids, and morphine is the opioid most commonly used. In addition to causing analgesia, morphine induces some degree of sedation, respiratory depression, constipation, urinary retention, nausea, and euphoria. It also produces vasodilation, which may cause hypotension, in part through the release of histamine. Fentanyl, a synthetic opioid that is approximately 100 times more potent than morphine, does not release histamine and therefore causes less hypotension. Hydromorphone, a semisynthetic morphine derivative, is more sedating than morphine and produces little euphoria.

830. (A) Morphine, fentanyl, and hydromorphone can be administered orally, subcutaneously, rectally, or intravenously. Opioids usually are given by the IV route to ICU patients, including those who are dying. These agents may be administered to inpatients and outpatients alike through the technique of PCA. Long-acting oral preparations of morphine and hydromorphone are available for outpatients. Fentanyl can be administered orally in the form of a lollipop. It can also be given by the transcutaneous route, which makes this agent particularly suitable for patients who have difficulty with oral medications.

831. (D) Many benefits of epidural anesthesia have been reported, including better suppression of surgical stress, more stable hemodynamics, better peripheral circulation, and reduced blood loss. A prospective, randomized study of 1021 abdominal surgery patients demonstrated that epidural opioid analgesia provides better postoperative pain relief compared with parenteral opioids. Furthermore, in patients undergoing abdominal aortic operations, overall morbidity and mortality were improved and intubation time and ICU length of stay were shorter. (Park, WY, Thompson JS, Lee KK. Effect of epidural anesthesia and analgesia in perioperative outcome: a randomized, controlled Veterans Affairs Cooperative Trial. *Ann Surg* 2001; 234:560-571)

832. **(A)** Atelectasis is most often seen in postsurgical or immobilized patients. As alveoli collapse, there is increased shunting with resultant hypoxemia. Additional findings are related to the degree of atelectasis and include diminished breath sounds and reduced lung volume, elevated hemidiaphragm, or consolidation on chest radiography. Associated fever usually abates with reinflation, but the collapsed alveoli are prone to bacterial colonization with the development of pneumonia. Treatment is aimed at reexpansion of collapsed alveoli. Maintenance of airway patency and pulmonary toilet are of primary importance. Pain management is pivotal to balance splinting with sedation and hypoventilation. Pneumonia is common in the ICU, particularly among ventilated patients and those with direct lung injury. The clinical presentation involves fever, leukocytosis, hypoxia, a distinct radiographic infiltrate, and purulent sputum with bacterial colonization. Respiratory support, pulmonary toilet, and antibiotics are the fundamentals of treatment.

CHAPTER 11

Behavioral and Psychological Aspects of Pain
Questions

833. Primary affective symptoms that are present with chronic pain

    (A) generally resolve when the pain is treated adequately
    (B) require treatment independent of the pain
    (C) are rare among the elderly
    (D) are always reactive or secondary to the pain
    (E) require thorough assessment by a psychopharmacologist

834. Which of the following include risk factors for completed suicide?

    (A) Age
    (B) Substance abuse
    (C) History of prior suicide attempts
    (D) Chronic medical conditions
    (E) All of the above

835. Tricyclic antidepressants

    (A) have been shown to assist with reducing neuropathic pain
    (B) have been shown to assist with chronic headache
    (C) should be closely monitored in depressed patients because of suicide risk and possible lethality of an overdose
    (D) have been infrequently used in the treatment of major depression
    (E) A, B, and C

836. Substance abuse risk assessment

    (A) is required as a minimum standard of care with chronic pain
    (B) is poorly conducted by most physicians
    (C) can reduce medico-legal risk when chronic opioid therapy is being considered
    (D) can be improved by use of brief, standardized screening questionnaires
    (E) all of the above

837. Patient self-report data is

    (A) highly reliable when a spouse is present in the interview
    (B) always subject to bias
    (C) often unreliable with assessment of substance abuse, unless toxic screening is used
    (D) more reliable when an anxiety disorder is present
    (E) all of the above

838. Spouse "oversolicitous" behavior

(A) can be assessed with the Minnesota Multiphasic Personality Inventory-2 (MMPI-2)

(B) can contribute to poor treatment outcome

(C) controls most of the variance in predicting disability and substance abuse

(D) is generally a reflection of positive social support, and should be reinforced

(E) all of the above

839. Somatization disorder

(A) commonly develops in the elderly, as a result of poor communication with health care providers

(B) precludes the presence of an organic disease or disorder

(C) develops in adolescence, with symptoms disappearing by the age of 35 years

(D) implies the patient is intentionally "making up" symptoms

(E) complicates the pain physician's ability to evaluate effectiveness of the treatment

840. Anxiety symptoms are common among most patients with chronic conditions, and

(A) structured anxiety questionnaires can replace time-consuming interview questions, providing they have sufficient reliability and validity

(B) anxiety symptoms with acute pain often abate after adequate treatment of the pain

(C) posttraumatic stress disorder is common when a history of domestic abuse is present

(D) anxiety symptoms rarely abate after adequate treatment of pain

(E) both B and C

841. With a work related spine injury, pain and disability are most dependent upon

(A) the level of the disc herniation

(B) the employee's appraisal of his work setting

(C) the patient's level of depression

(D) the adequacy of the patient's pharmacotherapy regimen

(E) all of the above

842. In general, a successful return to work with back pain is more likely if

(A) the patient is placed on light duty

(B) the return to work is rapid, ideally within 12 months of the injury

(C) ergonomic job modifications are made at the work-site

(D) time-release versus short-acting analgesics are employed

(E) psychological job counseling is instituted shortly after the injury

843. Biofeedback assisted relaxation has been shown to be effective in reducing frequency, duration, and severity of pain with

(A) myofascial pain conditions and migraine

(B) cluster headache

(C) trigeminal neuralgia

(D) postherpetic neuralgia

(E) all of the above

844. In general, compliance rates or "adherence" with pharmacotherapy recommendations is

(A) 70% if a chronic medical condition is present

(B) dependent upon the severity of the chronic condition

(C) greater with elderly patients

(D) dependent on the patient's intelligence level

(E) improved when the pain clinician is "emphatic," and readily accepts the patient's report of pain severity

845. Factors suggestive of a possible problematic course with chronic opioid therapy include

(A) tobacco use

(B) history of inpatient detoxification

(C) a high score on a standardized chronic opioid therapy–screening instrument

(D) comorbid psychiatric diagnosis such as posttraumatic stress disorder

(E) all of the above

846. A diagnosis of posttraumatic stress disorder is

(A) uncommon among pain patients who have domestic violence histories

(B) a risk factor in the development of a treatment-resistant chronic pain disorder

(C) not predictive of poor adherence when treating chronic pain conditions

(D) present in 70% of motor vehicle accidents who report neck pain after the first 12 months

(E) generally resolved within the first few weeks of a major trauma, provided that the patient has adequate treatment of acute pain

847. Patient pain ratings

(A) should be documented by the clinician during each visit

(B) are not particularly reliable

(C) are poor predictors of disability

(D) should be supplemented by other measures when chronic pain is present

(E) all of the above

848. Commonly used quality of life measures include

(A) Beck Depression Inventory and CES-D depression screening questionnaire

(B) Short Form-36 (SF-36) and the Sickness Impact Profile (SIP)

(C) Brief Pain Inventory

(D) Headache Disability Index

(E) MMPI-2

849. Psychological screening for spinal column stimulation should

(A) weigh the patient's realistic and unrealistic expectations for outcome

(B) exclude patients with a major depression, given a probable poor prognosis

(C) underscore the patient's likelihood for improved work capacity after successful implantation

(D) address possible malingering by the use of standardized psychologic testing

(E) all of the above

850. There is a greater likelihood of improved function and return to work when

(A) passive rehabilitation approaches are paired with biobehavioral approaches

(B) interventional approaches are paired with cognitive therapies

(C) active rehabilitation approaches are combined with cognitive therapies

(D) complimentary medicine approaches are combined with cognitive therapies.

(E) opioid therapy is combined with a light duty return-to-work schedule.

851. In part, factors associated with the placebo effect include

(A) patient and clinician expectations

(B) past learning and conditioning

(C) neurotransmitter responses

(D) credibility of the treatment intervention

(E) all of the above

852. A patient with chronic daily headache and myofascial neck pain improves after a series of trigger point injections. The effect could be attributed to

(A) the treatment intervention

(B) the natural course of the illness or "regression to the mean"

(C) placebo effect associated with the injections

(D) other concurrent treatment changes that may have occured, for example, patient terminated a prophylactic treatment in anticipation of the injection series

(E) all of the above

853. Pain support groups and online support organizations

(A) may reinforce the patient's somatic overconcern and promote disability behavior

(B) provide a valuable resource of information with chronic pain conditions, and help to minimize distress and tendency to feel isolated

(C) may provide the pain patient with critical evaluations of his/her health care provider

(D) are not a replacement for psychologic or psychiatric treatments

(E) all of the above

854. Historically, the traditional operant-conditioning–pain-rehabilitation programs

(A) expected the patient to increase activity levels until pain became severe

(B) measured level of pain as an integral component of assessment

(C) regarded as-needed analgesic consumption as a "pain behavior"

(D) established objective functional and recreational goals after the pain was adequately controlled

(E) all of the above

855. The Minnesota Multiphasic Personality Inventory (MMPI-2)

(A) is a brief, "clinician-friendly," self-report questionnaire that does not require interpretation by a clinical psychologist

(B) has rarely been challenged with respect to its utility in chronic pain settings, with most pain psychologists accepting the MMPI-2 as the testing instrument of choice

(C) is a 566 item true/false self-report instrument used to assist with the assessment of overall psychopathology

(D) has limited utility in clinical settings, primarily because of the lack of chronic pain normative data

(E) can assess whether a patient is malingering with respect to report of pain level

856. Which of the following are commonly employed cognitive behavioral techniques with pain conditions?

(A) Cognitive restructuring, problem solving, and dialectical behavior therapy

(B) Progressive muscle relaxation, autogenic training, and psychoanalytic psychotherapy

(C) Contingency management, stimulus generalization, and operant conditioning

(D) Surface electromyographic (EMG) biofeedback, thermal biofeedback, and muscle reeducation

(E) All of the above

857. A patient returns to work despite a fear of reinjury, and remains in the work setting until the fear gradually subsides. From a learning theory standpoint, this is considered

(A) punishment

(B) in vivo exposure

(C) negative reinforcement

(D) intermittent reinforcement

(E) systematic desensitization

858. Hypnosis is often used to

(A) reduce acute pain and relax the patient

(B) improve adherence

(C) treat posttraumatic stress disorder

(D) treat cluster headache

(E) both A and D

859. A patient is being considered for an implantable opioid pump. Which of the following can be considered a reasonable outcome, based upon current evidence-based reviews?

(A) Reduced side effects from oral opioid therapy

(B) Return to work and increase in recreational activity

(C) Reduced pain and depression

(D) Improved aerobic capacity and reduced side effects from opioids

(E) None of the above

860. "Mind-body" and structured "stress-management" programs often employ

(A) short-term, time-limited treatment techniques

(B) monitoring of stressors and precipitants of pain

(C) cognitive therapy to reduce perception of pain and control over all symptoms

(D) relaxation training

(E) all of the above

861. Cognitive behavioral treatments with pain in children might typically include all of the following EXCEPT

(A) enlisting parents to assess mediating stressors and reinforce positive coping skills

(B) structured play therapy

(C) relaxation training with possible adjunctive use of biofeedback

(D) rehearsal of positive cognitions

(E) efforts to return the child to school in order to minimize school phobia and disability behavior

862. Functional sleep disorders are common with chronic pain conditions, with as many as 80% of pain patients reporting problems with sleep. Behavioral approaches have consistently been shown to be superior to pharmacotherapy approaches. Which of the following is included in a behavioral approach to functional sleep disorder?

(A) Instruction in proper sleep hygiene and use of stimulus-control techniques

(B) Relaxation training and cognitive interventions

(C) Self-monitoring of sleep, with particular focus on sleep habits and anxiety symptoms

(D) Addressing common precipitants of poor sleep such as depression, inappropriate use of pharmacologic sleep aids, and/or substance use

(E) All of the above

863. Temporomandibular disorders have been most effectively treated by a combination of

(A) interventional and biobehavioral techniques

(B) biobehavioral and oral/dental/occlusal appliance therapy

(C) physical therapy and biobehavioral techniques

(D) low-dose chronic opioid therapy and thermal biofeedback

(E) none of the above

864. A patient presents with symptoms of chronic hand-arm pain, possibly neuropathic in origin, as well as a diagnosis of fibromyalgia with associated disability and depression. Which of the following is best treatment for this patient?

(A) Referral to cognitive therapy

(B) Multidisciplinary treatment, where behavioral interventions are integrated into the patient's care

(C) Interventional treatments, where appropriate, while concurrently referring the patient to a psychologist with a specialty in pain management

(D) Pharmacotherapy as a first-line treatment, with appropriate psychologic screening for risk factors if opioids are considered

(E) Treatment modalities that directly address the patient's presenting diagnosis, for example, a diagnosis of complex regional pain syndrome may require interventional procedures and/or neurostimulation, referral for behavioral treatment, and eventual referral to physical therapy

865. Addiction can co-occur with chronic pain disorders. If chronic pain and an addictive disorder co-occur, the patient

(A) can be effectively managed when the clinician primarily relies on interventional treatments

(B) requires referral for comanagement by an addiction specialist

(C) may show a decrease in addictive behavior, as many patients engage in addictive behavior because of inadequate treatment of pain

(D) requires an inpatient detoxification from the addictive substances prior to pain treatment

(E) should never be treated with chronic opioid therapy

866. In population-based studies, women suffering from pain

(A) typically do not report more severe and frequent pain than men

(B) may be at greater risk for specific pain disorders, for example, fibromyalgia, temporomandibular disorders, and migraine

(C) have been shown to be at greater risk because of endogenous and exogenous sex hormone changes

(D) may be subject to multiple psychosocial and cultural influences that impact on report of pain

(E) B, C, and D

867. A person's degree of belief that he/she can successfully manage aspects of their pain, including their pain level, is termed

(A) catastrophizing
(B) self-esteem
(C) cognitive coping skill
(D) self-efficacy
(E) locus of control

868. The construct of operant conditioning would apply to the following patient vignette:

(A) A worker has an acute back injury while lifting an object at work, experiences immediate pain and associated anxiety, and thereafter develops an unrealistic fear of any future lifting behavior

(B) A patient uses a short-acting opioid after an exacerbation of pain. He learns to take his pill when his pain reaches a certain level. His pill-taking behavior is initially reinforced by the effect of the analgesic or other nonspecific factors that contributed to his pain reduction

(C) A patient in physical therapy engages in her exercise "until I can't stand the pain," then discontinues the exercise, seeks bedrest, and rapidly feels better. She learns that escaping from physical therapy and lying down reduces her pain, and continues this behavior

(D) A patient becomes markedly anxious during the preparation for an interventional procedure, and the procedure is terminated prematurely owing to her anxiety. Upon returning to the pain clinic, the patient leaves the procedure room as her anxiety escalates. She has become phobic of interventional procedures

(E) Both B and C

869. There is empirical evidence to support

(A) the construct of a "pain prone personality"
(B) the concept that chronic pain is "masked depression"
(C) malingering as being rare, less than 1% with work injury-related chronic pain conditions
(D) the assumption that psychologic trauma may increase the likelihood of developing a treatment-resistant chronic pain disorder
(E) all of the above

870. A patient arrives at the pain center with persistent facial pain, secondary to a fall 6 months earlier. She has a history of other pain complaints, and reports that she follows with a counselor for "stress." When evaluating the

patient, the diagnostic interview content should include psychosocial questions that address

(A) depression and suicidal ideation

(B) substance use

(C) risk of domestic violence

(D) all of the above

(E) none of the above, while the patient should grant permission to the pain physician to speak with her counselor

871. Patients with cognitive impairments and pain

(A) may require administration of specific assessment tools relevant for their impairment, as standard pain assessment may be inadequate

(B) may be at risk for undertreatment of pain because of communication difficulties with the pain clinician

(C) are at higher risk for accidental injury

(D) do not necessarily have an intellectual disability

(E) all of the above

872. Adjunctive psychologic treatments for cancer pain might include

(A) cognitive therapies to improve patient's control over the medical treatment sequence

(B) autogenic relaxation training

(C) hypnosis

(D) brief family therapy

(E) all of the above

Answers and Explanations

833. **(B)** Reviews clearly suggest that affective symptoms require treatment independent of the patient's pain, either through pharmacotherapy, behavioral therapies, or both. Depression is common in chronic pain populations, with rates that exceed 50% within some populations. Unfortunately, physician adherence with respect to depression screening is poor. Risk of suicide can be significant with an untreated depression, and the elderly often fail to undergo adequate assessment. While consultation by a psychopharmacologist is desirable, many primary care physicians and other subspecialists elect to pharmacologically manage depression.

834. **(E)** While the ability to predict suicide is poor even among mental-health clinicians, the above illustrate commonly accepted risk facts. The presence of past suicide attempts is another predictor. The elderly, males, and those with chronic medical conditions are at great risk for suicide completion.

835. **(E)** While commonly used in pain practice, dosing of tricyclic antidepressants is rarely sufficient to cover comorbid major affective symptoms. Other commonly used antidepressant agents or proper dosing should be considered when significant affective symptoms are present, with close monitoring given the risk factors associated with an overdose.

836. **(E)** Substance abuse risk screening is generally considered required in all standard initial medical assessments, while physician adherence is poor. Serious substance abuse history and current substance abuse predicts to poor outcome with a range of medical treatments. Chronic pain patients may be at high risk for substance use disorders, and medico-legal risks may be present for physicians who fail to conduct adequate screening and refer the patient for treatment.

837. **(B)** The field has an inherent handicap because of the subjective nature of pain. Bias is always present with self-report, and reliability of pain ratings is poor. Presence of a significant other can greatly assist with validation of patient self-report, while the bias remains. Substance abuse assessment is necessary, self-report remains the only practical strategy, and toxic screening does not necessarily improve the veracity of the patient's report. Comorbid psychologic symptoms further compromise self-report. While assessment of pain level is necessary, additional assessment of other outcome variables remains important, that is, functional activities, return to work, medication adherence.

838. **(B)** The construct "oversolicitiousness" has been studied since the mid 1980s with the work of Andrew Block. The oversolicitious spouse is considered overly attentive to pain and disability behavior, potentially influencing the patient's report of pain and reinforcing pain behaviors. Several standardized assessment instruments address degree of spouse oversolicitiousness, such as the Multidimensional Pain Inventory. Therapy programs can incorporate treatments designed to modify spouse behavior and thereby improve the patient's treatment outcome, while other factors may control more of the variance with respect to overall pain level, disability, or other comorbid psychiatric symptoms.

839. **(E)** A diagnosis of somatization disorder is often missed in subspecialty practices. While the patient may present with a discrete pain complaint, comprehensive assessment and adequate record review may reveal a history of multiple somatic symptoms. The *Diagnostic and Statistical Manual of Mental Disorders* (Fourth Edition, Text Revision) (*DSM-IV-TR*) outlines criteria that include onset prior to age 30 years, and multiple unexplained symptoms persist with varying severity over many years. Patients are not "malingering" or feigning symptoms with this diagnosis. Comorbid disorders such as posttraumatic stress disorder and history of emotional trauma may be present. Patients may undergo questionable interventional or surgical procedures, and develop secondary iatrogenic problems. Other comorbid medical diagnoses may be missed, and ongoing assessment is compromised as a result of the patients impaired self-report. Patient resistance to psychologic intervention is great and outcomes for those who agree to treatment are generally poor. Coordinated management of the somatization disorder patient through primary care often is the mainstay, while pain specialists may assist with close communication among providers.

840. **(E)** Anxiety symptoms are common with all chronic pain and many acute pain conditions, while few pain patients meet psychiatric diagnostic criteria for an anxiety disorder, for example, posttraumatic stress disorder. In many cases, anxiety symptoms may abate when proper pain treatment occurs, either in acute or chronic pain. Some conditions do predict to a high likelihood of anxiety disorder, such as history of domestic abuse. Anxiety may persist in other chronic pain conditions and combined behavioral and pharmacologic treatments are often required. While many pain questionnaires address anxiety symptoms, screening questionnaires do not absolve the clinician from conducting an adequate interview assessment.

841. **(B)** While there are multiple factors associated with pain and disability and individual differences must be addressed, most investigations point toward the patient's appraisal of the work setting as a major factor influencing pain and disability, regardless of injury severity. Psychosocial factors associated with coping within a difficult work environment may be moderating factor. Investigators have not suggested malingering or feigning of pain as an explanation of these results.

842. **(B)** Timing appears to be a major factor with respect to successful return to work, with a rapid drop off in success after the 12-month mark. Despite widespread use, "light duty" strategies have shown mixed results, and greater success has been shown where no restrictions were proposed. The role of pharmacotherapy and return to work hasn't been adequately studied. While there may be a role for early psychologic counseling in some cases, data with respect to effect of counseling within this narrow time period are limited. Similarly, ergonomic modifications have shown limited effect, particularly in cases where chronic pain is present. When a patient's condition becomes more chronic, highly structured functional restoration rehabilitation approaches have shown the most promise with respect to return to work.

843. **(A)** EMG and thermal biofeedback involve the surface monitoring of physiological responses, with ongoing graphic visual or audio feedback to the patient. Relaxation training or cognitive techniques are employed to master control over the physiologic response, and additional practice techniques assist the patient to generalize the relaxation response to other settings. Studies suggest that adjunctive use of the biofeedback equipment offers benefit to some patients, and may be more effective with particular pain conditions. Positive outcomes have been demonstrated with migraine and various pain conditions considered as myofascial. Results with cluster headache are less promising, as are results with other specific neuropathic pain conditions. Nonetheless, a positive general relaxation effect has been shown with multiple pain conditions.

844. **(B)** Poor adherence is common with any chronic medical condition and worse when comorbid psychiatric disorders are presence. Adherence is defined as the extent to which the patient's behavior coincides with medical recommendations.

The term "compliance" has fallen in disfavor, as the term "adherence" assumes a more nonjudgmental assessment of the patient's behavior. Adherence is unrelated to age, sex, race, or intelligence. Notwithstanding extensive research on improving adherence, effects of various interventions have been modest with respect to changing difficult patient behavior. Within the field of pain medicine, particular attention has been pain to adherence when chronic opioid therapy is considered. Screening for risk factors and urine toxicology combined with structured treatment may result in improved adherence, while studies are still lacking. Adherence may be improved by simplified dosing schedules, increased frequency of office visits, reinforcing the importance of adherence when counseling the patient, and enlisting family members in the treatment plan. Where a language or cultural barrier is present, adherence may improve by enlisting skilled interpreters and clinicians who have an in-depth understanding of the particular cultural issues.

845. (E) Screening for chronic opioid therapy has received increasing attention, as risk factors have received closer scrutiny and outcomes have been poor with some patients. Among others, all of the above choices have been predictors of poor outcome. Several screening questionnaires have been developed with adequate reliability and validity, and these may assist the clinician in formulating an effective treatment plan. Examples include the SOAPP (Screener and Opioid Assessment for Patients with Pain) and DIRE (Diagnosis, Intractability, Risk and Efficacy Score) rating scale. Tobacco use, history of detoxification, and various comorbid psychiatric diagnoses may predict to a problematic course. Many State Medical Board Model Pain Policies suggest that special attention be paid to these at-risk patients when chronic opioid therapy is considered.

846. (B) Posttraumatic stress disorder (DSM-IV-TR) is classified as an anxiety disorder and often co-occurs with other psychiatric disorders. Posttraumatic stress disorder has been considered a risk factor with respect to development of treatment resistant chronic pain disorders. Patients may have frequent or recurrent periods of hyperarousal, and chronic symptoms may suggest a problematic course for pain treatment. While present in few motor vehicle accident victims after 1 year, other trauma precipitants such as early physical/sexual abuse or extensive domestic violence often result in chronic symptoms and a more complicated treatment course. Comanagement with a mental-health specialist is always recommended.

847. (E) Despite issues of reliability and the subjective nature of pain ratings, pain clinicians are required to record the patient's self-report, that is, the "fifth vital sign." Reliability is improved with increased frequency of ratings, and special populations may require a modification and/or improved description of the rating scale. Clinical relevance of ratings with chronic pain may be less than acute pain, as multiple problem areas are often present. Other adjunct assessments could include standardized measures for quality of life. The pain clinician can also supplement pain ratings through documentation of other objective indicators, for example, the patient may state that "I can now walk 20 minutes...I returned to work...I'm using medication as prescribed now...."

848. (B) While the other symptom-specific instruments are commonly used in pain, clinic settings, the SF-36 and SIP illustrate an example standardized instruments that are becoming increasingly important in health care settings as efforts are made to evaluate overall outcome.

849. (A) There do appear to be predictors of a problematic course with spinal column stimulation, while these tend to be the same predictors that suggest poor outcome with most pain treatments. Nonetheless, predictive validity studies have been few. Screening by a psychologist may help to better delineate possible predictors, and formal screening is often required by third party carriers. Realistic patient expectations may be particularly important with neurostimulation procedures. For example, spinal column stimulation may offer the patient pain relief, while structured rehabilitation approaches tend to show better outcome when goals such as return to work or improved function are targeted.

Patients with particular psychiatric conditions do not necessarily have a poor outcome if their symptoms can be readily treated, for example, major depression. Conversely, a diagnosis of somatization disorder or substance use disorder may predict a more difficult course of treatment. In some cases, problem areas can be identified and treated prior to embarking on neurostimulation, and outcome may be better.

850. **(C)** "Passive" rehabilitation approaches are considered to be less effective than "active" interventions when function or return to work are considered. Active approaches involving quota-based exercise may help the patient to reduce fear of pain and activity. Passive approaches sometimes rely on the patient being less involved, and may depend upon the clinician to provide the relief. Many active approaches have been coupled with cognitive therapies, resulting in a greater effect. Fewer definitive studies have addressed results of return to work with interventional procedures, opioid treatments, or complimentary therapies. While most investigations have been conducted with chronic back and neck populations, fibromyalgia and other conditions tend to show better functional improvement with more active versus passive rehabilitation approaches.

851. **(E)** Research on the placebo and nocebo effect is well-established in the pain field. A placebo effect can be as high as 100%, depending upon multiple variables. It's generally acknowledged that interventional treatments may have greater placebo effect than oral medications, and surgical approaches potentially have the greatest effect. While "noise" associated with reference to the placebo effect if often addressed in clinical trials, efforts to understand and "harness" the role placebo in clinical care has received growing attention. Investigations have revealed that clinicians tend to overestimate the impact of their treatments and underestimate the power of placebo or other nonspecific factors.

852. **(E)** Determining outcome based upon any particular treatment remains difficult with chronic pain conditions, and the effect on nonspecific or other treatment variables always must be considered.

853. **(E)** Studies of support organizations and volunteering suggest that these approaches may be a valuable resource for the pain patient, while the pain physician should use caution with respect to referral. Some organizations such as the American Chronic Pain Association provide admirable support and information, while fringe advocacy groups may increase the patient's distress and divert the patient from the most appropriate treatments.

854. **(C)** One of the first and most well known operant pain rehabilitation programs for chronic noncancer pain was established in Seattle Washington in the late 1970s under the guidance of Drs Wilbert Fordyce and John Loesser. On an intensive inpatient basis, patients were taught to increase function despite pain, recreational and other "well behaviors" were socially reinforced, and "pain behaviors" were ignored. Examples of pain behaviors included grimacing, pill consumption, or complaints of pain. Objective program goals were established prior to starting treatment. Functional outcomes were positive, and programs with varying levels of operant focus were developed throughout the country. Economic pressure forced programs to convert to outpatient services, and operant oriented "functional restoration programs" thrived into the late 1980s. Additional economic pressures ensued and most programs closed. Currently, there appears to be a resurgence of programs with this focus, given continued perceived need.

855. **(C)** The MMPI-2 has been widely administered in pain clinic settings as a general measure of psychopathology, while its use has declined over the last 15 years. Results provide an overall measure of psychopathology, while some clinicians with extensive training in the MMPI-2 argue that specific psychologic deficits can be ascertained from the results. The focus on psychopathology, its length (500+ items), and training requirements for interpretation have resulted in a reduction in its use. Other psychologic tests specifically developed for chronic pain have seen increasing use, while a long history of predictive validity studies suggests that the MMPI-2 will likely continue to be used in pain clinic settings.

856. **(A)** Cognitive therapies include the use of specific techniques targeted toward the patient's perception of pain or disability. Maladaptive thought patterns are altered or "restructured." Dialectical behavior therapy offers a similar, highly structured approach aimed at systematically modifying thoughts, often directed at disordered cognitions present with chronic depression or posttraumatic stress disorder. While most behavioral specialists agree that relaxation training, biofeedback, and operant strategies (contingency management, stimulus generalization, operant conditioning) have a large cognitive therapy component, these treatments generally are considered separate from standard cognitive approaches.

857. **(B)** In vivo exposure requires the patient to remain in the feared setting until the anxiety subsides. If the patient leaves at the height of the anxiety (or during the most severe pain), the patient may increase the severity of the phobia. Studies support a rapid return to work for work-injured patients in an effort to provide them with an in vivo exposure and reduce fear of activity. However, it's important that the patient have a "success," and remain in the work setting until the anxiety subsides. Ideally, the patient discovers that engaging in work tasks does not result in a reinjury. The worker may have intermittent exacerbations of pain, but also learns that pain subsides and does not result in greater physical "harm." The construct of punishment reduces behavior, while negative reinforcement increases behavior, for example, the patient terminates the aversive work setting by leaving. Systematic desensitization is a treatment method that generally requires to a graded exposure using guided imagery within a therapy setting. Work-simulation or work-hardening programs employ a similar principle by gradually reducing the patient's fear of work activity or increased pain. After achieving some level of relaxation and confidence, the clinician then introduces the patient to the in vivo work setting.

858. **(A)** Hypnotic analgesia has a long history as an adjunctive treatment for pain, with formal procedures for hypnosis dating back several hundred years. Some argue that the effects are similar to other standardized relaxation procedures, and self-hypnosis resembles many relaxation techniques. Positive effects have been shown with acute and chronic pain conditions. Studies addressing patient adherence suggest a role for multiple complex variables, and hypnosis has not been proposed as an important intervention for adherence. Other behavioral and pharmacologic strategies have shown much greater effect with conditions such as posttraumatic stress disorder or cluster headache.

859. **(A)** While implantable pumps have demonstrated effect with respect to reduced pain and reduced side effects from oral opioid therapy, objective gains with respect to improved function or change in emotional status are lacking. Psychologic techniques have been successfully employed to better prepare patients for implantable devices, most notably specific cognitive techniques.

860. **(E)** Mind-body and structured stress-management groups have been integrated into overall patient care, with promising results. These techniques may buttress rather than replace individual therapeutic approaches, especially in cases where chronic disability and more significant comorbid psychiatric disorders are present.

861. **(B)** Cognitive behavioral treatments for children with acute and chronic pain are typically short in duration and goal oriented. Pain and pain-related distress may be targeted, and functional activities may be reinforced. Involvement of the family or school can optimize outcome. While traditional play therapy approaches are common in child-treatment settings, the structure and short-term nature of cognitive therapy interventions would unlikely include this approach.

862. **(E)** Sleep disorders are exceedingly common among patients with chronic pain conditions, with prescription and over-the-counter sleep aids often providing limited benefit. Recent investigations have suggested that myofascial pain complaints may be precipitated or worsened by poor sleep, and disrupted sleep is well established as a precipitant of migraine headache.

863. **(B)** Defining temporomandibular disorders remain a problem, as with many chronic pain conditions. However, the role of myofascial factors is generally accepted, and recommendations from evidence-based reviews have consistently supported a role for cognitive and relaxation approaches. Dentists with an orofacial pain subspecialty also often manage these patients, and studies have shown the best effect with combined therapies. Opioid therapy, physical therapy, and various interventional procedures have been less well-studied with chronic temporomandibular disorders.

864. **(B)** When disability and depression are present with multiple chronic pain conditions, the minimum standard of care requires a multidisciplinary effort. Sequential efforts that start with pharmacotherapy or interventional treatments may extend the patient's period of disability and distress, and cross-discipline multidisciplinary coordination remains the standard of care. However, access to some specialty care may limit the pain physician's options, as psychological or rehabilitation services may be denied by an insurance carrier. Nonetheless, the data continue to support a multidisciplinary approach from the onset of the patient's care.

865. **(B)** The AAPM (American Academy of Pain Medicine)/APS (American Pain Society)/ASAM (American Society of Addiction Medicine) joint statement states that "addiction is a primary, chronic, neurobiological disease, with genetic, psychosocial, and environmental factors influencing its development and manifestations. It is characterized by behaviors that include one or more of the following: impaired control over drug use, compulsive use, continued use despite harm, and craving." The IASP (International Association for the Study of Pain) Core Curriculum further asserts that "adequate pain treatment will be difficult or may fail without concurrent treatment of addiction." Given the complexity of addictive disorders, comanagement is necessary. In many cases, addictive behavior can be managed on an outpatient basis. Opioid therapy is not an absolute contraindication in cases where the patient displays additive behavior, while care should be taken by close comanagement of the patient by other relevant specialists.

866. **(E)** Sex differences with respect to pain are well established, and recent animal studies appear to buttress these results. Women may report more frequent and severe pain than men, and hormonal factors, in part, may play a role. Psychosocial differences also appear to play a role. Conversely, women also have shown a more robust treatment effect than men with rehabilitation and multidisciplinary interventions.

867. **(D)** While all of the above constructs are addressed in cognitive treatment, self-efficacy is the defined construct. Self-efficacy is often associated with the early work of Albert Bandura, and researchers in the pain field have developed relevant assessment instruments. Self-efficacy is addressed clinically when the patient is trained to internalize the belief that he/she is capable and has the skills to managing exacerbations in pain, coordinating his/her medical care, or improve on some specific functional task.

868. **(E)** While all of the answer choices could include components of operant and classical (respondent) conditioning, choices (B) and (C) address the issue of reinforcement. In contrast, "classical" conditioning involves the pairing of a neutral (lifting, preparation for a procedure) with an immediate noxious (pain, anxiety) stimulus or pleasant stimulus. Often after one or repeated trials, reintroducing the "neutral" stimulus (a nerve block, a lifting episode) produces the unwanted response, that is, anxiety as outlined in a cases above. With respect to operant conditioning, a behavior is reinforced and thereby increases in frequency.

869. **(D)** The construct of a "pain prone personality" has largely been discredited, as has the construct of pain as a "masked depression." However, multiple psychosocial factors appear to be predictors of developing chronic pain disorders, while they are not necessarily causes. Rates of malingering, or consciously lying about disability and pain, appear to vary. Pain physicians are poor at assessing malingering, while most investigations agree that rates are higher in any circumstances where active adversarial/litigation is present. It is most important to note that malingering can occur when a legitimate medical or psychiatric condition is also present.

870. **(D)** The involvement of a mental-health specialist in the patient's care does not absolve the pain clinician of covering standard psychosocial interview questions within the assessment interview. State regulations also may require that the clinician address risk factors associated with domestic violence, and the above case would appear to suggest the presence of this risk. The pain clinician also must be aware or have access to resources for appropriate referral in cases where patients may be at risk.

871. **(E)** There are a range of conditions that require special attention by the pain clinician, for example, patients with dementia, head injuries, stroke, memory disorders, or developmental disabilities. These disorders can influence the patient's social and psychologic presentation, and their ability to communicate level of pain and impairment. Comanagement of similar patients with subspecialists in neurology, neuropsychology, occupational therapy, and related disciplines may maximize positive outcome.

872. **(E)** While acute and cancer pain conditions may require a modification of techniques, behavior-management strategies are often integrated into multidisciplinary treatment team management.

CHAPTER 12

Drug Abuse and Addiction
Questions

DIRECTIONS (Questions 873 through 883): Each of the numbered items or incomplete statements in this section is followed by answers or by completions of the statement. Select the ONE lettered answer or completion that is BEST in each case.

873. In performing urine drug testing (UDT), a physician must know all of the following, EXCEPT

   (A) the characteristics of the testing procedures, since many drugs are not routinely detected by all UDTs

   (B) that although no aberrant behavior is pathognomonic of abuse or addiction, such behavior should never be ignored

   (C) reliance on aberrant behavior to trigger a UDT will miss more than 50% of those individuals using unprescribed or illicit drugs

   (D) always prescribe "on-demand" for the patient until you are comfortable with the situation

   (E) a history of drug abuse does not preclude treatment with a controlled substance, when indicated, but does require a treatment plan with firmly defined boundaries

874. A 65-year-old man with cancer and multiple bony metastases complains of increasing requirement of intrathecal morphine. However, he also complains of increased nausea associated with the increased dose. All the workup with regards to carcinomatous spread failed to show any progression of the disease. Which of the following explanations is accurate?

   (A) The catheter is no longer in the intrathecal space and he is not receiving appropriate dosages

   (B) He is addicted to the drugs and requesting higher doses

   (C) He is physically dependent on the drug and is nauseated because of withdrawal symptoms

   (D) He has developed tolerance to the analgesics effects of intrathecal morphine

   (E) There is significant progression of the disease, which was unidentified by the evaluation

875. Which of the following is true regarding quality assurance?

   (A) Quality assurance, quality improvement, and quality management are interchangeable words

   (B) Quality assurance is internally driven, follows patient care, and has no end-points

   (C) Quality improvement is externally driven, focused on individuals, and works toward end points

   (D) Total quality of management, quality management and improvement, and continuous quality improvement are synonymous with quality assurance

   (E) A quality improvement program is different from quality assurance and focuses on patient care, process, and integrated analysis

876. Which of the following is true with typical detection times for urine testing of common drugs of abuse?

(A) Methadone, 2 to 4 days
(B) Chronic use of marijuana, 1 to 3 days
(C) Morphine, 15 days
(D) Cocaine, 15 days
(E) Benzodiazepines, 15 days

877. What is the mode of action for cocaine in the central nervous system?

(A) Increasing the reuptake of norepinephrine
(B) Blocking dopamine receptors
(C) Activating γ-aminobutyric acid (GABA) receptors
(D) Mediating its effect through dopamine cells in the ventral tegmentum
(E) Inhibiting acetylcholine esterase in the central nervous system

878. Which is the accurate statement on federal regulations?

(A) They are promulgated by the US Congress, CMS, and Office of Inspector General (OIG)
(B) They are promulgated by the Department of Justice (DOJ), Federal Bureau of Investigation (FBI), and OIG
(C) Courts may not promulgate any regulations, as it is the duty of the US Congress and Administration
(D) They are enforced by the US Congress
(E) They are enforced by local Medicare carriers

879. A 38-year-old white male with history of low back pain with radiation into the lower extremity with disc herniation demonstrated at L4-5 with nerve root compression, and electromyographic evidence of L5 radiculopathy was referred for consultation. You have examined the patient and decided to perform transforaminal epidural steroid injection at the L5 nerve root. This encounter is appropriately considered as follows:

(A) It is a consultation as the patient was referred by another physician for management
(B) It is a consultation as the patient was referred and your opinion was requested
(C) It is a new office visit since it is a known problem and the patient was referred to you for the treatment
(D) It is a consultation as you told the patient to return to the referring physician after completion of course of epidurals
(E) It is a consultation, as you do not plan on billing for another consultation within the next 3 years

880. Which of the following is schedule I substance?

(A) Buprenorphine
(B) Hydromorphone
(C) Heroin
(D) Cocaine
(E) Morphine

881. All of the following are accurate statements with managing opioid-dependent pregnant patients experiencing withdrawal symptoms when the drug is discontinued, EXCEPT

(A) methadone frequently is used to treat acute withdrawal from opioids
(B) current federal regulations restrict the use of methadone for the treatment of opioid addiction to specially registered clinics
(C) methadone may be used by a physician in a private practice for temporary maintenance or detoxification when an addicted patient is admitted to the hospital for an illness other than opioid addiction
(D) methadone may never be used by a private practitioner in an outpatient setting when administered daily
(E) methadone may be used by a private practitioner in an outpatient setting when administered daily for a maximum of 3 days

882. Your friend's daughter whom you have known for several years makes an appointment with you. During the visit, she tells you that she is a heroin addict and requests a prescription for hydrocodone. Your options in this situation are as follows:

(A) Immediately call her father and give hydrocodone

(B) Immediately tell father and give her methadone

(C) Start rapid detoxification in your office

(D) Provide her with a prescription for methadone maintenance

(E) Do not tell the father and do not give hydrocodone

883. Which of the following is true regarding opioid-induced constipation?

(A) Treat constipation

(B) Obtain a surgical consult to rule out complication

(C) Evaluate for drug abuse

(D) Start on transdermal fentanyl

(E) Start on methadone-maintenance program

DIRECTIONS: For Question 884 through 900, ONE or MORE of the numbered options is correct. Choose answer

(A) if only answer 1, 2, and 3 are correct

(B) if only 1 and 3 are correct

(C) if only 2 and 4 are correct

(D) if only 4 is correct

(E) if all are correct

884. What are the risks of malprescribing?

(1) Legal charges, probably jail time

(2) Conviction rate is currently almost 30%

(3) Felony conviction will likely prevent or at least severely limit future practice

(4) Duped and dated are highly viable defenses

885. Which of the following is (are) an accurate statement(s) with regards to function of Controlled Substances Act?

(1) It creates a closed system of distribution for those authorized to handle controlled substances

(2) The cornerstone of this system is the licensure of all those authorized by the State Medical Licensure Board to handle controlled substances

(3) Only the individuals and practices which dispense directly to the patients from their clinics are required to maintain a DEA license

(4) It requires maintaining complete inventory of controlled substances, only if the drugs are administered by physician, but not if dispensed to the patient

886. What are the pitfalls of opioid UDT?

(1) Tests for opiates are very responsive for morphine and codeine

(2) UDTs do not distinguish between morphine and codeine

(3) UDTs show a low sensitivity for semi-synthetic/synthetic opioids such as oxycodone

(4) A negative response excludes oxycodone and methadone use

887. What are the pitfalls of prescription practices?

(1) The four D's—deficient, duped, deliberate, dependent practitioner

(2) Never say "NO"—family, friends, patients

(3) Ignore complaints

(4) Focus on positive aspects of regulations and reimbursement

888. What are the risks of malprescribing related to practice management?

(1) Loss of provider status

(2) Insurers frequently report to Boards

(3) Plans may remove providers for overprescribing

(4) Insurers are unable to report to any type of national databank for malprescribing

889. *Diagnostic and Statistical Manual of Mental Disorder* (Fourth Edition) (*DSM-IV*) definition of substance abuse includes at least one of the following in 12 months:

(1) Maladaptive pattern leading to distress or impairment

(2) Recurrent failure to fill role

(3) Recurrent physically hazardous behavior

(4) Recurrent legal problems

890. Which of the following is (are) correct statement(s) regarding amphetamines in UDT?

(1) Tests for amphetamine/methamphetamine are highly cross-reactive

(2) Very predictive for amphetamine/methamphetamine use

(3) UDT will detect other sympathomimetic amines such as ephedrine and pseudoephedrine

(4) Further testing is not required

891. Which of the following is (are) the correct statement(s) about UDT for cocaine?

(1) Tests for cocaine react principally with cocaine and its primary metabolite, benzoylecgonine

(2) Tests for cocaine are nonspecific in predicting cocaine use

(3) Tests for cocaine have low cross-reactivity with other substances

(4) Cold medicines may test false-positive for cocaine

892. What precautions must a physician take in interpretation of UDT?

(1) Consult with laboratory regarding any unexpected results

(2) Never use results to strengthen physician-patient relationship and support positive behavior change

(3) Schedule an appointment to discuss abnormal/unexpected results with the patient; discuss in a positive, supportive fashion to enhance readiness to change/motivational enhancement therapy (MET) opportunities

(4) It is not necessary to document results and interpretation

893. Which of the following is (are) true about postoperative pain management in patients receiving methadone maintenance treatment?

(1) Continue maintenance treatment without interruption

(2) Immediately stop maintenance treatment

(3) Provide adequate individualized doses of opioid agonists, which must be titrated to the desired analgesic effect

(4) If opioids are administered in methadone maintenance patients, doses should be given less frequently and as needed

894. A 38-year-old white male with chronic low back pain and history of alcoholism, on a total of 200 mg of morphine per day, was admitted to the emergency room because he was acting agitated and confused. The emergency room physician notifies you of his admission. Which of the following identifies delirium tremens in differential diagnosis of this patient's condition?

(1) Clear sensorium

(2) Prominent tremor

(3) Auditory hallucination

(4) Dilated pupils with slow reaction to light

895. Which of the following is (are) true regarding the five schedules of controlled substances, known as schedules I, II, III, IV, and V?

(1) Schedule I substances have high potential for abuse and the substance has no currently accepted medical use in treatment in the United States

(2) Schedule I substances may be changed to a lower schedule if the safety of the drug is demonstrated even though there is a high potential for abuse and there is no accepted medical use in treatment

(3) Schedule II drugs have high potential for abuse and may lead to severe psychologic or physical dependence

(4) Schedule V drugs or substances have a high potential for abuse and may lead to physical or psychologic dependence

896. What are the characteristics of a drug-dependent (addict) practitioner?

(1) Starts by taking controlled-drug samples

(2) Never asks staff to pick up medications in their names

(3) Calls in scripts in names of family members or fictitious patients and picks them up himself

(4) Never uses another doctor's DEA number

897. Which is (are) the true statement(s) about marijuana UDT?

(1) UDTs provide reasonable reliability

(2) Marinol tests positive

(3) Protonix may test false-positive

(4) Marijuana may be positive 2 years after use

898. Which of the following is (are) the correct statement(s) for UDT?

(1) Thin-layer chromatography (TLC) is a relatively old technique, testing the migration of a drug on a plate or film, which is compared to a known control

(2) Gas chromatography (GC) is most sensitive and specific test, most reliable, and labor intensive/costly

(3) Enzyme immunoassay is easy to perform/highly sensitive, more sensitive than TLC, and less expensive than GC

(4) Rapid drug screens are not similar to other enzyme immunoassay tests and may be more expensive

899. Drug testing may be performed by any of the following:

(1) Hair samples

(2) Saliva testing

(3) Serum drug testing

(4) Urine drug screening

900. Which of the following is (are) accurate for addiction and dependence?

(1) Based on the Controlled Substances Act, the term "addict" means any individual who habitually uses any narcotic drug so as to endanger the public health and safety

(2) Based on *DSM-IV* definition, addiction means maladaptive pattern leading to distress or impairment

(3) *DSM-IV* definition of substance dependence includes tolerance, withdrawal, and continued use despite problems

(4) Federation of State Medical Board guidelines for the treatment of pain recommends use of controlled substances in patients with history of substance with no additional monitoring, referral, or documentation

Answers and Explanations

873. **(D)** In performing UDT, know the characteristics of testing procedures, since many drugs are not routinely detected by all UDTs. Although no aberrant behavior is pathognomonic of abuse or addiction, such behavior should never be ignored.

   Reliance on aberrant behavior to trigger a UDT will miss more than 50% of those individuals using unprescribed or illicit drugs. Never prescribe on-demand for the patient until you are comfortable with the situation. A history of drug abuse does not preclude treatment with a controlled substance, when indicated, but does require a treatment plan with firmly defined boundaries.

874. **(D)** The patient is most likely developing tolerance to the analgesic effects of the intrathecal morphine while continuing to complain of the adverse side effect of nausea as the intrathecal dose is increased. The mechanism by which tolerance develops is not known. The development of tolerance can be minimized by selecting the lowest effective narcotic dose; placing the catheter as close as possible to the cord level of the painful areas; giving multiple, small, divided doses rather than one or two large, daily boluses; and using low-dose continuous infusions whenever possible.

875. **(E)** A short tabular comparison of quality assurance versus quality improvement is given here:

Quality Assurance	Quality Improvement
Externally driven	Internally driven
Follows organizational structure	Follows patient care
Delegated to a few	Embraced by all
Focused on individuals	Focused on process
Works toward end points	Has no end points
"Assures" quality (perfection)	"Improves" quality
Divided analysis of effectiveness/efficiency	Integrated analysis

876. **(A)** A short tabular description of some common drugs of abuse and there typical detection time for urine testing is as follows:

Drug	Detection Time
Amphetamine or methamphetamine	2 to 4 d
Barbiturates (short-acting)	2 to 4 d
Barbiturates (long-acting)	Up to 30 d
Benzodiazepines	Up to 30 d
Cocaine (benzoylecgonine-cocaine metabolite)	1 to 3 d
Heroin or morphine	1 to 3 d
Marijuana (occasional use)	1 to 3 d
Marijuana (chronic use)	Up to 30 d
Methadone	2 to 4 d
Phencyclidine (occasional use)	2 to 7 d
Phencyclidine (chronic use)	Up to 30 d

877. **(D)** Cocaine acts by blocking reuptake of neurotransmitters (norepinephrine, dopamine, and serotonin) at the synaptic junctions, resulting in increased neurotransmitter concentrations. As norepinephrine is the primary neurotransmitter of the sympathetic nervous system it causes sympathetic stimulation and leads to vasoconstriction, tachycardia, mydriasis, and hyperthermia. Central nervous system stimulation

may appear as increased alertness, energy, and talkativeness, repetitive behavior, diminished appetite, and increased libido. Psychologic stimulation by cocaine produces an intense euphoria that is often compared to orgasm. Pleasure and reward sensations in the brain have been correlated with increased neurotransmission in the mesolimbic or mesocortical dopaminergic tracts (or both). Cocaine increases the functional release of dopamine, which activates the ventral tegmental–nucleus accumbens pathway, which seems to be major component of the brain reward system. Activation of this pathway is essential for the reinforcing actions of psychomotor stimulants.

878.   **(A)** Federal regulations are

Promulgated by	Enforced by
US Congress	Department of Justice (DOJ)
Centers for Medicare & Medicaid Services (CMS)	Federal Bureau of Investigation (FBI)
Office of Inspector General (OIG)	OIG
Local Medicare carriers	Courts

879.   **(C)**

Consultation

- An opinion is requested
- Patient is not referred

The three R's

- Request for opinion is received
- Render the service/opinion
- Report back to physician requesting your opinion

880.   **(C)** The Controlled Substances Act has divided drugs under its jurisdiction into five schedules. Schedule I drugs have a high potential for abuse and no accepted medical use in the United States. Examples of schedule I drugs include heroin, marijuana, lysergic acid diethylamide (LSD). Hydromorphone, heroin, morphine are schedule II drugs; buprenorphine is schedule III drug; and diazepam is schedule IV drug.

881.   **(D)**

A. Methadone frequently is used to treat acute withdrawal from opioids.

B. Current federal regulations restrict the use of methadone for the treatment of opioid addiction to specially registered clinics.

C Methadone may be used by a physician in private practice for temporary maintenance or detoxification when an addicted patient is admitted to the hospital for an illness other than opioid addiction. This includes evaluation for preterm labor, which can be induced by acute withdrawal.

D. Methadone may also be used by a private practitioner in an outpatient setting when administered daily for a maximum of 3 days while a patient awaits admission to a licensed methadone treatment program.

882.   **(E)**

A. A physician has to maintain patient's confidentiality. Further, she may be addicted to not only heroin, but hydrocodone. It is not certain at this point. She may be receiving hydrocodone from other sources.

B. A physician has to maintain patient's confidentiality. Further, she may be addicted to not only heroin, but hydrocodone. It is not certain at this point. She may be receiving methadone from other sources.

C. Rapid detoxification requires a special license.

D. Similarly, methadone maintenance treatment also requires special licensure.

E. The best option is to maintain confidentiality, protect the patient, and yourself.

883.   **(A)**

A. Constipation is the most frequent side effect of opioid therapy. Tolerance does not develop to this side effect. Therefore, as the dose of opioid increases, so does the potential for constipation. Frank bowel obstruction, biliary spasm, and ileus have occurred with opioid use. It is crucial to place patients on an active bowel regimen that includes laxatives, stool softeners, adequate fluids and exercise, and cathartics as needed to prevent the severe constipation that can occur with opioid use.

B. Surgical complications are unlikely.

C. Constipation is not a symptom of drug abuse.

D. Transdermal fentanyl may be an option if morphine titration fails. Constipation is similar.

E. Methadone maintenance is not indicated.

884. **(B)** Risks of malprescribing includes legal charges, probably jail time. Conviction rate is currently almost 90%. Felony conviction will likely prevent or at least severely limit future practice. Duped and dated aren't viable defense.

885. **(A)**

1. The CSA created a closed system of distribution for those authorized to handle controlled substances.

2. The system is the registration of all those authorized by the DEA to handle controlled substances.

3. Only the individuals and practices that dispense directly to the patients from their clinics are required to maintain a DEA license.

4. All individuals and firms that are registered are required to maintain complete and accurate inventories and records of all transactions involving controlled substances, as well as the security for the storage of controlled substances.

The attorney general may limit revocation or suspension of a registration to the particular controlled substance. However, the Board of Medical Licensure may also limit this indirectly by means of requesting the limitation by DEA and reaching an agreement with the practitioner.

886. **(A)** UDT method
Opioids: Pitfalls

- Tests for opiates are very responsive for morphine and codeine.
- Do not distinguish which is present.

- Show a low sensitivity for semisynthetic/synthetic opioids such as oxycodone.
- A negative response does not exclude oxycodone, or methadone use.

887. **(A)** The top 10 pitfalls of prescription practices are:

1. The four D's—deficient, duped, deliberate, dependent practitioner

2. Weak heart—pretend addiction doesn't exist

3. Never say "NO"—family, friends, patients

4. Poor documentation

5. No policies—no agreements

6. Ignore complaints

7. Focus on negative aspects of regulations and reimbursement

8. Not nice to investigators from the Board and DEA

9. Reckless disregard to law with prescription pads and regulations

10. Know it all—do it all

888. **(A)** Risks of malprescribing include loss of "provider" status; insurers frequently report to the Boards now; several plans have removed providers for "overprescribing"; and finally insurers can report to a separate national data bank, not available to public, but available to hospitals and other insurers.

889. **(E)** As per the *DSM-IV* definition for substance abuse at least one of the following should hold true in 12 months:

- Maladaptive pattern leading to distress or impairment.
- Recurrent failure to fill role.
- Recurrent physically hazardous behavior.
- Recurrent legal problems.
- Continued use despite social problems.
- Never met dependence criteria.

890. **(B)** UDT method
Amphetamines: Low specificity

- Tests for amphetamine/methamphetamine are highly cross-reactive.

- They will detect other sympathomimetic amines such as ephedrine and pseudoephedrine.
- Not very predictive for amphetamine/methamphetamine use.
- Further testing is required.

891. **(B)** UDT method
Cocaine: Very specific

- Tests for cocaine react principally with cocaine and its primary metabolite, benzoylecgonine.
- These tests have low cross-reactivity with other substances.
- Very specific in predicting cocaine use.

892. **(B)** UDT results
Consult with laboratory regarding any unexpected results:

- Schedule an appointment to discuss abnormal/unexpected results with the patient; discuss in a positive, supportive fashion to enhance readiness to change/motivational enhancement therapy (MET) opportunities.
- Use results to strengthen physician-patient relationship and support positive behavior change.
- Chart results and interpretation.

893. **(B)**

1. Continue maintenance treatment without interruption.
2. Maintenance treatment must be continued.
3. Provide adequate individualized doses of opioid agonists, which must be titrated to the desired analgesic effect.
4. Doses should be given more frequently and on a fixed schedule rather than as needed.

894. **(B)**

1. There is difficulty sustaining attention, disorganized thinking, and perceptual disturbances.
2. Acute alcoholic hallucinosis may start without a drop in blood alcohol concentration, and without delirium, tremor, or autonomic hyperactivity.

3. Hallucinations are usually auditory and paranoid and may last more than 10 days.
4. In delirium tremens, the patient is confused, with prominent tremor and psychomotor activity, disturbed vital signs, autonomic dysfunction with dilated pupils, and a slow reaction to light. Hallucinations are usually of the visual type.

895. **(B)**
1. and 2. Schedule I

The drug or other substance has a high potential for abuse.

The drug or other substances has no currently accepted medical use in treatment in the United States.

There is a lack of accepted safety for use of the drug or other substance under medical supervision.

3. Schedule II

The drug or other substance has a high potential for abuse.

The drug or other substances has no currently accepted medical use in treatment in the United States or a currently accepted medical use with severe restrictions.

Abuse of the drug or other substances may lead to severe psychologic or physical dependence.

Other
Schedule III

The drug or other substance has a potential for abuse less than the drugs or other substances in schedules I and II.

The drug or other substances has no currently accepted medical use in treatment in the United States.

Abuse of the drug or other substance may lead to moderate or low physical dependence or high psychologic dependence.

Schedule IV

The drug or other substance has a low potential for abuse relative to the drugs or other substances in schedule III.

The drug or other substance has a currently accepted medical use in treatment in the United States.

Abuse of the drug or other substances may lead to limited physical dependence or psychologic dependence relative to the drugs or other substances in schedule III.

4. Schedule V

The drug or other substance has a low potential for abuse relative to the drugs or other substances in schedule IV.

The drug or other substance has a currently accepted medical use in treatment in the United States.

Abuse of the drug or other substances may lead to limited physical dependence or psychologic dependence relative to the drugs or other substances in schedule IV.

896. **(B)** Drug dependent (addict)

- Starts by taking controlled drug samples.
- Asks staff to pick up medications in their names.
- Uses another doctor's DEA number.
- Calls in scripts in names of family members or fictitious patients and picks them up himself.

897. **(A)** UDT methods
THC: Marijuana: Moderate specificity

- Reasonable reliability
- Marinol: positive
- Protonix: false-positive

METABOLITES OF OPIOIDS

Morphine	M3G and M6G
Meperidine	Normeperidine
Levorphanol tartrate (Levo-Dromoran)	Long half-life
Hydromorphone	Hydromorphone-3-glucuronide (H3G)
Oxycodone	Noroxycodone, oxymorphone, oxycodols, and their respective oxides
Fentanyl	Extensive metabolism, primary by hepatic pathways
Codeine	Norcodeine Morphine
Hydrocodone	The conjugates of dihydrocodeine and nordihydrocodeine (both conjugated to approximately 65%) Dihydromorphone Hydromorphone Dihydrocodeine
Propoxyphene	Norpropoxyphene
Pentazocine	Metabolized almost exclusively in the liver

898. **(A)**

Thin-layer chromatography (TLC)
   Relatively old technique, testing the migration of a drug on a plate or film, which is compared to a known control

Gas chromatography: liquid and mass spectrometry (CGMS)
   Most sensitive and specific tests
   Most reliable
   Labor intensive/costly
      Several days to know results
      Used to confirm results of other tests

Enzyme immunoassay
   Easy to perform/highly sensitive
   More sensitive than TLC
   Less expensive than GC Common tests
      EMIT (enzyme multiplied immunoassay test)
      FPIA (fluorescent polarization immunoassay)
      RIA (radioimmunoassay)
      Screen only one drug at a time

Rapid drug screens
   Similar to other enzyme immunoassay tests
   May be more expensive

899. **(E)** Drug testing may be performed by any of the following:

- Urine drug screening
- Specific drug analysis (blood)
- Hair samples
- Saliva testing
- Serum levels

900. (B)

1. The term "addict" by CSA means any individual who habitually uses any narcotic drug so as to endanger the public morals, health, safety, or welfare, or who is so far addicted to the use of narcotic drugs as to have lost the power of self-control with reference to his or her addiction.

2. There is no definition for addiction in *DSM-IV*.

3. *DSM-IV* defines substance abuse with at least one of the following in a 12-month period.

- Maladaptive pattern leading to distress or impairment
- Recurrent failure to field role
- Recurrent physically undesirous behavior
- Recurrent legal problems
- Continued use despite social problems
- Never met dependence criteria

DSM-IV definition for substance dependence is as follows (need three of the following in a 12-month period):

- Tolerance
- Withdrawal
- Larger amounts/longer periods
- Efforts or desire to cut down
- Large amount of time using/obtaining/recovering
- Activities given up: social/work/recreation
- Continued use despite problems

An alternate definition for addiction is from the American Society of Addiction Medicine. It says addiction is a primary, chronic neurobiological disease with genetic, psychosocial and environmental factors affecting its course and presentation. Addiction is characterized by one or more of the following:

- Impaired control of drug use
- Compulsive use
- Craving
- Continued use despite harm

4. Federation of State Medical Board guidelines recommends several additional steps in patients with addiction or abuse.

CHAPTER 13

Cost, Ethics, and Medicolegal Aspects in Pain Medicine
Questions

DIRECTIONS: For Question 901 through 911, ONE or MORE of the numbered options is correct. Choose answer

(A) if only answer 1, 2, and 3 are correct
(B) if only 1 and 3 are correct
(C) if only 2 and 4 are correct
(D) if only 4 is correct
(E) if all are correct

901. What are the penalties under the False Claims Act?

(1) Three times the amount of damages suffered by the government
(2) A mandatory civil penalty of at least $5500 and no more than $11,000 per claim
(3) Submit 50 false claims for $50 each (liability between $282,500 and $557,500 in damages)
(4) Program exclusion

902. What are the steps to compliance of security standards for electronic patient records?

(1) Administrative safeguards
(2) Physical safeguard
(3) Technical safeguard
(4) Financial viability safeguard

903. Identify all accurate statements:

(1) The Emergency Medical Treatment and Active Labor Act (EMTALA) only applied to patients who are physically in a hospital's emergency department
(2) Physicians in a group practice may receive productivity bonuses without violating the Stark Self-Referral Rules if the bonuses are based on a physician's total number of patient encounters or relative value units (RVUs)
(3) You purchase a medical practice that is currently subject to a corporate integrity agreement (CIA), and the transfer of ownership will void the CIA
(4) According to the Department of Health and Human Services Office of Inspector General (OIG), having a compliance program without appropriate, ongoing monitoring is worse than not having a compliance program

904. Local medical review policy (LMRP) or local coverage determination (LCD) is utilized in all states. Which of the following is (are) true?

(1) LMRP or LCD is developed to assure beneficiary access to care
(2) Frequent denials indicate a need for development of LMRP or LCD
(3) A need for development of LMRP or LCD includes a validated widespread problem
(4) LMRPs or LCDs are the policies used to make coverage and coding decisions in the absence of specific statute, regulations, national coverage policy, and national coding policy or as an adjunct to a national coverage policy

905. True statements about *qui tam* (Whistleblower Act) are as follows:

(1) Suits are usually brought by employees

(2) If the government proceeds with the suit, the whistleblower receives 50% to 60% of settlement

(3) Individuals can bring suit against violators of federal laws on their own behalf as well as the government's

(4) If the government does not proceed and the individual continues, the individual receives 100% of the settlement

906. Identify true statement(s) differentiating consultation and referral visit:

(1) Written request for opinion or advice received from attending physician, including the specific reason the consultation is requested

(2) Patient appointment made for the purpose of providing treatment or management or other diagnostic or therapeutic services

(3) Only opinion or advice is sought. Subsequent to the opinion, treatment may be initiated in the same encounter if criteria are fulfilled

(4) Transfer of total patient care for management of the specified condition

907. What are some of the important aspects of documentation of medical necessity?

(1) Medicare will reimburse irrespective of the procedure, furnished, not for improvement function, but 20% pain relief

(2) The physician practice should be able to provide documentation such as a patient's medical records and physician's orders, to support the appropriateness of a service that the physician has provided

(3) Medicare concurs with physician opinion and patient request with respect to duration, frequency, and setting a procedure performed

(4) The physician practice should only bill those services that meet the Medicare standard of being reasonable and necessary for the diagnosis and treatment of a patient

908. What is (are) the correct statement(s) about a deficient (dated) practitioner?

(1) Too busy to keep up with CME

(2) Only aware of a few treatments or medications

(3) Prescribes for friends or family without a patient record

(4) Well aware of controlled-drug categories

909. Identify accurate statement(s) about clinical policies:

(1) They are expensive and labor intensive to develop and maintain

(2) The actual impact on the quality of care is nearly impossible to determine

(3) There are probable multiple indirect positive benefits of this effort with improved patient care and decreased practice variation

(4) They provide an inordinate amount of restrictions

910. What are the Federation of State Medical Board's guidelines for the treatment of pain?

(1) Use of controlled substances, including opiates may be essential in the treatment of pain

(2) Effective pain management is a part of quality medical practice

(3) Patients with a history of substance abuse may require monitoring, consultation, referral, and extra documentation

(4) MDs should not fear disciplinary action for legitimate medical purposes

911. Exclusion means which of the following for a provider?

(1) A prohibition from providing health care services for a period of time

(2) A prohibition from billing federal health programs for items or services

(3) A prohibition from practicing as a physician for a period of time

(4) A prohibition from receiving reimbursement from federal health care programs for items or services

Answers and Explanations

901. (E) Penalties under False Claims Act:

- Three times the amount of damages suffered by the government.
- A mandatory civil penalty of at least $5500 and no more than $11,000 per claim.
- Submit 50 false claims for $50 each (liability between $282,500 and $557,500 in damages).
- Program exclusion.

902. (A) The new rule on the security of electronic patient records boils down to three sets of standards that practices will need to implement step-by-step.

1. In the area of administrative safeguards we have the following:

   - Assess computer systems.
   - Train staff on procedures.
   - Prepare for aftermath of hackers or catastrophic events.
   - Develop contracts for business associates.

2. In the area of physical safeguard we have the following:

   - Set procedures for workstation use and security.
   - Set procedures for electronic media reuse and disposal.

3. In the area of technical safeguard we have the following:

   - Control staff computer log-in and log-out.
   - Monitor access of patient information.
   - Set up computers to authenticate users.

4. There is no financial viability safeguard.

903. (C)

1. EMTALA, also known as the patient antidumping law applies to an individual who requests examination or treatment and who is on hospital property (including off-campus clinics and hospital-owned ambulances that are not on hospital grounds). An individual in a non–hospital-owned ambulance on hospital property is also considered to have come to the hospital's emergency department.

2. Profit shares and productivity bonuses are permitted if they meet certain conditions. Physicians in a group practice, including independent contractors, may get shares of "overall profits" of the group or receive bonuses for services they personally perform—including incident-to-services—if such rewards are not based on referrals for any of the designated health services.

   Regardless of which type of reward is given, documentation that verifies how much was given and on what basis must be made available to investigators if requested.

   Overall profits are the profits from designated health services for the entire group or any part of the group that has at least five physicians. The profits are not based on referrals if only one of the following conditions is met:

   - The profits are divided per capita (per member or per physician, for example).
   - Designated health services revenue is distributed based on the way nondesignated health services revenue is distributed.

- Designated health service revenue is both less than 5% of the group's total income and is less than 5% of any physician's total compensation from the group.
- Overall profits are distributed in a reasonable and verifiable way that is unrelated to designated health service referrals.

Productivity bonuses are not based on referrals if

- It is based on a physician's total number of patient encounters or RVUs.
- It is not based in any way on designated health services.
- Designated health service revenue is both less than 5% of the group's total income and is less than 5% of any physician's total compensation from the group.
- It is distributed in a reasonable and verifiable way unrelated to designated health services DHS referrals.

3. and 4. Corporate integrity agreements (CIAs) are typically large, detailed and restrictive compliance plans that companies enter into as part of a deal with the Department of Health and Human Services Office of Inspector General (OIG). CIAs are intended to make sure that a company never again commits the kind of offenses against the Medicare program that landed it in trouble in the first place. There are strict reporting requirements and other rules a company must live up to once it agrees on a plan with OIG, but on the plus side, OIG allows the company to continue to do business with Medicare.

904. **(E)** LMRPs or LCDs are those policies used to make coverage and coding decisions in the absence of the following:

- Specific statute
- Regulations
- National coverage policy
- National coding policy
- As an adjunct to a national coverage policy

Development of LMRP—identification of need

- A validated widespread problem.
  - Identified or potentially high dollar and/or high volume services.
- To assure beneficiary access to care.
- LMRP development across its multiple jurisdictions by a single carrier.
- Frequent denials are issued or anticipated.

LMRP's reduce utilization and save money.

905. **(B)**

906. **(B)** Consultation versus referral visit (see Table below)

907. **(C)**

Reasonable and necessary service must be

- Safe and effective.
- Not experimental or investigational.

	Consultation	Referral Visit
Problem	Suspected	Known
Request language	"Please examine patient and provide me with your opinion and recommendation on his/her condition"	"Patient is referred for treatment or management of his/her condition"
Request	Written request for opinion or advice received from attending physician, including the specific reason the consultation is requested	Patient appointment made for the purpose of providing treatment or management or other diagnostic or therapeutic services
Report language	"I was asked to see Mr Jones in consultation by Dr Johnson"	"Mr Jones was seen following a referral from Dr Johnson"
Patient care	Only opinion or advice sought. Subsequent to the opinion, treatment may be initiated in the same encounter	Transfer of total patient care for management of the specified condition
Treatment	Undetermined course	Prescribed and known course
Correspondence	Written opinion returned to attending physician	No further communication (or limited contact) with referring physician is required
Diagnosis	Final diagnosis is probably unknown	Final diagnosis is typically known at the time of referral

- Appropriate, including the duration and frequency that is considered appropriate for the service, in terms of whether it is
  - Furnished in accordance with accepted standards of medical practice for the diagnosis or treatment of the patient's condition or to improve the function.
  - Furnished in a setting appropriate to the patient's medical needs and condition.
- Ordered and/or furnished by qualified personnel.
- One that meets, but does not exceed, the patient's medical need.

Documenting medical necessity

- The physician practice should be able to provide documentation such as a patient's medical records and physician's orders, to support the appropriateness of a service that the physician has provided.
- Only bill those services that meet the Medicare standard of being reasonable and necessary for the diagnosis and treatment of a patient.

908. **(E)** The following are correct statements about a deficient (dated) practitioner:

- Too busy to keep up with CME.
- Unaware of controlled-drug categories.
- Only aware of a few treatments or medications.
- Prescribes for friends or family without a patient record.
- Unaware of symptoms of addiction.
- Remains isolated with peers.
- Only education from reps.

909. **(A)** The following are correct statements about clinical policies:

- Expensive and labor intensive to develop and maintain.
- Actual impact on the quality of care is nearly impossible to determine.
- Probable indirect positive benefits of this effort like
  Increased acceptance of concept of "standards".
  Increased attention to our individual practices of medicine, especially over time.
  Decreased practice variation.
  Pay for performance.

910. **(E)** Federation of State Medical Board's guidelines for the treatment of pain include

- Use of controlled substances, including opiates may be essential in the treatment of pain.
- Effective pain management is a part of quality medical practice.
- Patients with a history of substance abuse may require monitoring, consultation, referral, and extra documentation.
- MDs should not fear disciplinary action for legitimate medical purposes.

911. **(C)** Exclusion means a provider is barred from receiving reimbursement from Medicare, Medicaid, or other federal health care programs. There are two types of exclusion: mandatory and permissive. Under mandatory exclusion, HHS must exclude—it has no choice. Under permissive exclusion, HHS has some discretion.

CHAPTER 14

Compensation and Disability Assessment
Questions

DIRECTIONS (Questions 912 through 938): Each of the numbered items or incomplete statements in this section is followed by answers or by completions of the statement. Select the ONE lettered answer or completion that is BEST in each case.

912. A concert pianist and a vice president of a major corporation have both suffered the loss of the second finger of the dominant hand. Which of the following statements is true regarding the condition of impairment or disability caused by the injury?

    (A) The concert pianist is more impaired than the vice president

    (B) The concert pianist and vice president are equally disabled

    (C) The concert pianist and vice president are both handicapped

    (D) The concert pianist is more disabled than the vice president

    (E) The concert pianist is more handicapped than the vice president

913. Identify the true statement with regards to a physician's role in impairment and disability evaluation:

    (A) Determine impairment; provide medical information to assist in disability determination

    (B) Provide a disability rating which is binding on the administrative law judge for social security and disability

    (C) In State Worker's Compensation Law, a physician's role is limited to determining only disability, not impairment

    (D) The World Health Organization (WHO) has specifically defined the role of the physician in impairment and disability

    (E) Physician's role in impairment and disability determination is independent, without input from employer and without consideration to job duties

914. Which of the following is true statement with reference to the Americans with Disability Act (ADA)?

    (A) The physician's input is not essential for determining any of the criteria under ADA

    (B) Conditions that are temporary and are not considered to be impairment under the ADA include pregnancy, old age, sexual orientation, sexual addiction, smoking, or current illegal drug use

    (C) To be deemed disabled for purposes of ADA protection, an individual needs to have only mild physical or mental impairment that does not limit major life activities

    (D) The person may be hypothetically or perceived to be disabled to be qualified under ADA

    (E) It is the physician's responsibility to identify and determine if reasonable accommodations are possible to enable the individual's performance of essential job activities in his or her employment

915. Which of the following is true regarding causation, apportionment, and worker's compensation?

(A) Determining medical causation requires detective work and witness of the accident

(B) For purposes of the *Guides to the Evaluation of Permanent Impairment*, causation means an identifiable factor, such as an accident that results in a medically identifiable condition

(C) The legal standard for causation in civil litigation and in worker's compensation is uniform across the United States

(D) Apportionment analysis in worker's compensation represents assignment of all factors

(E) The role of a physician in worker's compensation system is only to provide effective medical care but not be involved in other aspects of the care

916. Which of the following is true with regards to disability?

(A) It is a term that can be used interchangeably with the term "handicap"

(B) It is a condition that relates to the effects of a disease process or injury

(C) It is a condition that requires the use of an assistive device to perform activities of daily living

(D) It is expressed as a percentage of the body as a whole

(E) It is a condition that relates to function relative to work or other obligations

917. The CAGE questionnaire is used in case of

(A) mental retardation

(B) bipolar disorder

(C) major depression

(D) opioid abuse

(E) alcohol abuse

918. The "rules" that, in many cases, define which physician referrals are legal and which are not, are found in the following regulations:

(A) Stark regulations

(B) Antikickback statute

(C) Stark regulations and antikickback statute

(D) Stark regulations, antikickback statute, and Omnibus Budget Reconciliation Act (OBRA) of 1993

(E) Stark regulations, Health Insurance Portability and Accountability Act (HIPAA), and Balanced Budget Act (BBA)

919. Which of the following statements is correct?

(A) Patient may request that a provider amend a diagnosis that was submitted on a billing claim form

(B) A provider must act on a patient's request for amendment within 30 days, either deny or amend

(C) A provider does not agree with a patient's request for an amendment. The provider must make the amendment but can note disagreement in the amendment and inform the insurer

(D) Provider has to amend diagnosis in 30 days as provider may not deny the patient's requests

(E) Provider has no obligation even if the information on the claim was inaccurate

920. What are the consequences of downcoding?

(A) Compliance with guidelines may not be the most important aspect

(B) It is not necessary to assure proper coding of the level of service during downcoding

(C) Medicare will eventually reimburse all your downcoding after 5 years

(D) Downcoding is the largest area of loss of revenue for the practice

(E) Medicare may not investigate downcoding

921. Which is the accurate statement about billing and compliance?

(A) A physician may mark up durable medical equipment (DME) items under the physician self-referral Stark regulation in-office ancillary services exception

(B) If a practice which does not have a compliance plan discovers a billing error, it is not necessary for this practice to make a voluntary disclosure and a refund of the overpayment

(C) When a provider receives a payment from Medicare that should have gone to the patient, the provider should keep the payment

(D) Direct supervision is defined as "The physician is responsible overall, but is not necessarily present at the time of procedure"

(E) If an employee files a *qui tam* (whistleblower) suit against his or her employer, the employer may ask the employee to stay out of the work place and refrain from speaking to his or her co-workers until a full investigation has taken plan

922. A local clinical laboratory provides a phlebotomist free of charge to a doctor's office. The phlebotomist takes specimens from the physician's office to the laboratory. When the phlebotomist is not busy drawing blood, the phlebotomist assists the doctor's office personnel with filing of records and other clerical duties. What aspects of this scenario, if any, implicate the antikickback laws?

(A) Provision by the clinical laboratory of a phlebotomist free of charge to the physician

(B) Performance by the phlebotomist of clerical duties in the physician's office

(C) Phlebotomist taking specimens from physician's office to the laboratory

(D) All of the above

(E) None of the above

923. What do the physician self-referral Stark rules prohibit?

(A) They prohibit physicians from referring patients to hospitals where the physicians work

(B) They prohibit physicians from referring patients for designated health services

to entities in which the physicians have financial relationships, unless an exception applies

(C) They prohibit health care providers from billing for services of patients they refer to other providers

(D) They prohibit health care providers from receiving money from their services for any referrals to physical therapy

(E) The prohibit physicians performing cases in ambulatory surgery centers with physician ownership of 50% or more

924. Centers for Medicare and Medicaid Services (CMS) guidelines in a documentation of evaluation and management services recommend the use of the following:

(A) SOAP—subjective, objective, assessment, and plan

(B) SOAPER—subjective, objective, assessment, plan, education and return instructions

(C) SOAPIE—subjective, objective, assessment, plan, implementation, and evaluation

(D) SNOCAMP—subjective, nature of presenting problem, counseling, assessment, medical decision making, and plan

(E) Documentation involving elements, bullets, and level of care

925. Identify true statements about current procedural technology (CPT) and International Classification of Diseases (ICD-9) codes?

(A) ICD-9 is a systematic listing of procedure or service accurately defining and assisting with simplified reporting

(B) CPT is a systematic listing and coding of procedures and services performed by physicians

(C) ICD-9 identifies each procedure or service with a five-digit code

(D) CPT provides systematic listing of disease classification and provides alphabetic index to diseases

(E) CPT and ICD-9 both provide a tabular list of diseases

926. Which of the following factors will determine the number of drug-receptor complexes formed?

(A) Efficacy of the drug
(B) Receptor affinity for the drug
(C) Therapeutic index of the drug
(D) Half-life of the drug
(E) Rate of renal secretion

927. In response to a call from the patient's spouse informing the physician that the patient is abusing narcotics prescribed by the physician, the physician notes in the patient's medical record that the spouse called to report such information. The spouse is concerned that her husband would be extremely upset if he knew she called with the information. In an event that the husband requests a complete copy of his records, which of the following is correct statement?

(A) The physician is permitted to withhold the information
(B) The physician must provide entire chart immediately
(C) The physician must determine with 100% certainty that, wife will be harmed, to withhold the information
(D) The physician is required to provide oral information, but withhold written information
(E) The physician may provide this information only after spouse's death

928. Which of the following is a true statement applicable to a patient's request for a copy of his or her record?

(A) The physician is not required to give the patient any records that were not created or generated by the practice
(B) The provider is required to give a copy of all the records
(C) Designated record sets include only the medical records generated by the provider
(D) Medical records may be released only after patient has paid his bill in full
(E) Patient's access is limited to only certain areas of medical record

929. What are the ramifications of the antikickback statute on your practice?

(A) It is a felony—10 years imprisonment
(B) It is a crime to offer, solicit, pay, or receive remuneration, in cash or in kind, directly or indirectly, for referrals under a federally funded health care program
(C) Civil penalties—$500,000 per violation
(D) "Multipurpose" rule
(E) No safe harbors

930. The training requirements of needlestick safety include all of the following EXCEPT

(A) work hours
(B) ninety days after initial assignment
(C) at a cost to employee
(D) within 365 days after effective date of standard
(E) within 10 years of previous training

931. Identify accurate statement in the scenario where a health care provider fails to honor a patient's written request for an itemized statement of items or services within 30 days. What penalties may the provider face from the HHS (United States Department of Health and Human Services) Office of Inspector General (OIG)?

(A) Exclusion from Medicare program
(B) Civil monetary penalty of $5000
(C) Civil monetary penalty and exclusion
(D) Civil monetary penalty of $100 for each unfilled request
(E) Criminal penalty with 6-month prison time

932. What is the true statement about global fee policy?

(A) Global fee policy describes packaging or inclusion of certain services in allowance for a surgical procedure
(B) Global fee policy describes unbundling or combining multiple services into a single charge
(C) Global package includes preoperative and postoperative services for 120 days

(D) Global package includes initial evaluation if performed on the same day

(E) Global package includes all diagnostic tests

933. Pay for performance is being considered by Medicare and third-party payers. Identify accurate statements:

(A) Compensation incentives will not induce changes in the quality of services

(B) Outcome measures are easy to develop

(C) Compensation incentives rest on the economic field of agency theory (method of compensation induces conduct)

(D) Quality measures are already in place

(E) It is simple to finance incentives

934. For a service to be reasonable and necessary it must be

(A) safe

(B) experimental

(C) investigational

(D) patient can afford to pay

(E) furnished only in a hospital

935. Which of the following is an accurate statement about proper billing?

(A) Bill for items or services not rendered or not provided as claimed

(B) Submit claims for equipment, medical supplies, and services that are not reasonable and necessary

(C) Double bill resulting in duplicate payment

(D) Bill for noncovered services as if covered

(E) Knowingly do not misuse provider identification numbers, which results in improper billing

936. What are important aspects of the Needlestick Safety and Prevention Act of 2001?

(A) It has 24 areas of change

(B) Two terms were added to definitions

(C) It was enacted because of a total of more than 20 million needlesticks per year

(D) Risks of contracting disease were minimal

(E) Psychologic stress was the only issue

937. Multiple components of proper medical record documentation do not include the following:

(A) The reason for the patient's visit

(B) The indication of services provided

(C) The location of the services

(D) Itemized billing for services

(E) Plan of action including return appointment

938. Which of the following is an accurate statement describing legitimate professional courtesy?

(A) When a physician practice waives coinsurance obligations or other out-of-pocket expenses for other physicians or family members, but only based on their referrals

(B) When a hospital or other institution waives fees for services provided to their medical staff, but not employees

(C) When an organization waives fees based on proportion of referrals

(D) When a physician practice is able to collect full fee, by increasing charges proportionately

(E) When a physician practice waives all or part of a fee for services for office staff, other physicians or family members

DIRECTIONS: For Question 939 through 948, ONE or MORE of the numbered options is correct. Choose answer

(A) if only answer 1, 2, and 3 are correct

(B) if only 1 and 3 are correct

(C) if only 2 and 4 are correct

(D) if only 4 is correct

(E) if all are correct

939. Impairment is correctly characterized by the following definition(s):

(1) A loss, loss of use, or derangement of any body part, organ system, or organ function

(2) An alteration of an individual's capacity to meet personal, social, or occupational demands because of impairment

(3) An anatomical, physiological, or psychologic abnormality that can be shown by medically acceptable clinical and laboratory diagnostic techniques

(4) A barrier to full functional activity that may be overcome by compensating in some way for the causative impairment

940. Identify the true statement(s) describing functional restoration:

(1) Functional restoration is a monotherapy intended to return patients to work

(2) Functional restoration includes an interdisciplinary approach with physical therapy, occupational therapy, vocational rehabilitation, psychology, nursing, and physician

(3) Indications for functional restoration include temporary disability and ability to return to work following exercise program

(4) Phases of rehabilitation and functional restoration include initial reconditioning, comprehensive phase, and follow-up phase

941. Sedentary work is characterized by which of the following criteria?

(1) Lifting a maximum of 10 lb

(2) Carrying objects weighing up to 10 lb

(3) Requirement of occasional walking and standing, but mostly sitting

(4) Pushing and pulling of arm or leg controls

942. The Social Security Administration uses a number of criteria for determination of eligibility for disability benefits. The sequential evaluation for determination of benefits includes which of the following factors? (Nonexertional factors [evaluation of the applicant's cognitive capabilities] are part of the evaluation of residual functional capacity.)

(1) Age

(2) Educational background

(3) Previous work history

(4) Residual functional capacity

943. The following statement(s) is (are) true to describe the purposes of rehabilitation:

(1) To resolve deconditioning syndrome that developed from prolonged bed rest with loss of muscle strength, decreased flexibility, and increased stiffness

(2) To optimize outcome by restoring function and returning to activity

(3) To minimize potential or recurrence or reinjury

(4) Short periods of rest between activities help to exacerbate the deleterious effects of inactivity

944. Identify true statement(s) to assist in your practice by specialty designation of interventional pain management:

(1) Physician profiling or comparative utilization assessment

(2) 500% increase of practice expense calculation immediately

(3) Carrier advisory committee (CAC) membership

(4) 100% increase in physician's reimbursement

945. Which of the following statement(s) is (are) true with regards to the Controlled Substances Act of the Comprehensive Drug Abuse Prevention and Control Act of 1970?

(1) It is the legal foundation of the government's fight against the abuse of drugs and other substances

(2) It is a consolidation of numerous laws regulating the manufacture and distribution of narcotics, stimulants, depressants, hallucinogens, anabolic steroids, and chemicals used in the illicit production of controlled substances

(3) All the substances that are regulated under existing federal law are placed into schedule I of the five schedules

(4) Schedule I is reserved for the least dangerous drugs that have the highest recognized medical use

946. What does the following HIPAA compliance administrative simplification do?

(1) Increases costs associated with administrative and claims related transactions

(2) Establishes a national uniform standards for eight electronic transactions, and claims attachments

(3) Eliminates unique provider identifiers

(4) Establishes protections for the privacy and security of individual health information

947. What are true statements about fraud in medicine in the United States?

(1) Medicare fee for service error rate was 8% in 2004

(2) A GAO (US Government Accountability Office) audit reported that in the United States approximately 10% of every health care dollar is lost to fraud annually

(3) Estimated net improper payments of CMS for 2004 exceeded $50 billion

(4) Fraud and abuse cases include 60% public and 40% private cases

948. Which of the following statement(s) is (are) accurate?

(1) Voluntary disclosure program offers immunity to providers who come forward within 30 days of discovering an offence

(2) Providers must always repay all Medicare overpayments within 30 days

(3) Health care providers in medically underserved areas (MUAs) may automatically waive coinsurance and deductible payments

(4) Before the OIG issues a demand letter in a civil money penalty case, the government must have legally sufficient evidence for eight elements of civil monetary penalties offense

Answers and Explanations

912. (D) Both the concert pianist and the company vice president have impairment because of the loss of their digit. However, the concert pianist is significantly more disabled because the pianist will not be able to perform but the vice president will still be able to do the job. They are not significantly handicapped because they can still perform life's activities without the use of assistive devices or modification of the environment.

913. (A) Physicians' role

A. As per the *Guides to the Evaluation of Permanent Impairment*—Determine impairment; provide medical information to assist in disability determination.

B. As per Social Security Administration (SSA)—Determine impairment; may assist with the disability determination as a consultative examiner.

C. As per State Workers' Compensation Law—Evaluation (rating) of permanent impairment is a medical appraisal of the nature and extent of the injury or disease as it affects an injured employee's personal efficiency in the activities of daily living, such as self-care, communication, normal living postures, ambulation, elevation, traveling, and nonspecialized activities of bodily members.

D. As per WHO—Not specifically defined; assumed to be one of the decision makers in determining disability through impairment assessment.

E. Disability is determined based on job requirements and needs.

914. (B) The ADA defines disability as a physical or mental impairment that substantially limits one or more of the major life activities of an individual; a record of impairment, or being regarded as having an impairment.

A. The physician's input often is essential for determining the first two criteria and valuable for determining the third.

B. Conditions that are temporary are not considered to be severe, such as normal pregnancy, are not considered impairments under the ADA. Other nonimpairments include features and conditions such as hair or eye color, left-handedness, old age, sexual orientation, exhibitionism, pedophilia, voyeurism, sexual addiction, kleptomania, pyromania, compulsive gambling, gender identity disorders not resulting from physical impairment, smoking, and current illegal drug use or resulting psychoactive disorders.

C. A person needs to meet only one of the three criteria in the definition to gain the ADA's protection against discrimination.

To be deemed disabled for purposes of ADA protection, an individual generally must have a physical or mental impairment that substantially limits one or more major life activities. A physical or mental impairment could be any mental, psychologic, or physiological disorder or condition, cosmetic disfigurement, or anatomical laws that affect one or more of the following body systems: neurologic, special sense organs, musculoskeletal, respiratory, speech organs, reproductive, cardiovascular, hematologic, lymphatic, digestive, genitourinary, skin, and endocrine.

D. It is not necessary for a person to qualify under ADA to be disabled hypothetically or perceptionally.

E. It is the physician's responsibility to determine if the impairment results in functional limitations.

The physician is responsible for informing the employer about an individual's abilities and limitations. It is the employer's responsibility to identify and determine if reasonable accommodations are possible to enable the individual's abilities and limitations.

915. (B)

916. (E) Disability is the limiting, loss, or absence of the capacity of a person to meet personal, social, or occupational demands, or to meet statutory or regulatory requirements. Disability relates to function relative to work or other obligations and activities of daily living. It may be characterized as temporary, permanent, partial, or total. Methods of assessing functional performance include measurement of range of motion, strength, endurance, and work simulation. Disability is not synonymous with handicap. When an impairment is associated with an obstacle to useful activity, a handicap may exist; assistive devices or modifications of the environment are often required to accomplish life's basic activities.

917. (E) Four clinical interview questions, the CAGE questions, have proved useful in helping to make a diagnosis of alcoholism. The questions focus on cutting down, annoyance by criticism, guilty feeling, and eye-openers. The acronym "CAGE" helps the physician recall the questions:

"C"—Have you ever felt you should cut down on your drinking?

"A"—Have people annoyed you by criticizing your drinking?

"G"—Have you ever felt bad or guilty about your drinking?

"E"—Have you ever had a drink first thing in the morning to steady your nerves or to get rid of a hangover?

918. (C)

A. The "Stark I" regulations were published in the Federal Register on August 15, 1995. The "Stark II" law that was part of the Omnibus Budget Reconciliation Act of 1993, which expanded that application of Stark I rules to additional types of health care providers and to Medicaid. Note that regulations for this law were issued in two phases: phase I, released on Jan. 4, 2001, is final. Phase II, released on March 26, 2004, is effective from July 26, 2004.

B. The antikickback statute also addresses physician referrals.

C. Physician self-referrals are governed by Stark regulations and antikickback statute.

D. OBRA of 1993 includes Stark regulations.

E. HIPAA and BBA do not govern physician self-referrals.

919. (A) The privacy rule allows patients to request amendments of their records including amendments to billing records.

The provider is not obligated to make the amendment if the provider believes that the original information (the diagnosis in this scenario) was accurate as submitted. In fact, from a billing compliance standpoint the provider should not make the amendment if the original information was accurate and complete.

A provider is given 60 days to act on amendment requests and providers are always permitted to deny amendment requests when the information is accurate and complete when originally recorded.

920. (D) Downcoding

- Largest area of loss of revenue outside disbundling.
- Compliance with guidelines is important.
- Must assure proper coding of the level of service.

921. (A)

A. The DME must meet six requirements in order to be billed as in-office ancillary services:

- It is needed by the patient to move or leave the doctor's office, or is a blood glucose monitor.

- It is provided to treat the condition that brought the patient to the physician and in the "same building."

- It is given by the physician or another physician or employee in a group practice.

- The physician or group practice meets all DME supplier standards.

- The arrangement doesn't violate any billing laws or the antikickback statute.

- All other in-office ancillary requirements are met.

B. Providers only need to self-disclose to OIG in certain situations. They do not need to self-disclose every time they receive an overpayment from Medicare. However, every provider must learn when OIG views an overpayment as a deliberate attempt to defraud Medicare instead of the result of a harmless error.

If the circumstances surrounding the billing error resemble any of the situations described below, consider voluntary disclosure and return of the overpayment. Otherwise, a refund may be sufficient:

- The situation is the result of a willful disregard for fraud and abuse laws.

- The situation is a systematic problem that occurred over a long period of time.

- The provider has no such mechanisms as a compliance plan in place.

- The provider took no action once the problem was discovered.

C. Once a provider realized that he or she has received an overpayment, the provider is statutorily obligated to return it to Medicare. This includes instances where the provider receives an overpayment resulting from an unintended mistake on their part.

D. According to the CMS, there are three levels of supervision. General supervision means the procedure is furnished under the physician's overall direction and control, but the doctor's presence is not required during the procedure. (The physician remains responsible for training nonphysician personnel and for maintaining all necessary equipment and supplies.) Direct supervision means the physician must be present in the office suite and immediately available to furnish assistance and direction throughout the performance of a procedure. It does not mean that the physician must be present in the room when the procedure is performed. Finally personal supervision means a physician must be in attendance in the room during the performance of the procedure.

E. Whistleblowers who are discharged, demoted, suspended with or without pay, threatened, harassed or in any other manner discriminated against by their employers in the terms and conditions of employment are entitled to relief. That includes reinstatement with the same seniority, two times the amount of back pay, interest on the back pay and compensation for any damages, including attorney's fees.

922. **(B)** Don't accept anything from a clinical laboratory that you didn't pay fair market value for. OIG indicated it was aware of a number of deals between clinical laboratories and providers that could implicate the antikickback statute. When a laboratory offers or gives a referral source anything of value without receiving fair market value it can be viewed as an inducement to refer. It's also true when a potential referral source receives anything of value from the laboratory.

When permitted by state law, a laboratory can make available to a physician's office a phlebotomist who collects specimens from patients for testing by the outside laboratory. Although the simple placement of a laboratory employee in the physician's office isn't by itself necessarily an inducement forbidden by the antikickback statute, the statute does come into play when the phlebotomist performs additional tasks that are normally the responsibility of the physician's office staff. These tasks can include taking vital signs or other nursing functions, testing for the physician's office laboratory, or performing clerical services.

When the phlebotomist performs clerical or medical functions that aren't directly related to the collection or processing of laboratory specimens, OIG makes the deduction that the phlebotomist is providing a benefit in return for the physician's referrals to the laboratory. In this case, the physician, the phlebotomist and the laboratory may have exposure under the antikickback statute. This analysis also applies to the placement of phlebotomists in other health care settings, including nursing homes, clinics, and hospitals.

OIG also points out that the mere existence of a contract between a laboratory and a health care provider that prohibits the phlebotomist from performing services unrelated to specimen collection does not eliminate the concern over possible abuse, particularly if it's a situation where the phlebotomist is not closely monitored by his or her employer or where the contractual prohibition is not rigorously enforced.

923. **(B)** Stark regulations prohibit physicians from referring to an entity with which they or their immediate family members have a financial relationship for the furnishing of any of 11 designated Medicare-reimbursable health services if claims for those services are submitted to Medicare or Medicaid. Also, physicians may not bill Medicare or Medicare for such referred services. The 11 designated health services are as follows:

1. Clinical laboratory services.
2. Physical therapy services (including speech-language pathology services).
3. Occupational therapy.
4. Radiology and certain other imaging services.
5. Radiation therapy services and supplies.
6. Durable medical equipment and supplies.
7. Parenteral and enteral nutrients, equipment, and supplies.
8. Prosthetics, orthotics, prosthetic devices and supplies.
9. Home health services.
10. Outpatient prescription drugs.
11. Inpatient and outpatient hospital services (with exceptions).

A designated health service remains a designated service under Stark regulations even when it's billed as something else or bundled with other services. CMS has released an appendix to the Stark regulations detailing, by CPT and HCPCS (Healthcare Common Procedure Coding System) code, those services that are subject to the prohibition.

924. **(E)**

925. **(B)** CPT

1. Systematic listing and coding of procedures and services performed by physicians.
2. Procedure or service is accurately defined with simplified reporting.
3. Each procedure or service is identified with a five-digit code.

ICD codes classify diseases and a wide variety of signs, symptoms, abnormal findings, complaints, social circumstances, and external causes of injury or disease. Every health condition can be assigned to a unique category and given a code, up to six characters long. Such categories can include a set of similar diseases.

926. **(B)** Receptor affinity for the drug will determine the number of drug-receptor complexes formed. Efficacy is the ability of the drug to activate the receptor after binding has occurred.

Therapeutic index (TI) is related to safety of the drug. Half-life and secretion are properties of elimination and do not influence formation of drug-receptor complexes.

927. **(A)** The physician is permitted to withhold certain portions of a patient's record under limited circumstances including when the protected health information requested includes reference to another person and the physician has determined that access to the information is reasonably likely to cause substantial harm to the person who has provided the information.

Although the general rule is that a patient must be provided full access to his or her information. Certain exceptions to this rule apply in this scenario.

928. **(B)** Unless a limited exception applies, a health care provider must give a patient access to his or her records that are maintained in a designated record set. A patient is entitled to inspect and copy records that are maintained in a designated record set. A designated record set includes medical records maintained by or for the health care provider and includes any item, collection used or disseminated by or for a covered entity. There is no exception for records maintained by the provider but generated by others, and thus a provider is not permitted to withhold records held by the provider that have been created by another provider.

929. **(B)** It is a crime to offer, solicit, pay, or receive remuneration, in cash or in kind, directly or indirectly, for referrals under a federally funded health care program. The penalties of antikickback statute are

- Felony—Five years imprisonment.
- Civil penalties—$50,000 per violation.
- "One purpose" rule.
- Safe harbors—Safe harbors immunize certain payment and business practices that are implicated by the antikickback statute from criminal and civil prosecution under the statute. To be protected by a safe harbor, an arrangement must fit squarely in the safe harbor. Failure to comply with a safe harbor provision does not mean that an arrangement is *per se* illegal.

930. **(C)** Training requirements of needlestick safety include

- At no cost to employee
- During work hours
- At time of initial assignment
- Within 90 days after effective date of standard
- Within 1 year of previous training
- Shift in occupational exposure

931. **(D)** Under the Social Security Act Medicare patients have the right to submit a written request for an itemized statement to any physician, provider, supplier, or any other health care provider for any item or service provided to the patient by the provider.

After receiving a request, the provider has 30 days to furnish an itemized statement describing each item or service provided to the patient. Providers who fail to honor a request may be subject to a civil monetary penalty of $100 for each unfulfilled request. In addition, the provider may not charge the beneficiary for the itemized statements.

932. **(A)** Global fee policy is described as packaged or certain services are included in allowance for a surgical procedure. Bundling is described as combining multiple services into a single charge. Global package includes the following:

- Preoperative
- Procedure
- Postoperative

Global package does not include the following:

- Initial evaluation
- Unrelated visits
- Diagnostic test(s)
- Return trips to operating room
- Staged procedures

Global period is

- Major day prior, day of, and 90 days after
- Minor day of or day of and 10 days after

933. **(C)** Pay for performance

- Compensation incentives rest on the economic field of agency theory
  - Method of compensation induces conduct
- Compensation incentives will not induce changes in the quality of services
- Issues to consider in paying for performance:
  - How to measure quality
  - Vehicles for encouraging quality
  - What to reward
  - How to finance incentives

934. **(A)** For a service to be reasonable and necessary it must be

- Safe and effective.
- Not experimental or investigational.

- Appropriate, including the duration and frequency that is considered appropriate for the service, in terms of whether it is
  - Furnished in accordance with accepted standards of medical practice for the diagnosis or treatment of the patient's condition or to improve the function.
  - Furnished in a setting appropriate to the patient's medical needs and condition.
  - Ordered and/or furnished by qualified personnel.
  - One that meets, but does not exceed, the patient's medical need.

935. **(E)** Proper documentation summary says *never*

- Bill for items or services not rendered or not provided as claimed.
- Submit claims for equipment, medical supplies, and services that are not reasonable and necessary.
- Double bill resulting in duplicate payment.
- Bill for noncovered services as if covered.
- Knowingly misuse provider identification numbers, which results in improper billing.
- Unbundle (billing for each component of the service instead of billing or using an all-inclusive code).
- Upcode the level of service provided.

936. **(B)**

Needlestick Safety and Prevention Act of 2001—November 6, 2000
- Four areas of change
- Two terms added to definitions
- Why
  - Total of more than 600,000 needlesticks per year
  - Risk of contracting disease
  - Adverse side effects of treatments
  - Psychologic stress

Modification of definitions—area 1

- Relating to engineering controls
  - Definition: Includes all control measures that isolate or remove a hazard from the workplace.

- Examples: Blunt suture needles, plastic or Mylar wrapped capillary tubes, sharps disposal containers, and biosafety cabinets.

Modification of definitions—area 2

- Revision and updating of the exposure control plan
  - Review no less than annually
  - Reflect a new or modified task/procedure
  - Revised employee positions
  - Reflect changes in technology
  - Document consideration and/or implementation of medical devices

Modification of definitions—area 3

- Solicitation of employee input
  - Nonmanagerial employees who are responsible for direct patient care and potentially exposed to injury
  - Identification, evaluation, selection of effective engineering and work practice controls
  - Document employee solicitation in exposure control plan

Modification of definitions—area 4

- Record keeping
  - Sharps injury log
  - Type and brand of device involved
  - Department or work area of exposure incident
  - Explanation of how the incident occurred

937. **(D)** Proper medical record documentation includes the following:

- Why did the patient present for care?
- What was done?
- Where were the services rendered?
- When is the patient to return or what is the plan of action?
- Will there be follow-up tests or procedures ordered?

938. **(E)** The following are general observations about professional courtesy arrangements for physicians to consider:

- Regular or/and consistent extension of professional courtesy by waiving the entire fee for services rendered to a group of persons (including employees, physicians, or their family members) may not implicate any of OIG's fraud and abuse authorities if membership in the group receiving the courtesy is determined in a way that does not take into account directly or indirectly any group member's ability to refer to or otherwise generate federal health care program business for, the physician.

- Regular or consistent extension of professional courtesy by waiving otherwise applicable co-payments for services rendered to a group of persons (including employees, physicians, or their family members), would not implicate the antikickback statute if membership in the group is determined in a way that does not take into account directly or indirectly any group member's ability to refer to, or otherwise general federal health care program business for, the physician.

939. (B) Impairment definitions

As per *Guides to the Evaluation of Permanent Impairment*—A loss, loss of use, or derangement of any body part, organ system, or organ function.

As per WHO—Problems in body function or structure as a significant deviation or loss. Impairments of structure can involve an anomaly, defect, loss, or other significant deviation in body structures.

As per SSA—An anatomical, physiological, or psychologic abnormality that can be shown by medically acceptable clinical and laboratory diagnostic techniques.

As per State Workers' Compensation Law—Permanent impairment is any anatomic or functional loss after maximal medical improvement has been achieved and which abnormality or loss, medically, is considered stable or nonprogressive at the time of evaluation.

Permanent impairment is a basic consideration in the evaluation of permanent disability and is a contributing factor to, but not necessarily an indication of, the entire extent of permanent disability.

940. (C) Functional restoration is a comprehensive, multidisciplinary program intended primarily to correct disability in the patient with chronic low back pain who has demonstrated multiple barriers to recovery, including deconditioning, lack of motivation, psychologic dysfunction, and secondary gain issues. An interdisciplinary approach integrates physical therapy, occupational therapy, vocational rehabilitation, psychology, nursing, and the physician.

Indications

- Persistent disability despite completion of proper primary and secondary work-up and treatment
- Presence of barriers to recovery
- Deconditioning
- Lack of motivation
- Psychologic dysfunction
- Secondary gain issues
- Willingness to participate
- Willingness to comply

Elements

- Quantification of physical function
- Physical reconditioning of injured functional unit
- Work simulation and whole body coordination training
- Cognitive-behavioral disability management
- Fitness maintenance program with outcome assessment using objective criteria

Program content

- Initial medical evaluation
- Quantification of physical function
- Trunk range of motion
- Trunk strength
- Whole body task performance
- Assessment of symptom self-reports—pain and disability
- Psychologic evaluation
- Vocational assessment

Various phases of rehabilitation for functional restoration:

Initial reconditioning phase

- Focus: improving mobility, overcoming neuromuscular inhibition and pain sensitivity, and measuring cardiovascular endurance—up to 12 appointments over 4 to 6 weeks.
- Supervised stretching, aerobic, and light work simulation exercises for 2 hours twice per week.

Comprehensive phase

- 10 h/d, 5 d/wk, 3 weeks
- Vigorous stretching and aerobics classes
- Progressive resistive exercises twice a day under supervision of physical therapist
- Daily work—simulation of tasks, lifting drills, and position-tolerance training exercises similar to work hardening
- Classes on goal setting, work issues, stress management, and interpersonal skills development under direction of psychologist

941. **(B)** Sedentary work is defined as lifting 10 lb maximum, with occasional lifting or carrying of small, light objects. The work involves mostly sitting, with a small amount of walking or standing to perform job duties.

To perform light work, the employee must be able to lift up to 20 lb and carry up to 10 lb. Walking or standing may be required for significant periods of the work day. Pushing or pulling of arm or leg controls in the sitting or standing position are also classified as light work. For medium work, the employee must be able to lift 50 lb frequently and carry up to 25 lb. For heavy work, the employee must be able to lift up to 100 lb frequently and carry up to 50 lb. For very heavy work, objects more than 100 lb must be lifted and objects more than 50 lb are carried.

942. **(E)** To determine eligibility for Social Security funds, the applicant must undergo a sequential evaluation process that considers the applicant's ability to perform work despite any functional restrictions associated with physical impairment. Medical and psychologic variables are considered, along with the applicant's age, educational background, and previous work history. The applicant must undergo a medical evaluation to determine residual functional capacity. Both exertional factors (evaluation of the applicant's ability to perform work functions in several different work environments) and nonexertional factors (evaluation of the applicant's cognitive capabilities) are part of the evaluation of residual functional capacity.

943. **(A)** Purposes of rehabilitation are as follows:

To resolve deconditioning syndrome:

- Prolonged bed rest
- Flexibility
- Stiffness (loss of intrinsic muscle strength muscle strength, 10%-15% per week, 70% in 6 months)
- Cardiovascular fitness
- Disc nutrition
- Depression
- Short periods of rest between activities help to minimize the deleterious effects of inactivity

To optimize outcome by

- Restoring function
- Returning to activity
- Minimize potential recurrence or reinjury
- Rehabilitation continues beyond resolution of symptoms

To minimize need for surgical intervention:

- Failure of conservative care is the most common indication for surgery

944. **(B)** Interventional pain management-09 designation. The purpose of the designation is for

- Profiling
- Practice expense
- CAC membership

945. **(A)** The Controlled Substances Act (CSA), title 2 of the Comprehensive Drug Abuse Prevention and Control Act of 1970 is the legal foundation of the government's fight against the abuse of drugs and other substances. This law is a consolidation of numerous laws regulating the manufacture and distribution of narcotics, stimulants, depressants, hallucinogens, anabolic

steroids, and chemicals used in the illicit production of controlled substances.

All the substances that are regulated under existing federal law are placed into schedules I of the five schedules. This placement is based upon the substances' medicinal value, harmfulness, and potential for abuse or addiction.

Schedule I is reserved for the most dangerous drugs that have no recognized medical use. Schedule V is the classification used for the least dangerous drugs. The Act also provides a mechanism for substances to be controlled, added to a schedule, decontrolled, removed from control, rescheduled, or transferred from one schedule to another.

946. (C) HIPAA compliance—administrative simplification

1. Reduces costs associated with administrative and claims-related transactions
   - More than $30 billion in savings for more than 10 years.
2. Establishes a national uniform standards for eight electronic transactions, and claims attachments.
3. Established unique provider identifiers.
4. Establishes protections for the privacy and security of individual health information.
5. Implementation costs
   - More than $500 billion for more than 10 years.

947. (C) A GAO audit reported that in the United States approximately 10% of every health care dollar is lost to fraud annually:

- 10% = $100 billion of $1 trillion or $100,000 million
- In 2004—10% = $179.3 billion of $1.7934 of trillion or $1793.4 million
- By 2010—10% = $263.74 billion of $2.6374 trillion or $263,740 million

Fraud and abuse cases include 60% public and 40% private cases.

948. (D)

1. The voluntary disclosure program is designed to allow providers and others to come forward and admit health care fraud in exchange for the possibility of lenient treatment from the federal government. Providers already under investigation for fraud can also come forward to volunteer information. Making full disclosure to the investigative agency at an early stage generally benefits the individual or company, but there is no limit as to 30 days.

2. Normally, Medicare expects overpayments to be paid back in 30 days after the first demand letter. But if a lump sum refund would cause severe financial hardship, a provider can apply for an extended repayment plan (either through direct payments or deductions from the provider's future payments). For part B providers, here are the deadlines a provider may face for making payments (MCM 7160) (MIM 2224):
   - $5000 or less within 2 months
   - $5001 to $25,000 within 3 months
   - $25,001 to $100,000 within 4 months
   - $100,001 and above within 6 months

3. Regardless of their location, doctors, DME suppliers and other part B billers must make a good faith effort to collect the deductible and coinsurance payments owed by their Medicare patients—or face reimbursement cuts from CMS and possible Medicare suspension or exclusion. OIG sent out a fraud alert in 1990 targeting physicians and other suppliers who inappropriately waive co-payments or deductibles.

   The government also could hold a provider liable under the antikickback statute because routinely forgiving co-payments or deductibles may be considered an improper inducement for patients to buy Medicare items or services. Government penalties for illegal waivers can include imprisonment, criminal fines, civil damages and forfeitures, fines and exclusion from Medicare and Medicaid.

   Typically, if providers make a reasonable collection effort for coinsurance or deductibles, failure to collect payment isn't considered a reason for the carrier to reduce the charge or refer the provider to OIG or the Justice Department. A "reasonable collection effort" is one that is consistent with the effort a doctor's office typically makes to collect co-payments and deductibles. It must involve billing the patient and may include subsequent billings, collection letters, telephone calls or personal contacts, depending on the provider's usual practice. These efforts must be genuine, not token, collection efforts. A provider should check to see whether its local carrier or intermediary has defined a fair effort to collect, for instance, three bills in 120 days.

4. The OIG has identified eight elements of a civil money penalties offense:

- Any person
- Presents or causes to be presented
- To the United States or an agent of the United States
- A Claim
- For an item or service
- Not provided as claimed
- Which the person knows or has reason to know was not provided as claimed
- Materiality

CHAPTER 15

Rehabilitation
Questions

DIRECTIONS (Questions 949 through 964): Each of the numbered items or incomplete statements in this section is followed by answers or by completions of the statement. Select the ONE lettered answer or completion that is BEST in each case.

949. The Henneman size principle of therapeutic exercise says motor units are recruited in order of

    (A) increasing size, decreasing contraction strength, and diminishing fatigue

    (B) increasing size, increasing contraction strength, and diminishing fatigue

    (C) increasing size, increasing contraction strength, and escalating fatigue

    (D) decreasing size, increasing contraction strength, and diminishing fatigue

    (E) none of the above

950. What is an example of an open kinetic chain exercise?

    (A) Leg press

    (B) Knee extensions

    (C) Push up

    (D) Treadmill

    (E) Bench press

951. Which type of therapy has been found to reduce the risk of falls in the elderly?

    (A) Tai chi

    (B) Pilates

    (C) Yoga

    (D) Strength training

    (E) None of the above

952. Direct participants in interdisciplinary comprehensive pain management include all of the following, EXCEPT

    (A) vocational counselor

    (B) physical therapist

    (C) psychologist

    (D) general internal medicine physician

    (E) occupational therapist

953. Which of the following is true regarding aerobic training?

    (A) Persons placed on bedrest will experience a decrease in resting heart rate

    (B) Oxygen consumption (Vo_2) increases in proportion to the intensity of the exercise

    (C) For training to be effective, the duration of aerobic training must be at least 10 minutes at a stretch

    (D) Intensity of training must be within 40% to 85% of maximal Vo_2 (Vo_2 max) to be considered aerobic training

    (E) Patients placed at bedrest will experience an increase of Vo_2 max after 3 weeks.

954. All of the following are examples of core strengthening programs for spine rehabilitation, EXCEPT

    (A) lumbar stabilization

    (B) pilates training

    (C) yoga

    (D) abdominal exercises

    (E) all of the above

955. A typical exercise precaution that should be followed with a patient who has chronic osteoarthritis would be

(A) no exercise in patients with osteoarthritis of three or more joints

(B) no weight bearing on a limb with knee pain of 2 years' duration

(C) no ice when knee effusion occurs after exercise

(D) only low-impact exercises in a patient with severe osteoarthritis of both knees awaiting joint replacement surgery

(E) no stretching of a lower limb in a patient with osteoarthritis of the ankle who has a tight calf muscle

956. A patient presents to your office with T6 paraplegia. He was living independently until severity of neuropathic pain in his legs increased to 10/10. Now he can no longer go to work because the pain is so severe that he cannot concentrate at work. The fact that this patient cannot work is considered as

(A) impairment

(B) disability

(C) handicap

(D) physical capacity

(E) none of the above

957. A patient presents to the office with 2-week history of leg pain consistent with S1 radiculopathy. Magnetic resonance imaging (MRI) reveals a paracentral L5-S1 disc herniation. The pain is worsened with bending forward, driving, and lifting objects. A proper type of physical therapy exercise would be

(A) McKenzie method of physical therapy with extension exercises

(B) yoga

(C) Williams method of physical therapy with flexion exercises

(D) stationary bike

(E) no therapy

958. Which of the following is false regarding muscle tightness in the lower extremity?

(A) Gluteus maximus inflexibility may decrease lumbar lordosis causing increased forces on the lumbar spine

(B) The Ely test evaluates rectus femoris tightness

(C) Lumbar lordosis can be increased in iliopsoas tightness

(D) Anterior pelvic tilt may cause stress on the lumbar spine and can be caused by rectus femoris or hamstring tightness

(E) The Thomas test assesses tightness of the iliopsoas muscle

959. Which of the following statements regarding central pain is not correct?

(A) Patients with central pain are usually affected by a change in temperature

(B) More than 10% of patients with a stroke report significant central pain within the first year

(C) Central pain caused by a thalamic infarction is often a burning pain that may be described as agonizing and is on the side contralateral to the lesion

(D) Almost 90% of all central pain is caused by cerebral vascular accidents

(E) No singular pharmacologic, surgical or other treatment has been proven to be helpful in the long term

960. Achilles tendinosis is a chronic source of pain in many active adults. Which of the following interventions has been found to be helpful in the treatment of pain for this disease process?

(A) Nonsteriodal anti-inflammatory drugs

(B) Corticosteroid injections of the tendon

(C) Heel pads

(D) Topical laser therapy

(E) Ultrasonography

961. Chronic pain from fibromyalgia is characterized by the following statements, EXCEPT

(A) fibromyalgia affects women more often than men

(B) there is a suggestion that genetic factors contribute to the etiology of fibromyalgia

(C) mood and anxiety disorders are significant comorbidities in fibromyalgia

(D) patients with fibromyalgia may experience a range of other symptoms including irritable bowel or bladder syndromes

(E) cognitive disturbances are never part of fibromyalgia and suggest that there is an organic cause for the problem

962. The use of physical therapy that includes "directional preference" in the treatment of low back pain has not been shown to

(A) decrease the need for surgery
(B) decrease the use of medications
(C) be associated with greater improvements in pain control
(D) be as good as intensive dynamic strengthening
(E) be better than nondirectional exercises

963. Evaluation and treatment of anterior knee pain that is insidious in onset, bilateral, peripatellar, and most often problematic in repetitive load-bearing movements includes all the following, EXCEPT

(A) hamstring strengthening
(B) activity modification
(C) closed chain kinetic exercises
(D) patellar taping
(E) evaluation for apophysitis at the tibial tuberosity in adolescents

964. Which of the following is true regarding phantom limb sensations?

(A) Body parts that are sparsely innervated are most commonly represented
(B) Phantom sensations are unpleasant with burning and jabbing
(C) The incidence of phantom sensations decreases with age.
(D) The amputated limb phantom may feel shortened
(E) Phantom limb sensations require peripheral input

DIRECTIONS: For Question 965 through 979, ONE or MORE of the numbered options is correct. Choose answer

(A) if only answer 1, 2, and 3 are correct
(B) if only 1 and 3 are correct
(C) if only 2 and 4 are correct
(D) if only 4 is correct
(E) if all are correct

965. Which of the following physical examination maneuvers are not found to correlate with sacroiliac joint pain as confirmed by pain ablation with diagnostic injection with lidocaine under fluoroscopy, with at least 90% specificity?

(1) Patrick test
(2) Gaenslen test
(3) Compression test
(4) Distraction tests

966. In pain management, tissue structures are warmed via which of the following mechanism(s)?

(1) Conduction
(2) Convection
(3) Conversion
(4) Radiation

967. The SAID principle (specific adaptation to imposed demand) of therapeutic exercise for pain management includes the following:

(1) Stronger muscles develop with strength training
(2) Oxidative capacities of skeletal muscle decrease with aerobic training
(3) Pliability of connective tissue increases with flexibility exercises
(4) Circulation to the brain increases with aerobic training

968. Strength training consists of which type(s) of muscle contraction?

(1) Isometric
(2) Isotonic
(3) Isokinetic
(4) Isoconcentric

969. Which of these statements is (are) true regarding lumbosacral (LSO) supports?

(1) There was moderate evidence that LSO supports were effective for primary low back pain prevention

(2) There was moderate evidence that LSO supports were ineffective for primary low back pain prevention

(3) Lumbar supports are less effective in reducing back pain than no treatment

(4) Lumbar supports are more effective in reducing back pain than no treatment

970. A comprehensive, inpatient chronic pain treatment program advertises that they are CARF accredited treatment center. CARF is

(1) Commission on Activity with Rehabilitation Focus

(2) a certification for centers to show that they have better outcomes for pain reduction

(3) a certification for centers to show that they have better outcomes for return to work

(4) the rehabilitation accreditation commission

971. Which of these statements regarding exercise is false?

(1) Several studies indicate an increase in all-cause mortality with long-term regular exercise participation

(2) Physical activity is considered a major risk factor for the development of cardiovascular disease

(3) Both acute and chronic exercise can increase blood pressure in the long-term

(4) Most studies indicate that aerobic exercise training increases plasma triglycerides and may lower high-density lipoprotein (HDL) cholesterol

972. Physical effects of aquatic therapy include

(1) increase in cardiac output

(2) decrease in stroke volume

(3) offloading of immersed joints

(4) increased psychological stress due the aquatic exercise

973. The use of muscle relaxants in the rehabilitation of acute and chronic pain is common. Which of the following statements is (are) true regarding these drugs?

(1) Baclofen is a γ-aminobutyric acid analogue

(2) The active metabolite of cyclobenzaprine is meprobamate, which is a schedule intravenous controlled substance

(3) Tizanidine has been shown to be helpful in treating low back pain in several studies

(4) Skeletal muscle relaxants, like metaxalone and cyclobenzaprine, exert their effects directly on the muscle contractile mechanism in skeletal muscle

974. In acute musculoskeletal injury, which of the following is (are) direct effect(s) of using cold as a modality for treatment?

(1) Relieve pain

(2) Increase tissue repair

(3) Reduce hemorrhage

(4) Decrease risk of chromic pain

975. The following types of pain syndromes have been found to consistently respond to treatment with botulinum toxin A:

(1) Myofascial pain

(2) Chronic low back pain

(3) Headache

(4) Tennis elbow

976. Which of the following has been validated as effective in the treatment of neck pain?

(1) Soft collar

(2) Massage

(3) Cervical traction, mechanical traction

(4) Therapeutic exercises

977. In the treatment of a patient diagnosed with fibromyalgia syndrome, there is not a clear consensus on most therapies. Which of the following is (are) true regarding therapies for fibromyalgia?

(1) Ultrasound and massage are effective treatments for the deep muscle aches of fibromyalgia

(2) Recreational therapy can be an important aspect of return to socialization

(3) Occupational therapy is less likely to help return a patient to function than other forms of therapy

(4) Aerobic exercise is probably the most important therapeutic treatment for fibromyalgia

978. Which of the following regarding heat and cold therapies for pain is (are) true?

(1) Both heat and cold have direct effects on the muscle spindle

(2) Heat and cold are safe modalities and should be used extensively in the long term to get the best relief in chronic pain

(3) Both heat and cold can be helpful in treatment of muscle spasm

(4) Transcutaneous electrical nerve stimulation (TENS) has been consistently shown to be helpful in treating chronic muscle pains

979. Which of the following is (are) true regarding the treatment and rehabilitation of lateral epicondylitis (LE)?

(1) The use of extra corporeal shock wave therapy in LE has been validated and should be used early on in the disease process for best results

(2) Counterforce bracing in LE is a common treatment and has consistently been found to be of use

(3) Cold therapy has been found to be a helpful adjunct to treatment of LE

(4) Poor prognosis for recovery and return of function has been found with employment in manual jobs

Answers and Explanations

949. (C) Smaller, less powerful, fatigue resistant motor units, which contain slow-twitch muscle fibers, have the lowest firing threshold and are recruited first. Demands for larger forces are met by the recruitment of increasingly larger, more powerful, fatigable motor units. The largest motor units that contain the fast-twitch B fibers have the highest threshold and are recruited last.

950. (B) Open kinetic chain exercises are typically performed where the foot/leg or hand/arm is free to move, and non-weight bearing, with the movement occurring at the peripheral joint. Examples of these exercises would be knee extensions, straight leg raises, and biceps curl. In closed kinetic chain (CKC) exercise, the distal part of the limb-upper or lower, is fixed to the ground or to the wall or plate. Examples include leg press, push up, and running exercises. In bench press, the foot is on the floor so this too is a CKC exercise. CKC exercises are felt to be more "functional", since these exercises may mimic what patients do throughout the day or in an employment setting and thus are often favored. However, a mix of both types of exercises typically recommended.

951. (A)

A. Tai chi is an internal Chinese martial art often practiced with the aim of promoting health and longevity. Training consists of slow motion routines that groups of people practice together every morning in parks around the world, particularly in China. Many medical studies support its effectiveness as an alternative exercise and a form of martial arts therapy. Tai chi improves balance in persons of all ages.

B. Pilates is a physical fitness system developed in the early 20th century by Joseph Pilates. Pilates called his method "contrology," because he believed his method uses the mind to control the muscles. The program focuses on the core postural muscles which helps keep the body balanced and which are essential for providing support for the spine.

C. Yoga is a group of ancient spiritual practices originating in India. Yoga involves flexibility exercise combined with strength training, but also traditional chants and relaxation techniques that relax the mind and the body.

D. Strength training has been found to be effective in elderly patients but does not specifically reduce falls.

952. (D) While a family physician is important to provide medical information to the team, the team leader is most often a physician with sub-specialty qualifications in pain management. The team consists of professionals from a variety of therapeutic groups that work together with the patient to help them improve their function and manage their chronic pain. All of the above except the primary care physician can readily be found among the interdisciplinary team.

953. (D) When placed at bedrest, many detrimental changes occur to the cardiovascular system. People placed on bedrest will experience an increase in resting heart rate. Oxygen consumption (Vo_2) decreases in proportion to the intensity of the exercise. Patients will experience a 25% decrease in Vo_2 max after 3 weeks of bedrest. Additionally, during bedrest muscle breakdown occurs, osteoporosis occurs, and joint contractures can set in. Therefore, during acute pain episodes, it is imperative that patients are encouraged not to lie in bed for 24 hours.

954. (C)

A. Lumbar stabilization is a type of exercise that attempts to strengthen muscles in the abdomen and posterior spine (multifidus) by cocontracting the muscles in a position of "neutral spine." Neutral spine is a position where the spine hurts the least so exercise can take place.

B. Pilates is an exercise designed by Joseph Pilates to use machines to assist with strengthening of muscles of the abdomen and spine—the core muscles.

C. Yoga is an exercise of the mind and body. Positions are attempted that achieve maximum body stretch and relaxation. Strengthening is not a part of the program.

D. Abdominal muscles are part of the core. The core defined as muscles between the chest (nipple line) and the waist.

955. (D) The exercise program in patients with osteoarthritis must be adjusted to their tolerance level. Many patients are functionally impaired, obese, and are at high risk for developing medical complications such as type-2 diabetes or cardiovascular disease because of their inactivity. Thus, even if a patient is awaiting joint replacement because of chronic pain from osteoarthritis a period of physical activity before their surgery is warranted. Often protected weight-bearing, low-impact exercises, or exclusively aquatic exercises can allow the patient to tolerate sessions of physical therapy they otherwise could not tolerate.

956. (C)

A. The American Medical Association *Guides to the Evaluation of Permanent Impairment* define impairment as "a loss, loss of use, or derangement of any body part, organ system, or organ function." Thus in this case, the impairment would be the T6 injury.

B. The American Medical Association *Guides to the Evaluation of Permanent Impairment* define disability as "an alteration of an individual's capacity to meet personal, social, or occupational demands or statutory or regulatory requirements because of an impairment." Thus, the inability to walk would be a disability. Another example might be a finger injury. A lawyer might have no vocational disability but a pianist might have 100% disability from the same impairment.

C. Impairment is the functional consequence of the disability. Thus the inability to work, play a sport, or pay the rent would all be disabled.

D. Physical capacity is just the capacity of the body to operate.

957. (A)

A. Although individualized exercises also are performed, McKenzie exercises are most well known as a set of spinal extension exercises. The goal is to off-load the disk compression on the spinal nerve and reduce the pain in the leg. Often the pain "centralizes" to the lower back where is can be improved by other therapy methods. Although often practiced, little is written and even fewer studies have been performed to prove the effectiveness of the therapy. The study referenced above found improvement in leg pain in the short term (0-3 months) compared to other treatments but after 3 month, the benefit was no longer seen.

B. Yoga is a form of exercise where bending forward often occurs. This might worsen the symptoms. For chronic back pain, yoga has been found to be effective in a recent study.

C. Williams exercises are a set of flexion based exercises. Persons with acute paracentral disc herniations might get worse leg pain with flexion-type exercises. Flexion spine exercises can be beneficial in cases of stenosis or lateral disc herniations where flexion can result in offloading of neural structures.

D. Stationary bike is a flexion exercise. This can result in more pressure on the disc increasing the leg pain.

Although some studies suggest that physical therapy has no effect on painful disc herniations, many other studies find that therapy has a significant beneficial effect.

958. (D)

  A. Gluteus medius and hamstring inflexibility can lead to posterior pelvic tilt, decreasing lumbar lordosis.
  B. The Ely test evaluates the rectus femoris.
  C. Rectus femoris and iliopsoas tightness can cause anterior pelvic tilt, increasing lumbar lordosis.
  D. Increasing or decreasing lumbar lordosis can put stress on the lumbar spine.
  E. The Thomas test evaluates for iliopsoas muscle tightness while the Ely test evaluates the rectus femoris.

959. (B) Ninety percent of all cases of central pain are caused by cerebral vascular accidents but only 8% of all stroke patients will report central pain within the first year. The pain may be constant (85%) or intermittent (15%) and is primarily burning, prickling, aching, and lancinating. Thalamic strokes cause agonizing burning pain contralateral to the side of the lesion. Central pain is almost always affected by change in temperature and no one treatment has been found to be efficacious in the long term.

960. (A) Despite the controversy over the presence or lack of inflammation in Achilles tendonosis, there is weak evidence to support the use of oral nonsteroidal drugs for pain control. On the other hand there is weak evidence of lack of effect for heel pads, topical laser, heparin injections, and peritendinous corticosteroid injections. There is no well-designed study confirming the efficacy of ultrasound in treatment of this disease. Eccentric loading has been shown to be helpful.

961. (E) Fibromyalgia affects about 2% of the general population, affecting 3.4% of women and 0.5% of men. The symptoms include sleep disturbances, stiffness, anxiety, depression, cognitive disturbances, irritable bowel and bladder syndromes, headaches, paresthesias, and other less common symptoms. Fibromyalgia aggregates in families and congregates with major mood disorders in families, suggesting genetic factors may be involved in the etiology of fibromyalgia.

962. (A) McKenzie based exercises are often called directionally based exercises and have been thought to be better than regular physical therapy in the treatment of low back pain. Not all studies have agreed. Several large studies have evaluated this paradigm. In one case, intensive dynamic strengthening was found to be as good as the McKenzie method for treatment of subacute and chronic low back pain. Another large study showed directional preference exercises can decrease medication consumption by three-folds and give rapid significant pain control when compared to nondirectional therapy and opposite directional therapy. No study has evaluated the use of directional therapy in avoiding surgery.

963. (A) Patellofemoral pain syndrome (PFPS) is usually insidious in onset and often bilateral. It is most often associated with load-bearing exercises and repetition of the exercise. It is relatively benign, but in adolescents, one must consider the presence of a traction apophysitis of the tibial tuberosity. Closed kinetic chain exercises, patellar taping, and activity modification along with nonsteroidal anti-inflammatory drugs are the mainstays of treatment. Strengthening of the vastus medialis obliquus and other quadriceps muscles are important in the treatment and not strengthening of the hamstrings.

964. (D) Phantom limb sensation is an almost universal occurrence at some time during the first month following surgery.

  A. The strongest sensations come from body parts with the highest brain cortical representation, such as the fingers and toes. These highly innervated parts are also the areas of most persistent phantom limb sensation.
  B. Phantom sensations are either normal in character or as pleasant warmth and tingling. These are not painful.
  C. The incidence of phantom limb sensation increases with the age of the amputee. In children who have amputation before 2 years of age, the incidence of phantom limb sensation is 20%; the incidence of phantom limb sensation is nearly 100% when amputation occurs after 8 years of age.

D. The phantom limb may undergo the phenomenon known as telescoping, in which the patient loses sensations from the mid portion of the limb, with subsequent shortening of the phantom. Telescoping is most common in the upper extremity. During telescoping, the last body parts to disappear are those with the highest representation in the cortex, such as the thumb, index finger, and big toe. Only painless phantoms undergo telescoping, and lengthening of the phantom may occur if the pain returns. Thus, patients may feel that the amputated phantom limb shortened.

E. Phantom limb sensations do not appear to require peripheral nervous system input. Phantom limb sensations may be an attempt to preserve the self image and minimize distortion of the self image or may be a permanent inherited neural memory of postural patterns.

965. **(E)** Multiple published studies and meta-analysis of studies has found that the highest level of sensitivity and specificity for any physical examination test is 60%. The specific tests are as follows:

1. Patrick test—The hip is externally rotated, the foot is placed on the opposite knee, and gentle pressure is applied to the foot and ipsilateral anterior superior iliac spine (ASIS). Pain can then occur in either of the affected sacroiliac joint. Also called the flexion, abduction, and external rotation (FABER).

2. The goal of the Gaenslen test is to apply torsion to the joint. With one hip flexed onto the abdomen, the other leg is allowed to dangle off the edge of the table. Pressure should then be directed downward on the leg in order to achieve hip extension and stress the sacroiliac joint.

3. Apply compression to the joint with the patient lying on his or her side. Pressure is applied downwards to the uppermost iliac crest (iliac compression test).

4. Distraction can be performed to the anterior sacroiliac ligaments by applying pressure to the anterior superior iliac spine (iliac gapping test).

966. **(A)**

1. Conduction is the transfer of heat from on surface to another directly. Examples include heat packs or paraffin.

2. Convection in the most general terms refers to the movement of currents within fluids (ie, liquids, gases, and rheids). This would suggest movement of air or water across body surfaces. Examples include hydrotherapy or fluidotherapy.

3. Conversion is the transfer of heat via a change in energy which occurs with ultrasound, infrared lamps, and microwave treatments.

4. Radiation is energy in the form of waves or moving subatomic particles but is not used in therapy for pain management.

967. **(B)**

1. Many studies show muscle hypertrophy does occur with specific strength training.

2. Oxidative capacities of skeletal muscle increase with aerobic training.

3. Stretching exercises work to enhance flexibility and reduce stress on painful areas.

4. Brain function is not part of the SAID principle.

968. **(A)**

1. Isometric exercise refers to contraction that does not result in movement at the joint. Often these exercises are used in the acute injury setting when movement of the joint or spine causes extreme pain increase.

2. Isotonic exercise refers to an equivalent amount of weight being lifted throughout the range of motion (ROM) of the joint when contracting the muscle. This is the "traditional" exercise strength training that patients and nonpatients participate in. Machines such as nautilus or free weights may be used.

3. Isokinetic exercise or "equal speed" exercise is when the speed of movement remains constant. This goal is for maximum tension to be applied throughout the entire ROM of the joint/muscle contraction. Machines must be used for this type of exercise.

4. Concentric exercise is a shortening contraction—all three of the above exercises are examples of concentric exercise.

969. **(C)** The Cochrane back review systematically examined 13 trials. Five were randomized preventative trials. Two were nonrandomized trials. Six were randomized therapeutic trials. There was moderate evidence that LSO supports were ineffective for primary low back pain prevention. Although there was limited evidence that LSO supports were more effective than no treatment, there was no evidence that LSO supports were better than other treatments for low back pain.

970. **(D)** CARF (Commission on Accreditation of Rehabilitation Facilities) accredits a rehabilitation center if those services meet the standards outlined in the CARF standards manual. The CARF accreditation process certifies that the center meets the highest standards of quality but does not discuss or look at patient outcomes. A CARF accredited center meets certain minimum criteria set out to ensure that patients receive quality care expected in an interdisciplinary rehabilitation center.

971. **(E)**

1. Several studies indicate a decrease in all-cause mortality with long-term, regular exercise participation.
2. Physical inactivity is considered a major risk factor for the development of cardiovascular diseases.
3. Both acute and chronic exercise can decrease blood pressure in the long term.
4. Most studies indicate that aerobic exercise training decreases plasma triglycerides and may increase HDL cholesterol.

972. **(B)**

1. Water immersion results in lowering the pressure in the venous and lymphatic side of the circulatory system. This results in increased central venous pressure and right atrial distension. Thus with increase in central blood volume, the atrial pressure rises, the pulmonary arterial pressure rises, and the cardiac

volume increases. These changes all lead to an increase in stroke volume and increase in cardiac output with aquatic exercise.
2. Stroke volume increases with aquatic exercise.
3. As the body immerses in water, the water is displaced, creating a progressive off-loading of the immersed joints. A person who is immersed up to the pelvis has effectively offloaded 40% of their body weight. This allows the patient with chronic pain who may not have been able to exercise because of severe joint pain to exercise for a much longer period of time and in an upright position. It is hoped that the gains seen in the water can translate to the land.
4. The exercise program decreases stress on the mind and the body alike.

973. **(B)**

1. Baclofen is a γ-aminobutyric acid agonist analog, and it inhibits synaptic transmission in the spinal cord.
2. The active metabolite of carisoprodol, not cyclobenzaprine, is meprobamate, which is a schedule IV controlled substance.
3. Several studies have shown the efficacy of tizanidine in patients with musculoskeletal back pain with drowsiness being the main reason for discontinuation.
4. Skeletal muscle relaxants are poorly named as they have little or no effect on the skeletal muscle contractile mechanism.

974. **(B)** In acute musculoskeletal injuries cold is often used as part of the PRICE (protection, rest, ice, compression, and elevation) method. The effects of cold applied directly to the site of injury are to reduce hemorrhage and vasodilation, decrease local inflammatory response and edema, and to reduce pain. It may also decrease spasm associated with the injury.

975. **(C)** Studies on the use of botulinum toxin A (BTX-A) have been performed for the treatment of multiple problems in pain management. Most of the trials have been open label. The trials for myofascial pain and headaches have been mixed. Some of the discrepancies may have been regarding dosing and injection site. There

is no clear consensus for or against the use of BTX-A in either disease. Open label studies on chronic low back pain have been small but do seem to have a positive effect. A small report in 1999 showed efficacy of BTX-A in tennis elbow, but little further research has addressed this.

976. **(D)** In 2001, The Philadelphia Panel for Evidence Based Clinical Practice Guidelines on Selected Rehabilitation Interventions for Neck Pain reported on treatments for neck pain using the methods defined by the Cochrane collaboration. They found no evidence to include or exclude the use of thermotherapy, massage, electrical stimulation, mechanical cervical traction, and biofeedback in the treatment of neck pain. They did find that the only treatment with clinically important benefits was therapeutic exercises. Other studies have not found any benefit to any type of cervical orthosis for the treatment of neck pain.

977. **(C)**

1. Active, not passive, treatments have been found to be occasionally helpful in treatment of fibromyalgia. Passive treatments such as ultrasound, diathermy, and/or massage have no long-lasting benefit.

2. Often, recreational therapy is important to get the patient to move more freely and begin enjoying things again.

3. Occupational therapy can help optimize ergonomics gait, work, sleep, and play postures. As such they are very helpful in returning to functional activities.

4. Aerobic activity is the cornerstone of treatment for fibromyalgia. At least 20 minutes per day are recommended. The exact mechanism of its effectiveness is as of now unclear.

978. **(B)**

1. and 3. Pain from muscle spasms can be treated by affecting the muscle spindle. Spindle firing rates are affected by both heat and cold. These changes are both direct and indirect. Use of these modalities may help the muscle return to its normal resting length, but the precise mechanism of alleviating muscle spasm is still under investigation.

2. Heat and cold should be used with caution and to a limited extent in the rehabilitation of a chronic pain state.

4. Studies of TENS, acupuncture, and cold laser have left questions about their usefulness in reducing discomfort associated with chronic pain.

979. **(D)**

1. Extra corporeal shock wave therapy has had conflict reports of efficacy by a Cochrane review.

2. Counterforce bracing is the application of a non-elastic strap that supports the forearm in patients with LE. While some studies have shown efficacy in the treatment of LE, others have not.

3. A meta-analysis of all therapy modalities showed no evidence for long-term benefit for any physical modality.

4. Poor prognosis has been associated with high level of strain at work, high level of baseline pain, keyboarding, highly repetitive monotonous work, and manual jobs.

Suggested Reading

Chapter 2 [Pain Physiology]

Dougherty PM & Raja SN. Neurochemistry of somatosensory and pain processing. In: Benzon HT, Raja SN, Borsook D, Molloy RE, Strichartz G, eds. *Essentials of Pain Medicine and Regional Anesthesia.* 2nd ed. Philadelphia, PA: Elsevier Churchill-Livingstone; 2005:7-9.

Furst S. Transmitters involved in antinociception in the spinal cord—an analysis of descending and ascending pathways. *Brain Res Bull.* 1999;48(2):129-141(13).

Gohil K, Bell JR, Ramachandran J, Miljanich GP. Neuroanatomical distribution of receptors for a novel voltage-sensitive calcium channel antagonist, SNX-230 (ω-conopeptide MVIIC). *Brain Res.* 1994; 653:258-266.

Heavner JE, Willis ED. Pain pathways—anatomy and physiology. In: Raj PP, ed. *Practical Management of Pain.* 3rd ed. St. Louis, MO: Mosby; 2000:107-116.

Inturrisi CE, Jessel TM, Kelly TD. Pain and analgesia. In: Kandel ER, Schwartz JH, Jessell TM, eds. *Principles of Neuroscience.* 3rd ed. New York, NY: Elsevier; 1991.

Inturrisi CE. The role of N-methyl-D-aspartate (NMDA) receptors in pain and morphine tolerance. *Minerva Anestesiol.* 2005;71(7-8):401-403.

Kerr LM, Filloux F, Olivera BM, Jackson H, Wamsley JK. Autoradiographic localization of calcium channels with [125I] ω-conotoxin in rat brain. *Eur J Pharmacol.* 1988;146:181-183.

Li J, Simone DA, Larson AA. Windup leads to characteristics of central sensitization. *Pain.* 1999;79(1): 75-82.

McMahon SB, Koltzenburg M, eds. *Wall and Melzack's Textbook of Pain.* 5th ed. Philadelphia, PA: Elsevier Churchill-Livingstone; 2006.

Nassar MA, Stirling LC, Forlani A, et al. Nociceptor-specific gene deletion reveals a major role for Nav1.7 (PN1) in acute and inflammatory pain. *Proc Natl Acad Sci U S A.* 2004;101(34):12706-12711.

Petrenko AB, Yamakura T, Baba H, Shimoji K. The role of N-methyl-D-aspartate receptors (NMDARs) in pain: a review. *Anesth Analg.* 2003;97(4): 1108-1116.

Rauck RL, Wallace MS, Leong MS, et al. A randomized, double-blind, placebo-controlled study of intrathecal ziconotide in adults with severe chronic pain. *J Pain Symptom Manage.* 2006;31(5): 393-406.

Snutch TP. Targeting chronic and neuropathic pain: the N-type calcium channel comes of age. *NeuroRx.* 2005;2(4):662-670.

Tiengo MA, ed. *Neuroscience: Focus on Acute and Chronic Pain.* Springer-Verlag Italia; 2001. Gullo A, ed. *Topics in Anesthesia and Critical Care.*

Yaksh TL. Anatomy of the pain processing system. In: Waldman SD, ed. *Interventional Pain Management.* 2nd ed. Philadelphia, PA: W. B. Saunders; 2001: 11-20.

Yamakage M, Namiki A. Calcium channels—basic aspects of their structure, function and gene encoding; anesthetic action on the channels—a review. *Can J Anaesth.* 2002;49:151-164.

Chapter 3 [Pain Pathophysiology]

Bennetto L, Patel NK, Fuller G. Trigeminal neuralgia and its management. *BMJ.* 2007;334(7586): 201-205.

Body JJ. Breast cancer: bisphosphonate therapy for metastatic bone disease. *Clin Cancer Res.* 2006;12(20, pt 2):6258s-6263s.

Buchser E, Durrer A, Albrecht E. Spinal cord stimulation for the management of refractory angina pectoris. *J Pain Symptom Manage.* 2006;31(suppl 4): S36-S42.

Burbank KM, Stevenson JH, Czarnecki GR, Dorfman J. Chronic shoulder pain: part I. Evaluation and diagnosis. *Am Fam Physician.* 2008; 77(4):453-460.

Calmbach WL, Hutchens M. Evaluation of patients presenting with knee pain: part II. Differential diagnosis. *Am Fam Physician.* 2003;68(5):917-922.

Cohen SP, Raja SN. Pathogenesis, diagnosis, and treatment of lumbar zygapophysial (facet) joint pain. *Anesthesiology.* 2007;106(3):591-614.

Dworkin RH, Gnann JW Jr, Oaklander AL, Raja SN, Schmader KE, Whitley RJ. Diagnosis and assessment of pain associated with herpes zoster and postherpetic neuralgia. *J Pain.* 2008;9(1)(suppl 1):S37-S44.

Eisendrath SJ. Psychiatric aspects of chronic pain. *Neurology.* 1995;45(12) (suppl 9):S26-S34.

Evans S, Moalem-Taylor G, Tracey DJ. Pain and endometriosis. *Pain.* 2007;132 (suppl 1):S22-S25.

Farquhar C. Endometriosis. *BMJ.* 2007;334(7587): 249-253.

Fink E, Brenner G. Functional neuroanatomy and physiology of nociception. In: Loeser JD, ed. *Bonica's Management of Pain.* 4th ed. Philadelphia, PA: Lippincott Williams & Wilkins. In press.

Fink E, Oaklander AL. Diabetic neuropathy. *Pain Management Rounds.* 2005;2(3):1-6.

Illis LS. Central pain. *BMJ.* 1990;300(6735):1284-1286.

Jänig W, Baron R. Complex regional pain syndrome: mystery explained? *Lancet Neurol.* 2003;2(11):687-697.

Jung BF, Ahrendt GM, Oaklander AL, Dworkin RH. Neuropathic pain following breast cancer surgery: proposed classification and research update. *Pain.* 2003;104(1-2):1-13.

Kass SM, Williams PM, Reamy BV. Pleurisy. *Am Fam Physician.* 2007;75(9):1357-1364.

MacEvilly M, Buggy D. Back pain and pregnancy: a review. *Pain.* 1996;64(3):405-414.

Martin RF, Rossi RL. The acute abdomen. An overview and algorithms. *Surg Clin North Am.* 1997;77(6):1227-1243.

Meeus M, Nijs J. Central sensitization: a biopsychosocial explanation for chronic widespread pain in patients with fibromyalgia and chronic fatigue syndrome. *Clin Rheumatol.* 2007;26(4):465-473.

Miele VJ, Price KO, Bloomfield S, Hogg J, Bailes JE. A review of intrathecal morphine therapy related granulomas. *Eur J Pain.* 2006;10(3):251-261.

Mohammed I, Hussain A. Abrupt withdrawal from intrathecal baclofen: recognition and management of a potentially life-threatening syndrome. *Arch Phys Med Rehabil.* 2002;83(6):735-741.

Müller W, Schneider EM, Stratz T. The classification of fibromyalgia syndrome. *Rheumatol Int.* 2007;27(11):1005-1010.

Nair RJ, Lawler L, Miller MR. Chronic pancreatitis. *Am Fam Physician.* 2007;76(11):1679-1688.

Ossipov MH, Lai J, King T, Vanderah TW, Porreca F. Underlying mechanisms of pronociceptive consequences of prolonged morphine exposure. *Biopolymers.* 2005;80(2-3):319-24.

Sanchez-Del-Rio M, Reuter U, Moskowitz MA. New insights into migraine pathophysiology. *Curr Opin Neurol.* 2006;19(3):294-298.

Schofferman J, Reynolds J, Herzog R, Covington E, Dreyfuss P, O'Neill C. Failed back surgery: etiology and diagnostic evaluation. *Spine J.* 2003;3(5): 400-403.

Siccoli MM, Bassetti CL, Sándor PS. Facial pain: clinical differential diagnosis. *Lancet Neurol.* 2006;5(3):257-267.

Suresh E. Diagnosis of early rheumatoid arthritis: what the non-specialist needs to know. *J R Soc Med.* 2004;97(9):421-424.

Tallia AF, Cardone DA. Diagnostic and therapeutic injection of the ankle and foot. *Am Fam Physician.* 2003;68(7):1356-1362.

van Tulder M, Malmivaara A, Koes B. Repetitive strain injury. *Lancet.* 2007;369(9575):1815-1822.

Wang SM, Kain ZN, White PF. Acupuncture analgesia: II. Clinical considerations. *Anesth Analg.* 2008;106(2):611-621.

Wilbourn AJ. Thoracic outlet syndromes. *Neurol Clin.* 1999;17(3):477-497.

Wolfe F, Smythe HA, Yunus MB, et al. The American College of Rheumatology 1990 criteria for the classification of fibromyalgia. Report of the multicenter criteria committee. *Arthritis Rheum.* 1990;33(2): 160-172.

Woolf CJ. Dissecting out mechanisms responsible for peripheral neuropathic pain: implications for diagnosis and therapy. *Life Sci.* 2004;74(21):2605-2610.

Yale SH, Nagib N, Guthrie T. Approach to the vaso-occlusive crisis in adults with sickle cell disease. *Am Fam Physician.* 2000;61(5):1349-1356,1363-1364.

Chapter 5 [Diagnosis of Pain States]

Almekinders LC, ed. Knee injuries. *Soft Tissue Injuries in Sports Medicine.* 1996:244-289.

Boulton AJM, Malik RA. Diabetic neuropathy. *Med Clin North Am.* 1998;82(4):909-929.

Boureau F, Doubrere JF, Luu M. Study of verbal description in neuropathic pain. *Pain.* 1990;42:145-152.

Brown DL, ed. Interscalene block. *Atlas of Regional Anesthesia.* 2nd ed. Philadelphia, PA: Saunders; 1999: 23-29.

Canavan PK. Athletic injuries of the elbow. *Rehabilitation in Sports Medicine: A Comprehensive Guide.* Stamford, CT: Appleton & Lange; 1998: 229-236.

Finnerup N B, Jensen T S. Spinal cord injury pain—mechanisms and treatment. *Eur J Neurol.* 2004;11(2): 73-82.

Houten JK, Errico TJ. Paraplegia after lumbosacral nerve root block report of three cases. *Spine.* 2002; 2(1):70-75.

Loeser JD, ed. *Bonica's Management of Pain.* 3rd ed. Philadelphia, PA: Lippincott Williams & Wilkins; 2001.

Magee DJ. Cervical spine. *Orthopedic Physical Assessment.* 4th ed. Philadelphia, PA: W. B. Saunders; 2002: 161.

Price DD, Staud R. Neurobiology of fibromyalgia syndrome. *J Rheumatol Suppl.* 2005;32(suppl 75):29-37.

Raj PP, ed. *Pain Medicine: A comprehensive Review.* 2nd ed. Philadelphia, PA: Mosby; 2003.

Sammarco GJ, Cooper PS, eds. *Foot and Ankle Manual.* Philadelphia, PA: Lea and Febiger; 1998.

Somerville BW. Estrogen withdrawal migraine: duration of exposure of required and attempted prophylaxis by premenstrual estrogen administration. *Neurology.* 1975;25:239-244.

Waldman SD, ed. *Interventional Pain Management.* 2nd ed. Philadelphia, PA: W. B. Saunders; 2001.

Chapter 6 [Types of Pain]

Abdi S, Datta S, Trescot A, et al. Epidural steroids in the management of chronic spinal pain: a systematic review. *Pain Physician.* 2007;10:185-212.

Arnold LM, Lu Y, Crofford LJ, et al. A double-blind, multicenter trial was conducted that compared duloxetine to placebo in the treatment of fibromyalgia patients with or without major depressive disorder. *Arthritis Rheum.* 2004;50: 2974-84.

Arnold LM, Rosen A, Pritchett YL, et al. A randomized, double-blind, placebo-controlled trial of duloxetine in the treatment of women with fibromyalgia with or without major depressive disorder. *Pain.* 2005;119:5-15.

Ballas S. Pain management of sickle cell disease. *Hematol Oncol Clin North Am.* 2005;19;785-802.

Barrett AM, Lucero MA, Rebecca L, et al. Epidemiology, public health burden, and treatment of diabetic peripheral neuropathic pain: a review. *Pain Med.* 2007;8:S50-S62.

Benzon HT, Raja SN, Borsook D, Molloy RE, Strichartz G, eds. *Essentials of Pain Medicine and Regional Anesthesia.* 2nd ed. Philadelphia, PA: Elsevier Churchill-Livingstone; 2005.

Birch S, Jamison RN. Controlled trial of Japanese acupuncture for chronic myofascial neck pain: assessment of specific and nonspecific effects of treatment. *Clin J Pain.* 1998;14:248-255.

Bogduk N. *Clinical Anatomy of the Lumbar Spine and Sacrum.* 4th ed. Edinburgh, UK: Churchill Livingstone; 2005.

Bogduk N. Low back pain. *Clinical Anatomy of the Lumbar Spine and Sacrum.* 3rd ed. New York, NY: Churchill Livingstone; 1997: 187-214.

Boswell M, Trescott A, Datta S, et al. Interventional techniques: evidence-based practice guidelines in the management of chronic spinal pain. *Pain Physician.* 2007;10:7-111.

Boswell MV, Cole BE, eds. *Weiner's Pain Management: A Practical Guide for Clinicians.* 7th ed. Boca Raton, FL: Taylor and Francis Group, LLC; 2006.

Botwin KP, Castellanos R, Rao S, et al. Complications of Fluoroscopically Guided Interlaminar Cervical Epidural Injections. *Arch Phys Med Rehabil.* 2003;84:627-633.

Brenner GJ. Neural basis of pain. In: Ballantyne J, Fishman SM, Abdi S eds. *The Massachusetts General Hospital Handbook of Pain Management.* 2nd ed. Philadelphia, PA: Lippincott Williams & Wilkins; 2002:7-8.

Browner BD, Jupiter JB, Levine AM, Trafton PG, eds. *Skeletal Trauma: Basic Science, Management, and Reconstruction.* 3rd ed. Philadelphia, PA: W. B. Saunders; 2003.

Campbell JN, Basbaum AL, Dray A, Dubner R, Dworkin RH, Sang CN, eds. *Emerging Strategies for the Treatment of Neuropathic Pain.* Seattle, WA: IASP Press; 2006.

Canale ST. *Campbell's Operative Orthopaedics.* 10th ed. 2003: part VII, chap 25.

Goldman L, Ausiello D. *Cecil's Textbook of Medicine.* 22nd ed. Philadelphia, PA: Saunders (an imprint of Elsevier); 2004: part XVIII, chap 242.

Chen JT, Chen SM, Kuan TS, Chung KC, Hong CZ. Phentolamine effect on the spontaneous electrical activity of active loci in a myofascial trigger spot of rabbit skeletal muscle. *Arch Phy Med Rehabil.* 1998;79:790-794.

Clark SR, Bennett RM. Supplemental dextromethorphan in the treatment of fibromyalgia. A double blind, placebo controlled study of efficacy and side-effects. *Arthritis Rheum*. 2000;43:333.

Couppe C, Midttun M, Hilden J, Jorgensen U, Oxholm P, Fuglsang-Frederiksen A. Spontaneous needle electromyographic activity in myofascial trigger points in the infraspinatus muscle: a blinded assessment. *J Muscoskel Pain*. 2001;9(3):7-16.

Cummings TM, White A. Needling therapies in the management of myofascial trigger point pain: a systematic review. *Arch Phy Med Rehabil*. 2001;82: 986-992.

Finnerup NB, Jensen TS. Spinal cord injury pain—mechanisms and treatment. *Eur J Neurol*. 2004;11: 73-82.

Frontera WR, Silver JK. *Essentials of Physical Medicine and Rehabilitation*. Philadelphia, PA: Hanley & Belfus; 2002: part 2, sec I, chap 111.

Gam AN, Warming S, Larsen LH, et al. Treatment of myofascial trigger point with ultrasound combined with massage and exercise in a randomized controlled trial. *Pain*. 1998;77:73-79.

Gerwin R. A study of 96 subjects examined both for fibromyalgia and myofascial pain. *J Muscoskel Pain*. 1995;3(suppl 1):121.

Goetz CG, ed. *Textbook of Clinical Neurology*. 2nd ed. Philadelphia, PA: W. B. Saunders; 2003.

Gur A, Karakoc M, Nas E, et al. Cytokines and depression in cases with fibromyalgia. *J Rheumatol*. 2002;29(2):358-361.

Haldeman S, Carroll L, Cassidy J, et al. The bone and joint decade 2000-2010 task force on neck pain and its associated disorders: Executive summary. *Spine*. 2008;33(4S)(suppl):S5-S7.

Hansson PT, Fields HL, Hill RG, Marchettini P, eds. *Neuropathic Pain: Pathophysiology and Treatment*. Seattle, WA: IASP Press; 2001.

Harris RE, Clauw DJ, Scott DJ, et al. Decreased central mu-opioid receptor availability in fibromyalgia. *J Neurosci*. 2007;27(37):10000-10006.

Henriksson KG, Sorensen J. The promise of N-methyl-D-aspartate receptor antagonists in fibromyalgia. *Rheum Dis Clin North Am*. 2002;28: 343-351.

Holman AJ, Myers RR. A randomized, double-blind, placebo-controlled trial of pramipexole, a dopamine agonist, in patients with fibromyalgia receiving concomitant medications. *Arthritis Rheum*. 2005;52(8):2495-2505.

Hong CZ. Lidocaine injection versus dry needling to myofascial trigger point. *Am J Physi Medi Rehab*. 1994;73:256-263.

Hubbard DR, Berkoff GM. Myofascial trigger points show spontaneous needle EMG activity. *Spine*. 1993;18:1803-1807.

Huntoon MA. Anterior spinal artery syndrome as a complication of transforaminal epidural steroid injections. *Seminars in Pain Medicine*. 2004;2(4):204-207.

International Headache Society. International classification of headache disorders. Second edition. *Cephalalgia*. 2004;24(suppl 1):8-160.

Jankovic D, Wells C. *Regional Nerve Blocks*, 2nd ed, Berlin, Germany: Blackwell; 2001: 232.

Kang YK, Russell IJ, Vipraio GA, et al. Low urinary 5-hydroxyindole acetic acid in fibromyalgia syndrome: evidence in support of a serotonin-deficiency pathogenesis. *Myalgia*. 1998;1:14-21.

Little A, Edwards J, Feldman E. Diabetic neuropathies. *Pract Neurol*. 2007;7(2):82-92.

Loeser JD, ed. *Bonica's Management of Pain*. 3rd ed. Philadelphia, PA: Lippincott Williams & Wilkins; 2001.

Manchikanti L, Manchikanti K, Cash K, et al. Age-related prevalence of facet-joint involvement in chronic neck and low back pain. *Pain Physician*. 2008;11(1):67-75.

McMahon SB, Koltzenburg M, eds. *Wall and Melzack's Textbook of Pain*. 5th ed. Philadelphia, PA: Elsevier Churchill-Livingstone; 2006.

Moldofsky H. Management of sleep disorders in fibromyalgia. *Rheum Dis Clin North Am*. 2002;28:353-365.

Moss J, Glick D. The autonomic nervous system. In: Miller RD, ed. *Miller's Anesthesia*. 6th ed. Philadelphia, PA: Elsevier Churchill-Livingstone; 2005: sec II, chap 16.

Nachemson A, Jonsson E, eds. *Neck and Back Pain: The Scientific Evidence of Causes, Diagnosis, and Treatment*. Philadelphia, PA: Lippincott Williams & Wilkins; 2000.

Porter RW. Spinal stenosis and neurogenic claudication. *Spine*. 1996;21(17):2046-2052.

Raj P. *Practical Management of Pain*, 3rd ed. St. Louis, MO: Mosby; 2000.

Raj PP, ed. *Pain Medicine: A Comprehensive Review*. 2nd ed. Philadelphia, PA: Mosby; 2003.

Simons DG, Hong CZ, Simons LS. Endplate potentials are common to midfiber myofascial trigger points. *Am J Phys Med Rehabil*. 2003;81:212-222.

Sjaastad O, Fredriksen TA, Pfaffenrath V. Cervicogenic headache: diagnostic criteria. *Headache.* 1998;38:442-445.

Spitzer WO, Skovron ML, Salmi LR, et al. Scientific monograph of the Quebec Task Force on whiplash-associated disorders: redefining "whiplash" and its management. *Spine.* 1995;20(8S):1S-73S.

Sykes N, Fallon MT, Patt RB. *Clinical Pain Management: Cancer Pain.* London, UK: Arnold; 2003.

Travell J. Myofascial trigger points: clinical view. In: Bonica JJ, Albe-Fessard D, eds. *Advances in Pain Research and Therapy.* New York, NY: Raven Press; 1976:919-926.

Waldman SD, ed. *Pain Management.* vol. 1. Philadelphia, PA: Elsevier; 2007.

Wall PD, Melzack R. *Textbook of Pain.* 4th ed. Edinburgh, UK: Churchill Livingstone; 1999.

Wallace DJ, Linker-Israeli M, Hallegua D, et al. Cytokines play an aetiopathogenetic role in fibromyalgia: a hypothesis and pilot study. *Rheumatology.* 2001;40:743-749.

Wallace M, Staats P, eds. *Pain Medicine & Management: Just the Facts.* New York, NY: McGraw-Hill; 2005.

Wilson PR, Stanton-Hicks M, Harden NR eds. *CRPS: Current Diagnosis and Therapy.* Seattle, WA: IASSP Press; 2005.

Wolfe F, Smythe HA, Yunus MB, et al. The American College of Rheumatology 1990 criteria for the classification of fibromyalgia. Report of the multicenter criteria committee. *Arthritis Rheum.* 1990;33(2):160-172.

Wood PB, Schweinhardt P, Jaeger E, et al. Fibromyalgia patients show an abnormal dopamine response to pain. *Eur J Neurosci.* 2007;25(12):3576-3582.

Chapter 7 [Pain Assessment]

McMahon SB, Koltzenburg M, eds. *Wall and Melzack's Textbook of Pain.* 5th ed. Philadelphia, PA: Elsevier Churchill-Livingstone; 2006.

Raj PP. *Pain Medicine: A Comprehensive Review.* 2nd ed. Philadelphia, PA: Mosby; 2003.

Raj PP, ed. *Practical Management of Pain.* 3rd ed. St. Louis, MO: Mosby; 2000.

Chapter 8 [Pain Management Techniques]

Abdi S, Datta S, Trescot AM, et al. Epidural steroids in the management of chronic spinal pain: a systematic review. *Pain Physician.* 2007;10(1):185-212.

Ackerman WE 3rd, Ahmad M. The efficacy of lumbar epidural steroid injections in patients with lumbar disc herniations. *Anesth Analg.* 2007;104(5):1217-22.

Ahadian FM. Pulsed radiofrequency neurotomy: advances in pain medicine. *Curr Pain Headache Rep.* 2004;8:34-40.

Amoils SP. The Joule Thomson cryoprobe. *Arch Opthalmol.* 1967:78(2):201-207.

Ballantyne JC, Fishman SM, Abdi S. *The Massachusetts General Hospital Handbook of Pain Management.* 3rd ed. Philadelphia, PA: Lippincott Williams & Wilkins: 2005.

Bogduk N, Macintosh J, Marsland A. Technical limitations to the efficacy of radiofrequency neurotomy for spinal pain. *Neurosurgery.* 1987;20(4):529-535.

Buonocore M, Bonezzi C, Barolet G. Neurophysiological evidence of antidromic activation of large myelinated fibers in lower limbs during spinal cord stimulation. *Spine.* 2008;33(4): E90-E93.

Buvanendran A, Lubenow TJ. Efficacy of transverse tripolar spinal cord stimulator for the relief of chronic low back pain from failed back surgery. *Pain Physician.* 2008;11(3):333-338.

Cohen SP, Abdi S. Lateral branch blocks as a treatment for sacroiliac joint pain: a pilot study. *Reg Anesth Pain Med.* 2003;28(2):113-119.

Cohen SP, Larkin T, Abdi S, Chang A, Stojanovic M. Risk factors for failure and complications of intradiscal electrothermal therapy: a pilot study. *Spine.* 2003;28(11):1142-1147.

Cohen SP, Larkin T, Fant GV, Oberfoell R, Stojanovic MP. Does needle insertion site affect diskography results? A retrospective analysis. *Spine.* 2002; 27(20):2279-2283; discussion 2283.

Cohen SP, Larkin TM, Barna SA, Palmer WE, Hecht AC, Stojanovic MP. Lumbar discography: a comprehensive review of outcome studies, diagnostic accuracy, and principles. *Reg Anesth Pain Med.* 2005;30(2):163-183.

Cohen SP, Raja SN. Pathogenesis, diagnosis, and treatment of lumbar zygapophysial (facet) joint pain. *Anesthesiology.* 2007;106(3):591-614.

Cooper IS, Lee AS. Cryostatic congelation: a system for producing a limited, controlled region of cooling or freezing of biologic tissues. *J Nerv Ment Dis.* 1961;133:259-263.

Deer T, Masone J. Selection of spinal cord stimulation candidates for the treatment of chronic pain. *Pain Med.* 2008;9(S1):82-92.

Deer TR, Raso LJ. Spinal cord stimulation for refractory angina pectoris and peripheral vascular disease. *Pain Physician.* 2006;9(4):347-352.

Deer TR. Spinal cord stimulation for the treatment of angina and peripheral vascular disease. *Curr Pain Headache Rep.* 2009;13(1):18-23.

Falowski S, Celii A, Sharan A. Spinal cord stimulation: an update. *Neurotherapeutics.* 2008;5:86-99.

Forward KR, Fewer HD, Stiver HG. Cerebrospinal fluid shunt infections. A review of 35 infections in 32 patients. *J Neurosurg.* 1983;59(3):389-394.

Govind J, King W, Bailey B, Bogduk N. Radiofrequency neurotomy for the treatment of third occipital headache. *J Neurol Neurosurg Psychiatry.* 2003;74(1):88-93.

Hansen HC, McKenzie-Brown AM, Cohen SP, et al. Sacroiliac joint interventions a systematic review. *Pain Physician.* 2007;10:165-184.

Harke H, Gretenkort P, Ladlef HU, et al. Spinal cord stimulation in sympathetically maintained complex regional pain syndrome type I with severe disability. A prospective clinical study. *Eur J Pain.* 2005;9(4):363-373.

Holsheimer J, Struijk JJ, Tas NR, et al. Effects of electrode geometry and combination on nerve fibre selectivity in spinal cord stimulation. *Med Biol Eng Comput.* 1995;33(5):676-682.

Kapur S, Mutagi H, Southall J, et al. Long-term outcome of spinal cord stimulation in late complex regional pain syndrome. *Reg Anesth Pain Med.* 2006;31(5)(suppl 1):46.

Kapural L, Mekhail N, Hayek SM, Stanton-Hicks M, Malak O, Occipital nerve electrical stimulation via the midline approach and subcutaneous surgical leads for treatment of severe occipital neuralgia: a pilot study. *Anesth Analg.* 2005, 101(1): 171-174

Kapural L, Narouze SN, Janicki TI, et al. Spinal cord stimulation is an effective treatment for chronic intractable visceral pelvic pain. *Pain Med.* 2006;7(5):440-443.

Kapural L, Rakic M. Spinal cord stimulation for chronic visceral pain secondary to chronic non-alcoholic pancreatitis. *J Clin Gastroenterol.* 2008; 42(6):750-751.

Kemler MA, de Vet HC, Barendse GA, et al. Effect of spinal cord stimulation for chronic complex regional pain syndromes type I: five-year final follow-up of patients in a randomized controlled trial. *J Neurosurg.* 2008;108(2):292-298.

Klomp HM, Steyerberg EW, van Urk H, et al. Spinal cord stimulation is not cost-effective for non-surgical management of critical limb ischaemia. *Eur J Vasc Endovasc Surg.* 2006;31(5):500-508.

Kumar K, Nath RK, Toth C. Spinal cord stimulation is effective in the management of reflex sympathetic dystrophy. *Neurosurgery.* 1997;40(3):503-508.

Kumar K, Taylor RS, Jacques L, et al. Spinal cord stimulation versus conventional medical management for neuropathic pain: a multicenter randomized controlled trial in patients with failed back surgery syndrome. *Pain.* 2007;132(1-2):179-188.

Lloyd JW, Barnard JD, Glynn CJ. Cryoanalgesia. A new approach to pain relief. *Lancet.* 1976;2(7992): 932-934.

Malanga GA. Lumbosacral facet syndrome. http://www.emedicine.com/sports/TOPIC65.H TM#MULTIMEDIA, Published July 15, 2008, Updated: July 15, 2008. Accessed March 29, 2009.

Manjunath PS, Jayalakshmi TS, Dureja GP, et al. Management of lower limb complex regional pain syndrome type 1: an evaluation of percutaneous radiofrequency thermal lumbar sympathectomy versus phenol lumbar sympathetic neurolysis—a pilot study. *Anesth Analg.* 2008;106:647-649.

Mayer RD, Howard FM. Sacral nerve stimulation: neuromodulation for voiding dysfunction and pain. *Neurotherapeutics.* 2008;5:107-113.

Mekhail NA, Aeschbach A, Stanton-Hicks M, et al. Cost benefit analysis of neurostimulation for chronic pain. *Clin J Pain.* 2004;20:462-468.

Melzack R, Wall PD. Mechanisms: a new theory. A gate control system modulates sensory input from the skin before it evokes pain perception and response. *Science.* 1965;150(699):971-979.

Nauta HJ, Soukup VM, Fabian RH, et al. Punctate midline myelotomy for the relief of visceral cancer pain. *J Neurosurg Spine.* 2000;92: 125-130.

North R, Prager J, Barolat G, et al. Practice parameters for the use of spinal cord stimulation in the treatment of chronic neuropathic pain. *Pain Med.* 2007;8(S4):S200-S275.

Oakley JC, Prager JP. Spinal cord stimulation: mechanisms of action. *Spine.* 2002; 27(22):2574-2583.

Oakley JC. Spinal cord stimulation: patient selection, technique, and outcomes. *Neurosurg Clin N Am.* 2003;14(3):365-380.

Prager J, Jacobs M. Evaluation of patients for implantable pain modalities: behavioral assessment. *Clin J Pain.* 2001;17(3):206-214.

Qin C, Lehew RT, Khan KA et al. Spinal cord stimulation modulates intraspinal colorectal visceroreceptive transmission in rats. *Neurosci Res.* 2007;58(1):58-66.

Raj P, Lou L, Erdine S, et al. *Radiographic Imaging for Regional Anesthesia and Pain Management.* Marrickville, N.S.W: Churchill Livingstone; 2003.

Rathmell JP, Aprill C, Bogduk N. Cervical transforaminal injection of steroids. *Anesthesiology.* 2004; 100(6):1595-1600.

Sayson SC, Ramamurthy S, Hoffman J. Incidence of genitofemoral nerve block during lumbar sympathetic block: comparison of two lumbar injection sites. *Reg Anesth.*1997; 22(6):569-574.

Shealy CN. Percutaneous radiofrequency denervation of spinal facets: treatment for chronic back pain and sciatica. *J Neurosurg.* 1975;43:448-451.

Simonpoulos TT, Malik AB, Sial KA, et al. Radiofrequency lesioning of the L2 ramus communicans in managing discogenic low back pain. *Pain Physician.* 2005;8:61-65.

Slappendel R, Crul BJ, Braak GJ, et al. The efficacy of radiofrequency lesioning of the cervical spinal dorsal root ganglion in double-blinded, randomized study: no difference between 40 degrees C and 67 degrees C treatments. *Pain.* 1997;73:159-163.

Slipman CW, Derby R, Simeone FA, et al. *Interventional Spine an Algorithmic Approach.* Saunders Elsevier, USA; 2007.

Sluijter M, Racz G. Technical aspects of radiofrequency. *Pain Pract.* 2002;2(3):195-200.

Smith TJ, Staats PS, Deer T, et al. Randomized clinical trial of an implantable drug delivery system compared with comprehensive medical management for refractory cancer pain: impact on pain, drug-related toxicity, and survival. *J Clin.* 2002;20(19):4040-4049.

Stanton-Hicks M, Salamon J. Stimulation of the central and peripheral nervous system for the control of pain. *J Clin Neurophysiol.* 1997;14(1):46-62.

Stanton-Hicks M. Complex regional pain syndrome: manifestations and the role of neurostimulation in its management. *J Pain Symptom Manage.* 2006; 31(suppl 4):S20-S24.

Stojanovic MP, Dey D, Hord ED, Zhou Y, Cohen SP. A prospective crossover comparison study of the single-needle and multiple-needle techniques for facet-joint medial branch block. *Reg Anesth Pain Med.* 2005;30(5):484-490.

Stojanovic MP, Vu TN, Caneris O, Slezak J, Cohen SP, Sang CN. The role of fluoroscopy in cervical epidural steroid injections: an analysis of contrast dispersal patterns. *Spine.* 2002;27(5):509-514.

Stojanovic MP. Stimulation methods for neuropathic pain control. *Curr Pain Headache Rep.* 2001;5(2): 130-137.

Tekin I MIrzai H, Erbuyun K, et al. A comparison of conventional and pulsed radiofrequency denervation in the treatment of chronic facet joint pain. *Clin J Pain.* 2007;23:524-529.

Tracy JP, Gaeta R. Neurolytic blocks revisited. *Curr Pain Headache Rep.* 2008;12:7-13.

Tran KM, Frank SM, Raja SN, El-Rahmany HK, Kim LJ, Vu B. Lumbar sympathetic block for sympathetically maintained pain: changes in cutaneous temperatures and pain perception. *Anesth Analg.* 2000;90(6):1396-1401.

Trescot A. Cryoanalgesia in interventional pain management. *Pain Physician.* 2003;6:345-360.

Vallejo R, Benyamin RM, Kramer J, et al. Pulsed radiofrequency denervation for the treatment of sacroiliac joint syndrome. *Pain Med.* 2006;7(5): 429-434.

Wall PD, Sweet WH. Temporary abolition of pain in man. *Science.* 1967;155(758):108-109.

Warfield CA, Bajwa ZH. *Principles and Practice of Pain Medicine.* 2nd ed. New York, NY: McGraw-Hill; 2004.

Chapter 9 [Complementary and Alternative Medicine]

Agency for Health Care Policy and Research. *Chiropractic in the United States: Training, Practice, and Research.* Rockville, MD: Agency for Health Care Policy and Research; 1998: AHCPR publication no. 98-N002.

Astin JA, Shapiro SL, Eisenberg DM, et al. Mind-body medicine: state of the science, implications for practice. *J Am Board Fam Pract.* 2003;16(2): 131-147.

Barnes P, Powell-Griner E, McFann K, Nahin R. CDC advance data report #343. Complementary and alternative medicine use among adults: United States, 2002. NCCAM Press Release. May 27, 2004.

Barrett BP, Brown RL, Locken K, et al. Treatment of the common cold with unrefined Echinacea: a randomized, double-blind, placebo-controlled trial. *Ann Intern Med.* 2002;137(12):939-946.

Daniel O Clegg, Domenic J Reda, Crystal L Harris, et al. Glucosamine, chondroitin sulfate, and the two in combination for painful knee osteoarthritis. *N Engl J Med.* 2006;354(8):795-808.

Eisenberg DM, Davis RB, Ettner SL, et al. Trends in alternative medicine use in the United States, 1990-1997, results of a follow-up national survey. *JAMA.* 1998;280(18):1569-1575.

Ernst E, White A. Life-threatening adverse reactions after acupuncture? A systematic review. *Pain.* 1997;71:123-126.

Fugh-Berman A. Echinacea for the prevention and treatment of upper respiratory infections. Seminars in Integrative Medicine. 2003;1(2):106-111.

Haldeman S, Rubinstein SM. Cauda equina syndrome in patients undergoing manipulation of the lumbar spine. *Spine.* 1992;17(12):1469-1473.

Hufnagel A, Hammers A, Schonle PW, et al. Stroke following chiropractic manipulation of the cervical spine. *J Neurol.* 1999;246(8):683-688.

Hui KK, Liu J, Makris N, et al. Acupuncture Modulates the Limbic System and Subcortical Gray Structures of the Human Brain: Evidence from fMRI Studies in Normal Subjects. *Hum Brain Mapp.* 2000;9(1):13-25.

Jeret JS, Bluth M. Stroke following chiropractic manipulation: report of 3 cases and review of the literature. *Cerebrovasc Dis.* 2002;13(3):210-213.

Jonas WB, Kaptchuk TJ, Linde K. A critical overview of homeopathy. *Ann Intern Med.* 2003;138(5):393-399.

Lang EV, Benotsch EG, Fick LJ, et al. Adjunctive non-pharmacological analgesia for invasive medical procedures: a randomised trial. *Lancet.* 2000;355(9214):1486-1490.

Luskin FM, Newell KA, Griffith M, et al. A review of mind/body therapies in the treatment of musculoskeletal disorders with implications for the elderly. *Altern Ther Health Med.* 2000;6(2):46-56.

Ma SX. Neurobiology of acupuncture: toward CAM. *Evid Based Complement Alternat Med.* 2004;1(1):41-47.

Melchart D, Weidenhammer W, Streng A, et al. Prospective investigation of adverse effects of acupuncture in 97,733 patients. *Arch Intern Med.* 2004;164(1):104-105.

Mundy EA, DuHamel KN, Montgomery GH. The efficacy of behavioral interventions for cancer treatment-related side effects. *Semin Clin Neuropsychiatry.* 2003;8(4):253-275.

National Center for Complementary and Alternative Medicine (NCCAM), Basic CAM information. nccam.nih.gov/health.

Rutledge JC, Hyson DA, Garduno D, et al. Lifestyle modification program in management of patients with coronary artery disease: the clinical experience in a tertiary care hospital. *J Cardiopulm Rehabil.* 1999;19(4):226-234.

Senstad O, Leboeuf-Yde C, Borchgrevink C. Frequency and characteristics of side effects of spinal manipulative therapy. *Spine.* 1997;22(4):435-440.

Shekelle PG, Adams AH, Chassin MR, et al. Spinal manipulation for low-back pain. *Ann Intern Med.* 1992;117(7):590-598.

Smith MJ, Logan AC. Naturopathy. *Med Clin North Am.* 2002;86(1):173-184.

Solomon PR, Adams F, Silver A, Zimmer J, DeVeaux R. Ginkgo for memory enhancement: a randomized controlled trial. *JAMA.* 2002;288(7):835-840.

Taylor JA, Weber W, Standish L, et al. Efficacy and safety of Echinacea in treating upper respiratory tract infections in children: a randomized controlled trial. *JAMA.* 2003;290(21):2824-2830.

Vickers A, Zollman C. ABC of complementary medicine. The manipulative therapies: osteopathy and chiropractic. *BMJ.* 1999;319(7218):1176-1179.

Wetzel MS, Eisengerg DM, Kaptchuk TJ. Course involving complementary and alternative medicine at U.S Medical School. *JAMA.* 1998;280(9):784-787.

Zhang WT, Jin Z, Cui GH, et al. Relations between brain network activation and analgesic effect induced by low versus high frequency electrical acupoint stimulation in different subjects: a functional magnetic resonance imaging study. *Brain Res.* 2003;982(2):168-178.

Chapter 10 [Interdisciplinary Pain Management]

Mason RJ, Broaddus VC, Murray JF, Nadel JA, eds. *Murray and Nadel's Textbook of Respiratory Medicine.* 4th ed. Philadelphia, PA: Saunders; 2005.

McMahon SB, Koltzenburg M, eds. *Wall and Melzack's Textbook of Pain.* 5th ed. Philadelphia, PA: Elsevier Churchill Livingstone; 2006.

Raj P, ed. *Practical Management of Pain.* 3rd ed. St. Louis, MO: Mosby; 2000.

Wallace M, Staats P. *Pain Medicine & Management: Just the Facts.* New York, NY: McGraw Hill; 2005.

Chapter 11 [Behavioral and Psychological Aspects of Pain]

Arnstein P, Vidal M, Wells-Federman C, et al. From chronic pain patient to peer: benefits and risks of volunteering. *Pain Manag Nurs.* 2002;3:94-103.

Asmundson GJ, Jacobson, SJ, Allerdings M, Norton GR. Social phobia in disabled workers with chronic musculoskeletal pain. *Behav Res Ther.* 1996;34:939-943.

Barsky AJ. Amplification, somatization, and the somatoform disorders. *Psychosomatics.* 1992;33(1):28-34.

Belgrade MJ, Cassandra D, Schamber D, Lindgren BR. The DIRE Score: Predicting Outcomes of Opioid Prescribing for Chronic Pain. *J Pain.* 2006;7(9):671-681.

Blanchard EB, Hickling EJ. *After the Crash: Psychological Assessment and Treatment of Survivors of Motor Vehicle Accidents.* 2nd ed. Washington, DC: American Psychological Association, USA; 2004.

Block, AR. Investigation of the response of the spouse to chronic pain behavior. *Psychosom Med.* 1981;43(5):415-422.

Boothby JL, Thorn BE, Overduin LY, Ward LC. Catastrophizing and perceived partner response to pain. *Pain.* 2004;109(3):500-506.

Breau LM, Camfield CS, McGrath PJ, Finley GA. Risk factors for pain in children with severe neurological impairments. *Dev Med Child Neurol.* 2004; 46(6):364-371.

Butler SF, Budman SH, Fernandez K, Jamison RN. Validation of a screener and opioid assessment measure for patients with chronic pain. *Pain.* 2004;112:65-75.

Caudill M, Schnable R, Zuttermeister P, et al. Decreased clinic use by chronic pain patients: response to behavioral medicine intervention. *Clin J Pain.* 1991;7(4):305-310.

Charlton JE. *Core Curriculum for Professional Education in Pain.* Seattle, WA: IASP Press; 2005.

Dworkin RH, Turk DC, Farrar JT, et al. Core outcome measures for chronic pain clinical trials: IMMPACT recommendations. *Pain.* 2005;113(1-2):9-19.

Edwards LC, Pearce SA, Turner-Stokes L, Jones A. The pain beliefs questionnaire: an investigation of beliefs in the causes and consequences of pain. *Pain.* 1992;51(3):267-72.

Fishbain DA. The association of chronic pain and suicide. *Semin Clin Neuropsychiatry.* 1999;4(3):221-227.

Gatchel RJ, Turk DC, eds. *Psychosocial Factors in Pain: Clinical Perspectives.* New York, NY: Guilford Press; 1999.

Jacox AK, Carr DB, Payne R, et al. *Management of Cancer Pain. Clinical Practice Guideline No. 9 (AHCPR Pub. No. 94-0592).* Rockville, MD: Agency for Health Care Policy and Research; 1994.

Jansen DEMC, Krol B, Groothoff JW, Post D. People with intellectual disability and their health problems: a review of comparative studies. *J Intellect Disabil Res.* 2004;48:93-102.

Jessup BA, Gallegos X. Relaxation and biofeedback. In: Wall PD, Melzack R, eds. *Textbook of Pain.* 3rd ed. Edinburgh, UK: Churchill Livingstone; 1994: 1321-1336.

Kapteyn A, Smith JP, van Soest A. *Dynamics of Work Disability and Pain.* IZA Discussion Papers 2057, Institute for the Study of Labor (IZA): 2006.

Karjalainen K, Malmivaara A, van Tulder M, et al. Multidisciplinary rehabilitation for fibromyalgia and musculoskeletal pain in working age adults. *Cochrane Database of Systematic Reviews.* 1999, Issue 3. Art. No.: CD001984. DOI: 10.1002/14651858.CD001984.

Keefe FJ, Lefebvre JC, Egert JR, Affleck G, Sullivan MJ, Caldwell DS. The relationship of gender to pain, pain behavior, and disability in osteoarthritis patients: the role of catastrophizing. *Pain.* 2000;87(3):325-334.

Keefe FJ, Rumble ME, Scipio CD, Giordano LA, Perri LM. Psychological aspects of persistent pain: current state of the science. *J Pain.* 2004;5(4):195-211.

Kori SH, Miller RP, Todd DD. Kinesiophobia. A new view of chronic pain behavior. *Pain Management.* 1990;19:35-43.

Kulich RJ, Andrew L. Psychological assessment and behavioral treatment of chronic pain. In: Ballantyne J, ed. *Massachusetts General Hospital Pain Handbook.* 3rd ed. Philadelphia, PA: Lippincott Williams & Wilkins; 2005.

Kulich RJ, Mencher P, Bertrand C, Maciewicz R. Post traumatic stress disorder: assessment and treatment: clinical and forensic issues. *Curr Rev Pain, Current Science.* 2000;4:36-48.

Lande S, Kulich RJ, eds. *Managed Care and Pain.* Glenview, IL: American Pain Society; 2000.

Mailis-Gagnon A, Furlan AD, Sandoval JA, Taylor R. Spinal cord stimulation for chronic pain. *Cochrane Database of Systematic Reviews.* 2004;3 (Art. No.: CD003783. DOI: 10. 1002/14651858. CD003783.pub2).

Main C, Wood PL, Hollis S, et al. The distress and risk assessment method; a simple patient classification to identify distress and evaluate the risk of poor outcome. *Spine.* 1992;17:42-52.

McCracken LM, Gross RT, Sorg PJ, Edmands TA. Prediction of pain in patients with chronic low back pain: effects of inaccurate prediction and pain-related anxiety. *Behavior Research Therapy.* 1993;31(7),647-652.

McCracken LM, Zayfert C, Gross RT. The Pain Anxiety Symptoms Scale: a multimodal measure of pain-specific anxiety. *Behavior Therapist.* 1993;16:183-184.

McCracken LM. Social context and acceptance of chronic pain: the role of solicitous and punishing responses. *Pain.* 2005;113:155-159.

McDonald HP, Garg AX, Haynes RB. Interventions to enhance patient adherence to medication prescriptions: scientific review. *JAMA.* 2002;288(22): 2868-2879.

Mercado AC, Carroll LJ, Cassidy D, Cote P. Passive coping is a risk factor for disabling neck or low back pain. *Pain.* 2005;117(1-2):51-57.

Morin CM, Culbert JP, Schwartz SM. Nonpharmacological interventions for insomnia: a meta-analysis of treatment efficacy. *Am J Psychiatry.* 1994; 151:1172-1180.

Nicolaisis C, Curry M, Benson, M. Gerity M. Violence, mental health, and physical symptoms in an academic internal medicine practice. *J Gen Intern Med.* 2004;19:819-827.

Polatin PB, Kinney RK, Gatchel RJ, Lillo E, Mayer TG. Psychiatric illness and chronic low-back pain. The mind and the spine—which goes first? *Spine.* 1993;18:66-71.

Prochaska JO, DiClemente CC, Norcross JC. In search of how people change. Applications to addictive behaviors. *Am Psychol.* 1992;47(9): 1102-1114.

Rogers R, Bender SD. Evaluation of malingering and deception. In: Goldstein AM, Weiner IB, eds. *Handbook of Psychology.* 2003: 109. *Forensic Psychology,* vol 11. Wiley, USA.

Rosenstiel AK, Keefe FJ. The use of coping strategies in chronic low back pain patients: relationship to patient characteristics and current adjustment. *Pain.* 1983;17(1):33-44.

Rudy TE, Turk DC, Kubinski JA, Zaki HS. Differential treatment response of TMD patients as a function of psychological characteristics. *Pain.* 1995;61:103-112.

Rush AJ, Beck AT, Kovacs M, Hollon S. Comparative efficacy of cognitive therapy and pharmacotherapy in the treatment of depressed outpatients. *Cognit Ther Res.* 1977;1:17-37.

Savage S, Covington EC, Gilson AM, GourlayD, Heit HA, Hunt JB. *Public Policy Statement on the Rights and Responsibilities of Healthcare Professionals in the use of Opioids for the Treatment of Pain.* American Pain Society; March 2004: http://www.ampainsoc.org/advocacy/rights.htm. Accessed on March 29, 2009.

Schatman, ME, Campbell A. *Chronic Pain Management: Guidelines for Multidisciplinary Program Development.* New York, NY: Informa Healthcare; 2007.

Schwartz MS. *Biofeedback: A Practitioner's Guide.* 2nd ed. New York, NY: Guilford Press; 1995.

Schwarzer R, Jerusalem M. Generalized self-efficacy scale. In: Weinman J, Wright S, Johnson M, eds. *Measures in Health Psychology: A User's Portfolio, Causal and Control Beliefs.* Windsor, UK: NFER Nelson; 1995: 35-37.

Sullivan MJ, Thorn B, Haythornthwaite, JA, et al. Theoretical perspectives on the relation between catastrophizing and pain. *Clin J Pain.* 2001;17(1): 52-64.

Turk DC, Flor H. Pain greater than pain behaviors. The utility of the pain behavior construct. *Pain.* 1987;31:277-295.

Turk DC, Gatchel RJ, eds. *Psychological Approaches to Pain Management: A Practitioner's Handbook.* New York, NY: Guilford Press; 2002.

Turk DC, Melzack R. *Handbook of Pain Assessment.* 2nd ed. New York, NY: Guilford Press; 2005.

Turk DC, Okifuji A. Detecting depression in chronic pain patients: adequacy of self-reports. *Behavior Research Therapy.* 1994;32:9-16.

Turner JA. Nonspecific treatment effects. In: Loeser JD, ed. *Bonica's Management of Pain*. 3rd ed. Philadelphia, PA: Lippincott Williams & Wilkins; 2001: 1649-1656.

Waddell G, Burton AK, Main CJ. *Screening for Risk of Long-Term Incapacity: A Conceptual and Scientific Review*. London, UK: Royal Society of Medicine Press; 2003.

Wilson L, Dworkin SF, Whitney C, LeResche L. Somatization and pain dispersion in chronic temporomandibular disorder pain. *Pain*. 1994; 57(1):55-61.

Chapter 12 [Drug abuse and Addiction]
Chapter 13 [Medicolegal Issues]
Chapter 14 [Compensation and Disability Assessment]

Cocchiarella L, Andersson GBJ. *AMA Guides to the Evaluation of Permanent Impairment*. USA: AMA Press; 2004.

Manchikanti L. Recent developments in evaluation and management services. *Pain Physician*. 2000;3:403-421.

Chapter 15 [Rehabilitation]

Akuthota V, Nadler SF. Core strengthening. *Arch Phys Med Rehabil*. 2004;85(3)(suppl 1):S86-S92.

Arnold L. Duloxetine and Other Antidepressants in the Treatment of Patients with Fibromyalgia. *Pain Medicine*. 2007; 8 (S2): S63-S74.

Busanich BM, Verscheure SD. Does McKenzie therapy improve outcomes for back pain? *J Athl Train*. 2006;41(1):117-119.

Chou LH, Akuthota V, Drake DF, Toledo SD, Nadler SF. Sports and performing arts medicine. 3. Lower-limb injuries in endurance sports. *Arch Phys Med Rehabil*. 2004;85(3)(suppl 1):S59-S66.

DeLisa JA, Gans BM, Walsh NE, Bockenek WL, Frontera WR, eds. *Physical Medicine and Rehabilitation Principles and Practice*. Philadelphia, PA: Lippincott Williams & Wilkins: 2005.

Foye PM, Sullivan WJ, Sable AW, Panagos A, Zuhosky JP, Irwin RW. Industrial medicine and acute musculoskeletal rehabilitation. 3. Work-related musculoskeletal conditions: the role for physical therapy, occupational therapy, bracing, and modalities. *Arch Phys Med Rehabil*. 2007;88(3)(suppl 1):S14-S17.

Harden RN. Muscle pain syndromes. *Am J Phys Med Rehabil*. 2007;86(suppl):S47-S58.

Henneman E, Clamann HP, Gillies JD, Skinner RD. Rank order of motoneurons within a pool: law of combination. *J Neurophysiol*. 1974;37(6):1338-1349.

Hord and Shannon. Phantom pain. In: Raj PP, ed. *Practical Management of Pain*. 3rd ed. Raj P. St. Louis, MO: Mosby; 2000: 212-213.

Jellema P, van tulder MW, van Poppel MN, Nachemson AL, Bouter LM. Lumbar supports for prevention and treatment of low back pain: a systematic review within the framework of the Cochrane Back Review Group. *Spine*. 2001;26:377-86.

Lang AM. Botulinum toxin type A therapy in chronic pain disorders. *Arch Phys Med Rehabil*. 2003;84(3)(suppl 1):S69-S73.

Panagos A, Sable AW, Zuhosky JP, Irwin RW, Sullivan WJ, Foye PM. Industrial medicine and acute musculoskeletal rehabilitation. 1. Diagnostic testing in industrial and acute musculoskeletal injuries. *Arch Phys Med Rehabil* 2007;88(3)(suppl 1): S3-S9.

Slipman CW, Sterenfeld EB, Chou LH, Herzog R, Vresilovic E. The predictive value of provocative sacroiliac joint stress maneuvers in the diagnosis of sacroiliac joint syndrome. *Arch Phys Med Rehabil*. 1998;79(3):288-292.

Stanos SP, Prather H, Press JM, Young JL. Physical Medicine and Rehabilitation Approaches to Pain Management. In: Benzon HT, Raja SN, Borsook D, Molloy RE, Strichartz G, eds. *Essentials of Pain medicine and Regional Anesthesia*. 2nd ed. Philadelphia, PA: Churchill-Livingstone Elsevier; 2005: 197-208.

Sullivan WJ, Panagos A, Foye PM, Sable AW, Irwin RW, Zuhosky JP. Industrial medicine and acute musculoskeletal rehabilitation. 2. Medications for the treatment of acute musculoskeletal pain. *Arch Phys Med Rehabil*. 2007;88(3)(suppl 1):S10-S13.

Index